Imaging for Students

Imaging for Students

THIRD EDITION

David A. Lisle FRANZCR
Consultant Radiologist at Holy Spirit Northside, Brisbane Private, and
St Andrew's War Memorial Hospitals, Brisbane; Visiting Radiologist at
Redcliffe District Hospital, Redcliffe; Associate Professor of Medical Imaging at
the University of Queensland Medical School, Brisbane, Australia

Hodder Arnold
A MEMBER OF THE HODDER HEADLINE GROUP

First published in Great Britain in 1995 by Arnold
Second edition 2001
This third edition published in 2007 by
Hodder Arnold, an imprint of Hodder Education and a member of the Hodder Headline Group,
338 Euston Road, London NW1 3BH

http://www.hoddereducation.com

Distributed in the United States of America by
Oxford University Press Inc.,
198 Madison Avenue, New York, NY10016
Oxford is a registered trademark of Oxford University Press

Whilst the advice and information in this book are believed to be true and accurate at the date of going to press, neither the author nor the publisher can accept any legal responsibility or liability for any errors or omissions that may be made. In particular (but without limiting the generality of the preceding disclaimer) every effort has been made to check drug dosages; however it is still possible that errors have been missed. Furthermore, dosage schedules are constantly being revised and new side-effects recognized. For these reasons the reader is strongly urged to consult the drug companies' printed instructions before administering any of the drugs recommended in this book.

British Library Cataloguing in Publication Data
A catalogue record for this book is available from the British Library

Library of Congress Cataloging-in-Publication Data
A catalog record for this book is available from the Library of Congress

ISBN-10 0 340 92591 4
ISBN-13 978 0 340 92591 1

1 2 3 4 5 6 7 8 9 10

Commissioning Editor: Sara Purdy
Project Editor: Jane Tod
Production Controller: Lindsay Smith
Cover Designer: Laura DeGrasse
Indexer: June Morrison

Typeset in Goudy 10/14 pts by Charon Tec Ltd (A Macmillan Company), Chennai, India
www.charontec.com
Printed and bound in India by Replika Press Pvt Ltd

What do you think about this book? Or any other Hodder Arnold title?
Please visit our website at www.hoddereducation.com

To my wife Lyn and our daughters Victoria,
Charlotte and Margot

Contents

Preface

Despite over 30 years of rapid technological development and growing clinical demand, the specialty of Radiology or Medical Imaging continues to receive scant attention in most medical curricula. The aims of this, the third edition of *Imaging for Students*, remain the same as for the previous two editions. The first of these aims is the ability to interpret radiographs, or X-rays, in order to diagnose common conditions such as pneumonia, cardiac failure, intestinal obstruction and perforation, fractures and dislocations. Second, I hope to impart some understanding of how the various imaging modalities work, including associated hazards. It is also important for students to have some idea about more invasive tests and procedures and how these may impact on the patient.

Finally, it is more vital than ever for students to understand the appropriate ordering of more sophisticated and costly imaging examinations. The pace of technological advance in medical imaging has far outpaced the ability of clinical research to keep up and there is a trend for technologies to be introduced into clinical practice before clinical efficacy or cost effectiveness has been established. These trends are troubling for a number of reasons. First among these is the increasing level of radiation exposure, largely due to the more frequent use of computed tomography (CT) for common clinical problems.

The economic costs of modern medical imaging are expanding at a disconcerting rate. Despite the widespread availability of expensive technologies, the history and clinical examination are still the foundation stones of medical practice. More often than not a correct diagnosis may be achieved with history and examination plus a few simple blood tests and a plain X-ray, where indicated. Too often, sophisticated tests are ordered to add a layer of 'certainty' that in fact does nothing or little to alter the management of the patient. Conversely,

where a clinical problem demands assessment with CT or magnetic resonance imaging (MRI), there is often no point ordering less sophisticated tests first. In the current climate of overstretched health budgets, the appropriate use of medical imaging is more important than ever.

A major, and often forgotten consequence of modern medical imaging is the incidental finding. Modern ultrasound, CT and MRI scanners are highly sensitive and incidental findings are common. A major radiology journal recently devoted an entire issue to 'incidentalomas'. In my opinion, a patient who has been put through one or more extra examinations to investigate a harmless incidental finding found on a test that was not justified in the first place has been done a great disservice by the medical profession. Radiologists may, of course, refuse to perform tests that seem unwarranted. This is not as easy as it may seem, as the radiologist is not always privy to all of the pertinent information about an individual patient. In practical day-to-day medical practice it is the responsibility of the referring doctor to ensure that the potential benefits of an imaging investigation outweigh its risks.

With these considerations in mind several changes and updates have been added to the new edition. Chapter 1 is an introduction to the various imaging modalities. The bare essentials are provided here, with an ear for the kinds of questions students often ask me, questions such as 'What do the terms T1 and T2 mean?' and 'Why is MRI so noisy?'. Chapter 2 gives an overview of common hazards of medical imaging, including the increasingly important issue of radiation exposure. The titles of Chapters 3 and 6 are self-explanatory: 'How to read a chest X-ray' and 'How to read an abdomen X-ray'. Chapter 11 covers the more common fractures as well as an introductory section on the basics of skeletal radiography. Chapter 13 is largely concerned with interpretation of spine radiographs in trauma.

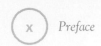

The remainder of the book is divided into broad clinical headings. Examples of normal radiographs and CT scans have been added. The major change in these chapters is the addition of much more clinical information. This has drawn on evidence-based guidelines and appropriateness criteria, where these are available.

My hope is that the information in these chapters will help students to sort out not only which test is appropriate, but whether imaging is required at all.

David A. Lisle
Brisbane, March 2006

Acknowledgements

As with previous editions many people have assisted me in the preparation of this book. My thanks go to the following for helping me find images: Michael Cheers, Jim Coates, Craig Collins, Neville Collins, Aaron Hall, Allison Hayes, Todd Malone, Lynda-Jane Michel, Ken Mitchell, Paul Monsour, Jane Reasbeck, Paul Rigby, John Shipstone, Richard Slaughter, Carmel Smith and Catherine Yantsch. Thanks also to Jane Tod, Fiona Goodgame, Clare Weber and Clare Patterson at Arnold Publishers for their continued trust and support. Finally, my eternal gratitude goes to my family without whom none of it is possible or worthwhile.

Education is an admirable thing, but it is well to remember from time to time that nothing that is worth knowing can be taught.

Oscar Wilde (1856-1900)

Introduction to medical imaging

X-RAY IMAGING

CONVENTIONAL RADIOGRAPHY (X-RAYS; PLAIN FILMS)

X-rays are a form of electromagnetic radiation. The frequency and energy of X-rays are much greater than visible light. They are produced in an X-ray tube by focusing a beam of high-energy electrons on to a tungsten target. They are able to pass through the human body and on to X-ray film thus producing an image (Fig. 1.1). X-ray films are held in cassettes of varying size depending on the part of the body to be examined. After an X-ray exposure is made the films are processed in a darkroom or more commonly in free-standing daylight processors. The resulting image is commonly known as an 'X-ray'. The common terms 'chest X-ray' and 'abdomen X-ray' are widely accepted and commonly abbreviated to CXR and AXR, respectively. More correct terms for an X-ray image are 'radiograph' or 'plain film'.

As a beam of X-rays passes through the human body some of the X-rays are absorbed or scattered producing reduction or attenuation of the beam. The degree of X-ray beam attenuation is largely dependent on the density and atomic number of the various tissues. Tissues of high density cause more X-ray beam attenuation. X-rays turn X-ray film black. Therefore, less-dense tissues and structures appear darker than tissues of higher density. Similarly, materials of high atomic number cause more X-ray beam attenuation than those of low atomic number.

Five principal densities are recognized on plain radiographs (Fig. 1.2). They are listed here in order of increasing density:

1 Air/gas: black, e.g. lungs, bowel and stomach.
2 Fat: dark grey, e.g. subcutaneous tissue layer, retroperitoneal fat.
3 Soft tissues/water: light grey, e.g. solid organs, heart, blood vessels, muscle and fluid-filled organs such as bladder.
4 Bone: off-white.
5 Contrast material/metal: bright white.

An object will be seen with conventional radiography if its borders lie beside tissue of different density. For example, the heart border is seen because it lies against aerated lung, which is less dense. When lung consolidation occurs, such as in pneumonia, the lung density approaches that of soft tissue. Consolidated lung lying against the heart border will therefore obscure that border. A good example is consolidation or collapse of the right middle lobe causing loss of definition of the right heart border (Fig. 1.3). These comments apply to all radiographically visible anatomical interfaces in the body.

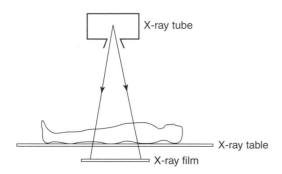

Fig. 1.1 *Conventional radiography.*

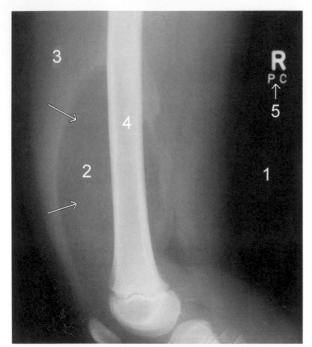

Fig. 1.2 *The five principal radiographic densities. This radiograph of a benign lipoma (arrows) in a child's thigh demonstrates the five basic radiographic densities: (1) air; (2) fat; (3) soft tissue; (4) bone; (5) metal.*

FLUOROSCOPY

Fluoroscopy refers to the technique of examination of the anatomy and motion of internal structures by a constant stream of X-rays. The term 'fluoroscopy' is derived from the ability of X-rays to cause fluorescence. The original fluoroscopes were rather primitive and consisted of an X-ray tube, fluorescent screen and X-ray table. The radiologist directly viewed the image on the fluorescent screen. The images were very faint; examinations were performed in a darkened room by a radiologist with dark-adapted vision. Dark-adaptation was achieved by wearing red goggles for 30 minutes.

Fluoroscopy was revolutionized in the 1950s by the development of the image intensifier. The image intensifier converts X-rays into images that are usually viewed via a closed circuit television chain (Fig. 1.4). Images may be recorded as X-ray spot films performed during screening or electronically from television cameras in digital format.

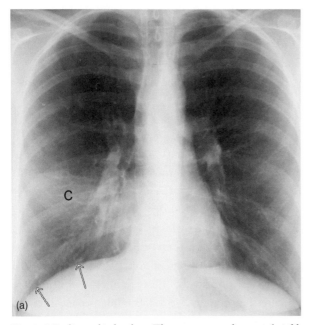

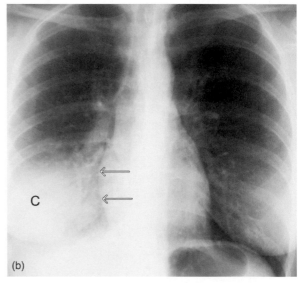

Fig. 1.3 *Radiographic borders. The presence or absence of visible radiographic borders can assist in the diagnosis and localization of pathology as illustrated in these two examples. (a) Consolidation of the right middle lobe (C) obscures the right heart border. The diaphragm can still be seen (arrows). (b) Consolidation of the right lower lobe (C) obscures the diaphragm. The right heart border can still be seen (arrows).*

Uses of fluoroscopy include:

- Barium studies of the gastrointestinal tract.
- Angiography and interventional radiology.
- General surgery (operative cholangiography, colonoscopy, etc.).
- Orthopaedic surgery: reduction and fixation of fractures, joint replacements, etc.
- Airway screening in children for tracheomalacia, and diaphragm screening.

DIGITAL SUBTRACTION IMAGING

Digital subtraction imaging (DSI) is a process whereby a computer removes unwanted information from a radiographic image. It is particularly useful for angiography, referred to as DSA. The principles of digital subtraction are illustrated in Fig. 1.5.

COMPUTED AND DIGITAL RADIOGRAPHY

Diagnostic imaging is currently undergoing a 'digital revolution'. Radiographic images may now be produced digitally using one of two processes, computed radiography (CR) and digital radiography (DR). Both methods use an X-ray tube, as described above. Instead of using X-ray film, CR employs cassettes that contain a photostimulable phosphor. After the X-ray exposure is performed the cassette is inserted into a laser reader. A fine laser beam passes across the phosphor in the cassette dislodging light photons. The number of photons dislodged is in proportion to the amount of X-rays that have hit the phosphor. An analogue-digital converter (ADC) produces a digital image. Digital radiography uses a detector screen containing silicon detectors. These detectors produce an electrical signal when exposed to X-rays. This signal is analysed to produce a digital image.

Computed radiography is generally more portable and versatile than DR. The latter is most widely used in mammography and dental radiography. Both methods remove the need for the chemicals used in processing X-ray films. More important are the many inherent advantages of digital imaging. These include the ability to perform various manipulations on the images after they have been taken, including magnification of areas of interest, alteration of density and accurate measurements of distances and angles (Fig. 1.6).

PICTURE ARCHIVING AND COMMUNICATION SYSTEMS

Many hospital X-ray departments now employ large computer storage facilities and networks known as

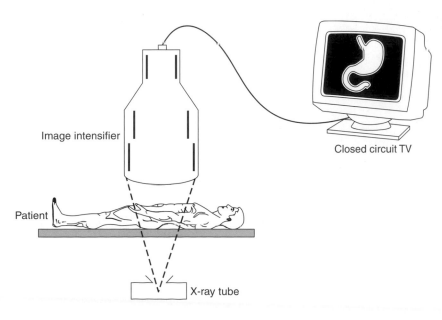

Image intensifier

Closed circuit TV

Patient

X-ray tube

Fig. 1.4 *Fluoroscopy.*

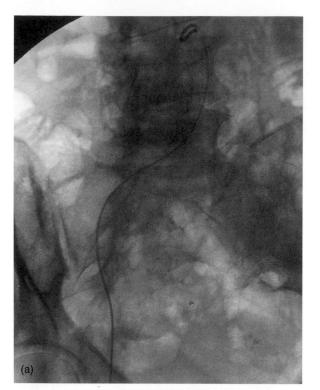

(a)

picture archiving and communication systems (PACS). Images obtained by CR and DR may be stored digitally, removing the need for bulky X-ray packets and large X-ray storage rooms in hospitals. The PACS also allow instant recall and display of a patient's radiographs and scans. These can be displayed on monitors in the wards or theatre as required.

CONTRAST MATERIALS

The ability of conventional radiography and fluoroscopy to display a range of organs and structures may be enhanced by the use of various contrast materials. The most common contrast materials are based on barium or iodine. Barium and iodine are high atomic number materials that strongly absorb X-rays and are therefore seen as dense white on radiography.

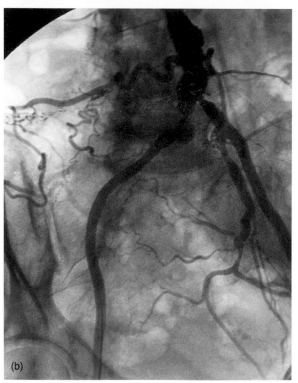

(b)

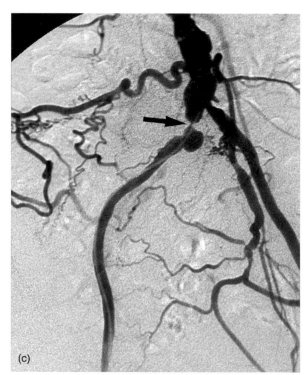

(c)

Fig. 1.5 *Digital subtraction angiography (DSA). (a) Mask image performed before injection of contrast material. (b) Contrast material injected producing opacification of the arteries. (c) Subtracted image. The computer subtracts the mask from the contrast image leaving an image of contrast filled arteries unobscured by overlying structures. Note a stenosis of the right common iliac artery (arrow).*

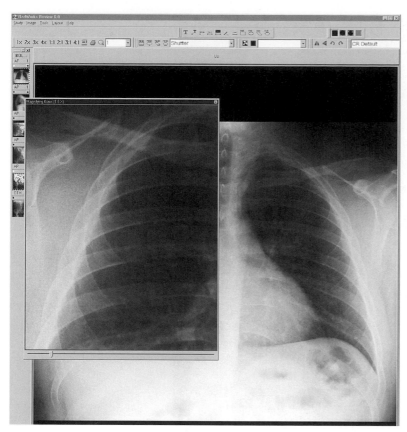

Fig. 1.6 *Computed radiography. With computed radiography images may be reviewed and reported on a computer workstation. This allows various manipulations of images as well as application of functions such as measurements of length (see Fig. 3.4) and angle measurements (see Fig. 13.18). This example shows a 'magnifying glass' function, which provides a magnified view of a selected part of the image.*

GASTROINTESTINAL CONTRAST MATERIALS

Contrast materials may be swallowed or injected via nasogastric tube to outline the upper gastrointestinal tract and small bowel, or may be introduced via an enema tube to demonstrate the large bowel. Gastrointestinal contrast materials are usually based on barium, which is non-water-soluble. Occasionally a water-soluble contrast material based on iodine is used for imaging of the gastrointestinal tract. A single contrast barium study is one where a hollow viscus such as the stomach or bowel is filled with barium. The outline of the organ can be appreciated, although not its mucosal surfaces (Fig. 1.7). If gas is then used to dilate the organ, the mucosal surfaces can be seen coated with barium. This is 'double contrast' (Fig. 1.8). The majority of barium meals and enemas are performed in double contrast as it provides much better mucosal detail than single contrast. For double contrast barium meals gas-forming compounds are swallowed along with the barium. In double contrast barium enemas air is pumped into the bowel after coating of the mucosal surfaces with barium. Single contrast studies using barium only may be performed in children, and occasionally in the very elderly.

IODINATED CONTRAST MATERIALS

Water-soluble contrast materials may be injected into veins, arteries, and various body cavities and systems. The radiographic contrast of these water-soluble contrast materials is based on the high atomic number of iodine. These compounds are therefore known as iodinated contrast materials. Iodinated contrast materials are

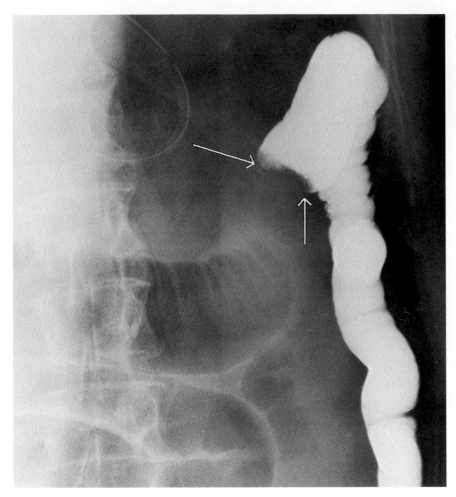

Fig. 1.7 *Single contrast barium enema showing an obstructing tumour (arrows) in the distal transverse colon.*

used in radiography to visualize various body systems and organs as follows:

- Arteries: injection into arterial system – arteriography or angiography (Fig. 1.5).
- Kidneys, ureters and bladder: intravenous injection followed by renal excretion – intravenous pyelography (IVP).
- Joints: injection into various joints including shoulder, hip and knee – arthrography.
- Outline of nerve roots and spinal cord: injection into thecal sac – myelography.
- Salivary glands: injection into salivary gland duct – sialography.

Iodinated contrast materials are also used to enhance tissue contrast in computed tomography scanning (see below). For notes on adverse reactions to iodinated contrast materials please see Chapter 2.

COMPUTED TOMOGRAPHY

COMPUTED TOMOGRAPHY PHYSICS AND TERMINOLOGY

Computed tomography (CT) is an imaging technique whereby cross-sectional images are obtained with the use of X-rays. The patient passes through a gantry that rotates around the level of interest. The gantry has an X-ray tube on one side and a set of detectors on the other. Information from the detectors is analysed by

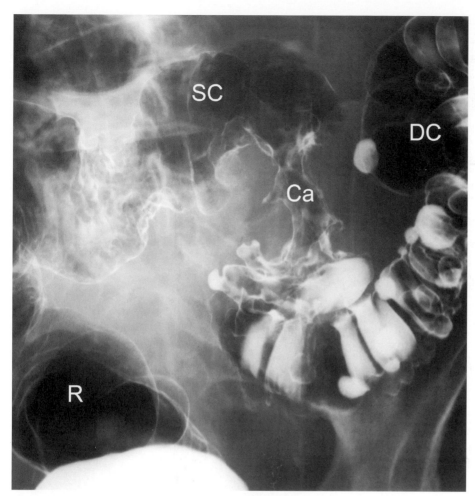

Fig. 1.8 *Double contrast barium enema showing a carcinoma (Ca) of the sigmoid colon (SC). The carcinoma produces localized narrowing of the bowel in the shape of an apple-core. Note also the rectum (R) and descending colon (DC).*

computer and displayed as an image (Fig. 1.9). Owing to the use of computer analysis, a much greater array of densities can be displayed than on conventional X-ray films. This allows differentiation of solid organs from each other and from pathological processes such as tumour or fluid collections. It also makes CT extremely sensitive to the presence of minute amounts of fat, calcium or contrast material.

As with plain radiography, high-density objects cause more attenuation of the X-ray beam and are therefore displayed as lighter grey than objects of lower density. White and light-grey objects are therefore said to be of 'high attenuation'; dark-grey and black objects are said to be of 'low attenuation'. Furthermore, the image information can be manipulated by the computer to display the various tissues of the body. This is called 'altering the window settings'. For example, in chest CT where a wide range of tissue densities is present, a good image of the mediastinal structures shows no lung details. By setting a lung window the lung parenchyma is seen in remarkable detail, though the mediastinal structures are poorly differentiated (Fig. 1.10).

Intravenous iodinated contrast material is used in CT for a number of reasons, as follows:

- Differentiation of normal blood vessels from abnormal masses, e.g. hilar vessels versus lymph nodes (Fig. 1.11).
- To make an abnormality more apparent, e.g. liver metastases (Fig. 8.2, page 121).

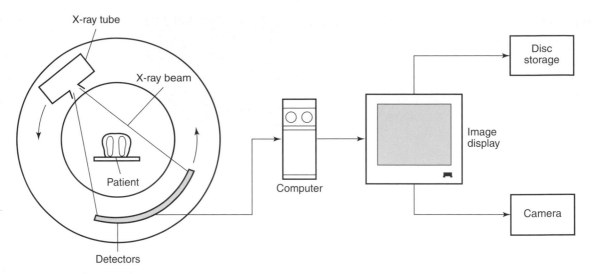

Fig. 1.9 *Computed tomography.*

- To demonstrate the vascular nature of a mass and thus aid in characterization (Figs 8.3 and 8.4, page 122).
- CT angiography (see Chapters 5 and 14).

Oral contrast material is also used for CT of the abdomen to allow differentiation of normal enhancing bowel loops from abnormal masses or fluid collections (Fig. 1.12). For detailed examination of the pelvis and distal large bowel administration of rectal contrast material is occasionally used.

The first CT scanners in the 1970s were used only for examination of the head because of their small size. With the development of larger scanners in the 1980s CT was applied to all areas of the body. With the development of helical CT and then multidetector CT through the 1990s many more CT applications have been developed as outlined below.

MULTIDETECTOR ROW CT

Helical (spiral) CT scanners became available in the early 1990s. These machines differ from conventional

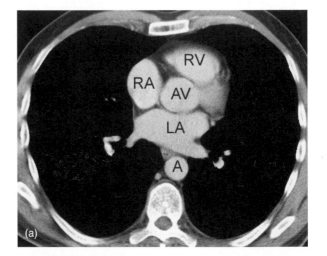

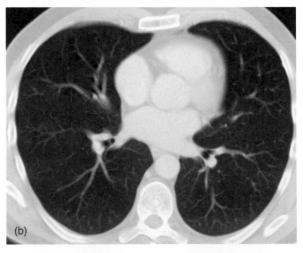

Fig. 1.10 *Computed tomography windows. (a) Mediastinal windows showing mediastinal anatomy: right atrium (RA), right ventricle (RV), aortic valve (AV), aorta (A), left atrium (LA). (b) Lung windows showing lung anatomy.*

scanners in that the tube and detectors rotate without stops as the patient passes through on the scanning table. In this way, a continuous set of data is obtained which has a helical configuration (Fig. 1.13a).

The major advantages of helical scanning over conventional scanning are:

- Increased speed of examination.
- Rapid examination at optimal levels of intravenous contrast concentration.
- The continuous volumetric nature of data allows accurate high-quality three-dimensional (3D) reconstruction.

Multidetector row CT (MDCT), also known as multi-slice CT (MSCT), was developed in the mid- to late-1990s. MDCT builds on the concepts of helical CT in that a circular gantry holding the X-ray tube on one side and detectors on the other rotates continuously as the patient passes through. The difference is that instead of a single row of detectors multiple detector rows are used (Fig. 1.13b). The initial MSCT scanners used two or four rows of detectors. In a four-row scanner, four sections (or 'slices') are obtained with each rotation of the gantry. At the time of writing 16- and 64-row scanners are widely available. Multidetector row CT allows the acquisition of overlapping fine sections of data, which, in turn, allows the reconstruction of highly accurate and detailed 3D images as well as sections in any desired plane. Four-row scanners opened up many new and varied applications of CT including:

- Repair of fractures in complex areas: acetabulum, foot and ankle, distal radius and carpus.
- Display of complex anatomy for planning of cranial and facial reconstruction surgery (Fig. 1.14).
- CT angiography: coronary, cerebral, carotid (Fig. 1.15), pulmonary, renal, visceral, peripheral.
- Coronary artery calcium scoring.
- CT colography (virtual colonoscopy).

The newer 16- and 64-row machines allow accurate imaging of rapidly moving structures. This has opened up the field of cardiac CT, including CT coronary angiography.

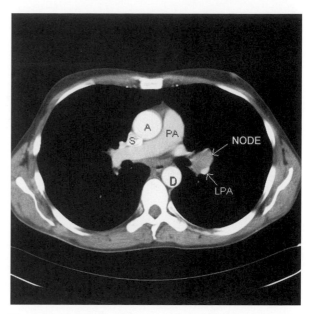

Fig. 1.11 *Intravenous contrast. An enlarged left hilar lymph node is differentiated from enhancing vascular structures: left pulmonary artery (LPA), main pulmonary artery (PA), ascending aorta (A), superior vena cava (S) and descending aorta (D).*

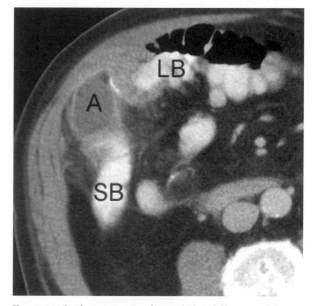

Fig. 1.12 *Oral contrast. An abscess (A) is differentiated from contrast-filled small bowel (SB) and large bowel (LB).*

LIMITATIONS AND DISADVANTAGES OF CT

Disadvantages of CT relate to its use of ionizing radiation, hazards of intravenous contrast material, lack of portability of equipment, and its relatively high cost. Radiation dose is a particularly important issue and is discussed in Chapter 2.

ULTRASOUND

ULTRASOUND PHYSICS AND TERMINOLOGY

Ultrasound (US) imaging uses ultra-high-frequency sound waves to produce cross-sectional images of the body. The basic component of the US probe is the piezoelectric crystal. Excitation of this crystal by electrical signals causes it to emit ultra-high-frequency sound waves (the piezoelectric effect). Sound waves are reflected back to the crystal by the various tissues of the body. These sound waves act on the piezoelectric crystal in the ultrasound probe to produce an electric signal, again by the piezoelectric effect. Analysis of this electric signal by a computer produces a cross-sectional image (Fig. 1.16, page 13).

Assorted body tissues produce various degrees of sound wave reflection and are said to be of different echogenicity. A tissue of high echogenicity reflects more sound than a tissue of low echogenicity. The terms hyperechoic and hypoechoic are used to describe tissues of high and low echogenicity respectively. In an ultrasound image, hyperechoic tissues are shown as white or light grey and hypoechoic tissues are seen as dark grey (Fig. 1.17, page 13). Examples of hyperechoic tissues include fat-containing masses and liver haemangiomas; lymphoma and fibroadenoma of the breast are examples of hypoechoic tissues.

Pure fluid reflects virtually no sound and is said to be anechoic. Fluid is seen on US images as black. Furthermore, because virtually all sound is transmitted through a fluid-containing area, tissues distal to such an area receive more sound and hence appear lighter. This effect is known as acoustic enhancement and is seen in tissues distal to the gallbladder, the urinary bladder and simple cysts. The reverse effect occurs with areas of sharply increased echogenicity where distal tissues receive

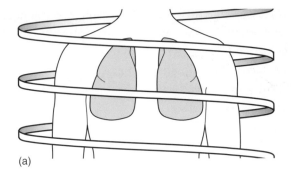
(a)

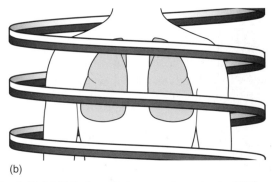
(b)

Fig. 1.13 *(a) Helical or spiral computed tomography (CT). (b) Multidetector row or multislice CT (MDCT). (Images courtesy of Michael Cheers, Siemens Ltd., Medical Solutions.)*

little sound and are thus perceived as black. This phenomenon is known as acoustic shadow and is seen distal to gas-containing areas, as well as gallstones, renal stones and other areas of calcification.

DOPPLER US

Anyone who has heard a police or ambulance siren speed past will be familiar with the Doppler effect, which describes the influence of a moving object on sound waves. An object travelling towards the listener causes sound waves to be compressed giving a higher frequency; an object travelling away from the listener gives a lower frequency.

The Doppler effect has been applied to US imaging. Flowing blood causes an alteration to the frequency of sound waves returning to the US probe. This frequency change or shift is calculated allowing quantification of blood flow (Fig. 1.18, page 13).

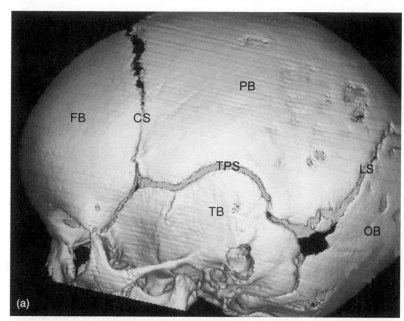

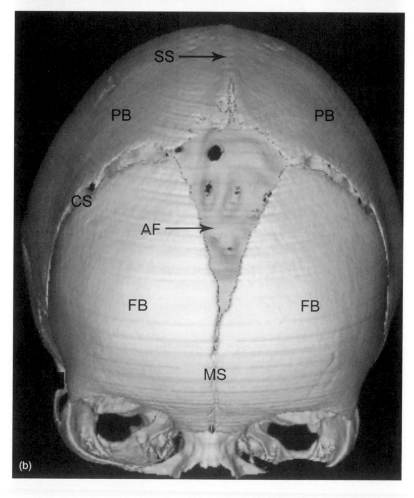

Fig. 1.14 *Three-dimensional (3D) reconstruction of an infant's skull showing a fused sagittal suture. Normal sutures are seen on 3D computed tomography (CT) as lucent lines between skull bones. Note the lack of a normal lucent line at the position of the sagittal suture indicating fusion of the suture. (a) Lateral view showing the frontal bone (FB), parietal bone (PB), temporal bone (TB), occipital bone (OB), coronal suture (CS), temporoparietal suture (TPS) and lambdoid suture (LS). (b) Frontal view also shows the metopic suture (MS), anterior fontanelle (AF) and fused sagittal suture (SS).*

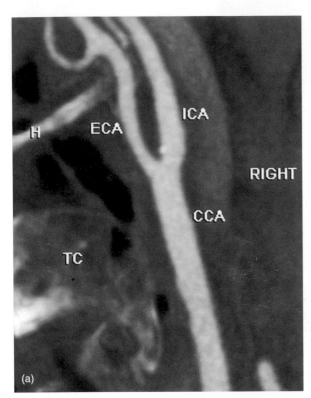
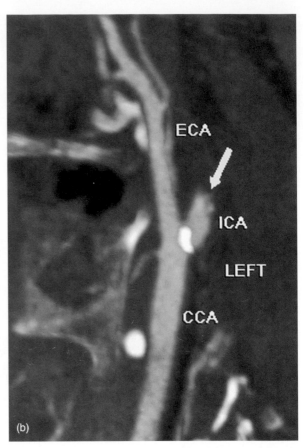

Fig. 1.15 *Computed tomography angiography (CTA). (a) Right side: a reconstruction in the sagittal plane shows the common carotid artery (CCA), internal carotid artery (ICA), external carotid artery (ECA), as well as the hyoid bone (H) and thyroid cartilage (TC). (b) Left side: CTA shows total occlusion of the left internal carotid artery.*

Colour Doppler is an extension of these principles, in that blood flowing towards the transducer is coloured red, blood flowing away from the transducer is coloured blue. The colours are superimposed on the cross-sectional image allowing instant assessment of direction of flow. Colour Doppler is particularly useful in echocardiography and for identifying very small vessels such as the calf veins, or arcuate arteries in the kidneys. It is also used to confirm blood flow within organs (e.g. testis to exclude torsion) and to assess the vascularity of tumours.

The combination of conventional two-dimensional US imaging with Doppler US is known as Duplex US (Fig. 1.19). As outlined in Chapters 5 and 14, Duplex US is an important technique in the examination of arteries and veins.

INTRACAVITARY SCANNING

An assortment of probes is now available for imaging various body cavities and organs. Transvaginal scanning allows more accurate assessment of gynaecological problems and of early pregnancy up to about 12 weeks gestation. Transrectal probes are used to assess the prostate gland and guide biopsy. Small US probes can be attached to endoscopes for assessment of tumours of the upper gastrointestinal tract as well as rectal tumours. Echocardiography can be performed

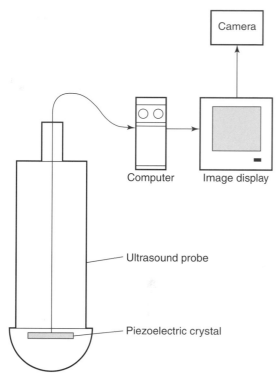

Fig. 1.16 *Ultrasound (US). The piezoelectric crystal in the US probe is used to both transmit and receive the US waves. The returned signal is analysed by computer and displayed as an image.*

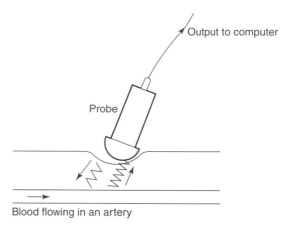

Fig. 1.18 *Doppler ultrasound. Blood flow is toward the ultrasound probe. The returning signal is of higher frequency. The frequency shift between the emitted and returning ultrasound signals is analysed by computer and displayed as a graph.*

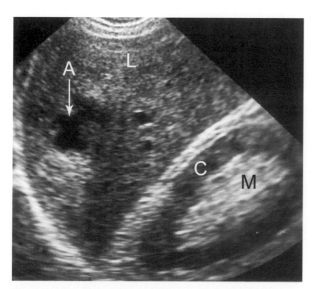

Fig. 1.17 *An abscess in the liver demonstrates tissues of varying echogenicity. Note the anechoic fluid in the abscess (A), moderately echogenic liver (L), hypoechoic renal cortex (C) and hyperechoic renal medulla (M).*

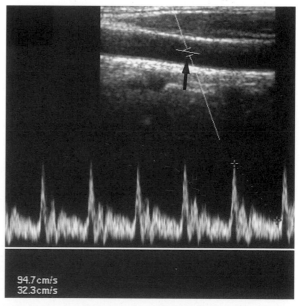

Fig. 1.19 *Duplex ultrasound. The Doppler sample gate is positioned in the artery (arrow) and the frequency shifts displayed as a graph. Peak-systolic and end-diastolic velocities are calculated and displayed on the image in centimetres per second.*

via an endoscopic probe sited in the oesophagus. This removes the problem of overlying ribs and lung, which can obscure the heart when performing conventional echocardiography.

HIGH-FREQUENCY SCANNING

The use of high-frequency probes has opened up the area of musculoskeletal ultrasound (Fig. 1.20). This technique has found greatest application in the shoulder joint, specifically in the assessment of the rotator cuff. Most muscles and tendons of the body can also be examined for rupture, inflammation, tumour, etc. In general surgery, high-frequency US has increased the accuracy of small parts imaging such as thyroid and parathyroid. Intraoperative US also uses high-frequency probes directly applied to the organ of interest, including liver and pancreas.

USES AND ADVANTAGES OF US

The principal advantage of US is the lack of ionizing radiation. This is a particular advantage in the assessment of pregnancy and in paediatrics. Other advantages include relatively low cost and portability of equipment. Ultrasound scanning is applicable to the solid organs of the body including liver, kidneys, spleen and pancreas. It has a long-established and extensive role in obstetrics and gynaecology. High-frequency, smaller probes are used for US examination of the thyroid, breast and

testes, as well as the musculoskeletal system. Used in conjunction with Doppler, US is has found a wide variety of cardiovascular applications including echocardiography, assessment of carotid, renal, mesenteric and peripheral arteries for stenosis and assessment of deep veins for thrombosis or incompetence.

DISADVANTAGES AND LIMITATIONS OF US

Ultrasound cannot penetrate gas or bone. Hence, lesions lying behind or within gas or bone cannot be visualized. Therefore, US is not used for pulmonary conditions, and bowel gas may obscure structures deep in the abdomen such as the pancreas or renal arteries. Bone lesions are not usually amenable to assessment with US. Similarly, the intracranial contents of an adult cannot be examined because of the overlying skull vault.

SCINTIGRAPHY (NUCLEAR MEDICINE)

PHYSICS OF SCINTIGRAPHY AND TERMINOLOGY

Scintigraphy refers to the use of gamma radiation to form images following the injection of various radiopharmaceuticals. The key word to understanding scintigraphy is 'radiopharmaceutical'. The 'radio' part refers to the radionuclide, i.e. the emitter of gamma rays. The most commonly used radionuclide in clinical practice is technetium, written in this text as ^{99m}Tc, where 99 is the atomic mass, and the small 'm' stands for metastable. Metastable means that the technetium atom has two basic energy states: high and low. As the technetium passes from the high-energy state to the low-energy state, it emits a packet of energy in the form of a gamma ray, which has energy of 140 keV (Fig. 1.21). The gamma rays are detected by a gamma camera that converts the absorbed energy of the radiation to an electric signal. This signal is analysed by a computer and displayed as an image (Fig. 1.22).

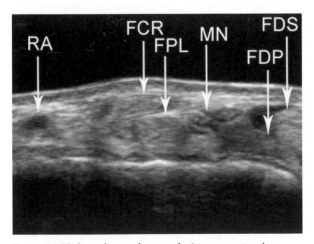

Fig. 1.20 *High-resolution ultrasound. A cross-sectional image at the level of the carpal tunnel shows the radial artery (RA) and the median nerve (MN) as well as the following tendons: flexor carpi radialis (FCR), flexor pollicis longus (FPL), flexor digitorum superficialis (FDS) and flexor digitorum profundus (FDP).*

The 'pharmaceutical' part of radiopharmaceutical refers to the compound to which the radionuclide is bound. This compound will vary depending on the area to be examined. For example, diphosphonate compounds such as methylene diphosphonate (MDP) are taken up by osteoblasts. Technetium is attached to MDP to form a radiopharmaceutical written as ^{99m}Tc-MDP. Areas of high osteoblastic activity in 'active' bone lesions such as bone metastases or osteomyelitis have increased uptake of ^{99m}Tc-MDP. These lesions are therefore detected as areas of increased gamma radiation or 'hot spots'. Areas of low uptake are referred to as photon-deficient or 'cold'.

For other applications technetium may be attached to red blood cells by injection of stannous pyrophosphate for a labelled red blood cells study. This technique is used in cardiac studies to search for sites of bleeding especially in the gastrointestinal tract, and occasionally

to characterize haemangiomas in the liver. For some applications a pharmaceutical is not required. Free technetium (referred to as pertechnetate) is used for thyroid scanning and in other less common applications such as Meckel's diverticulum. Other commonly used radionuclides include gallium (^{67}Ga) citrate, thallium (^{201}Tl), indium (^{111}In) and iodine (^{131}I). Gallium scanning is used in a number of clinical situations. Gallium is bound to plasma proteins, most strongly to transferrin. It is also taken up by white blood cells. Scanning is performed at 24, 48 and occasionally 72 hours post-injection. The most common indications for gallium scanning are to localize occult infection in a patient with pyrexia of unknown origin and in the staging and follow-up of lymphoma (Fig. 1.23). Thallium (^{201}Tl) is used in cardiac scanning, indium (^{111}In) in labelled white cell studies and iodine (^{131}I) in thyroid scanning.

The main advantages of scintigraphy are:
- Scintigraphy is highly sensitive. For example, early osteomyelitis may not be visible on plain films for 7–10 days, while scintigraphy will be positive at the time of presentation.
- Functional information is provided as well as anatomical information. For example, diethylene-triamine pentaacetic acid (DTPA) renal scans provide information on renal function, as well as renal size and drainage of the collecting systems.

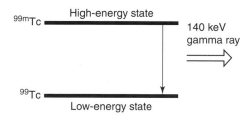

Fig. 1.21 *Gamma ray production. The metastable atom ^{99m}Tc passes from a high-energy to a low-energy state and releases gamma radiation with a peak energy of 140 keV.*

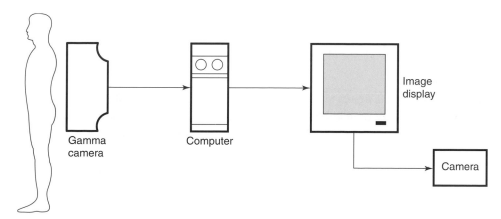

Fig. 1.22 *Scintigraphy (nuclear medicine).*

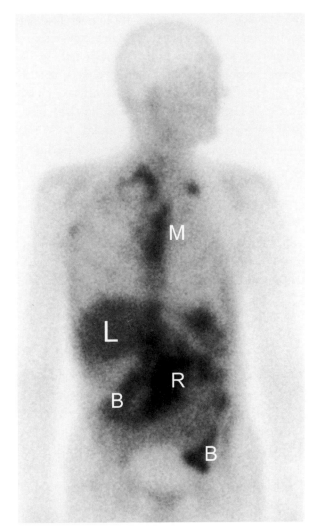

Fig. 1.23 *Gallium scintigraphy: lymphoma. Abnormal uptake of gallium indicating lymphadenopathy in the mediastinum (M) and retroperitoneum (R), as well as normal physiological uptake in liver (L) and bowel (B).*

SINGLE PHOTON EMISSION COMPUTED TOMOGRAPHY

Single photon emission computed tomography (SPECT) is a technique whereby the computer is programmed to analyse data coming from a single depth within the patient. In this way, cross-sectional scans analogous to plain tomography are obtained. This technique allows greater sensitivity in the detection of subtle lesions overlain by other active structures. A common example is the detection of pars interarticularis defects in the lower spine (Fig. 1.24). The main applications of

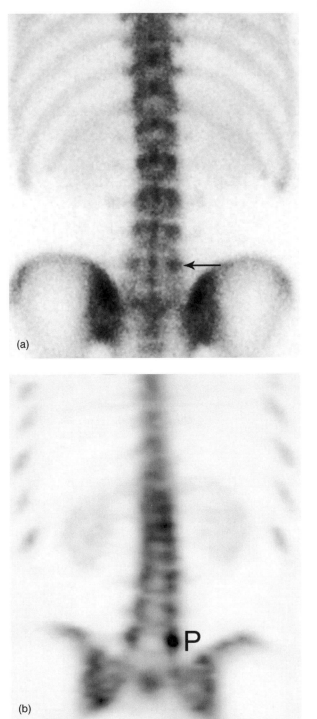

Fig. 1.24 *Single photon emission computed tomography (SPECT). (a) Scintigraphy in a man with lower back pain shows a subtle area of mildly increased activity (arrow). (b) A SPECT scan in the coronal plane shows an obvious focus of increased activity in a pars interarticularis defect (P).*

SPECT are in bone scanning, ^{201}Tl cardiac scanning, and in cerebral perfusion studies.

POSITRON EMISSION TOMOGRAPHY

Positron emission tomography (PET) is a relatively new imaging technique that is gaining increasing acceptance, particularly in the fields of oncology and cardiology. It requires radionuclides that decay by positron emission. Positron emission occurs when a proton-rich unstable isotope transforms protons from its nucleus into neutrons and positrons. Positron-emitting isotopes are produced in a cyclotron.

Positron-emission tomography is based on principles similar to other fields of scintigraphy whereby a radionuclide is attached to a biological compound to form a radiopharmaceutical, which is injected into the patient. The most commonly used radionuclide in PET scanning is fluorodeoxyglucose (FDG), which is 2-deoxyglucose labelled with the positron-emitter fluorine-18 (^{18}F). Positrons emitted from the ^{18}F in FDG collide with negatively charged electrons. The mass of both particles is converted into two 511 keV photons (i.e. high-energy gamma rays) which are emitted in opposite directions to each other. This event is known as annihilation (Fig. 1.25).

The PET camera consists of a ring of detectors that register the annihilations. Fluorodeoxyglucose is an analogue of glucose and therefore accumulates in areas of high glucose metabolism. An area of high concentration of FDG will have a large number of annihilations and will be shown on the resulting image as a 'hot spot'. Normal physiological uptake of FDG occurs in the brain (high level of glucose metabolism), myocardium and in the renal collecting systems, ureters and bladder. Less intense normal uptake of FDG may be seen in liver, spleen, bone marrow and salivary glands, with more variable uptake in the gastrointestinal tract.

The current roles of PET imaging may be summarized as follows:
- Oncology:
  (i) Differentiate benign and malignant masses, e.g. solitary pulmonary nodule;
  (ii) Primary tumour staging, especially for breast carcinoma, melanoma, non-small cell carcinoma of the lung and Hodgkin's disease (Fig. 1.26);
  (iii) Detect tumour recurrence, especially in areas where changes from surgery or radiotherapy make CT difficult to interpret, e.g. colorectal carcinoma.
- Cardiac: non-invasive assessment of myocardial viability in patients with coronary artery disease.
- Central nervous system:
  (i) Characterization of dementia disorders;
  (ii) Localization of seizure focus in epilepsy.

POSITRON-EMISSION TOMOGRAPHY–CT FUSION IMAGING

As with other types of scintigraphy, a problem with PET is its non-specificity. Put another way, 'hot spots' on PET may have multiple causes with false positive findings commonly encountered. This non-specificity may be reduced by close correlation with anatomical information. This has led to the development of PET–CT fusion imaging. As suggested by the name PET–CT fusion imaging combines the functional and metabolic information of PET with the precise cross-sectional anatomy

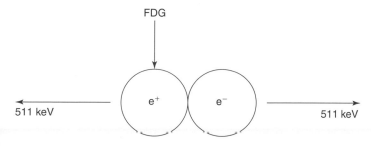

Fig. 1.25 *Annihilation. A positron (e^+) emitted by an FDG molecule encounters an electron (e^-). The two particles annihilate converting their mass into energy in the form of two 511 keV gamma rays, which are emitted in opposite directions.*

FDG

511 keV ← e^+ e^- → 511 keV

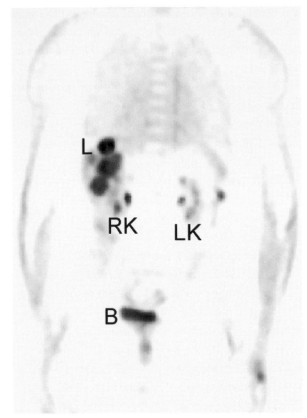

Fig. 1.26 *Positron-emission tomography (PET): liver metastases. A coronal PET image shows normal activity in the kidneys (RK and LK) and bladder (B). Multiple round areas of increased activity in the right upper abdomen indicate multiple metastases in the liver (L).*

of CT. As well as reducing the number of false positive scans, PET–CT fusion imaging increases the accuracy of follow-up of malignancy, especially differentiating tumour recurrence from post-radiotherapy fibrosis.

LIMITATIONS AND DISADVANTAGES OF SCINTIGRAPHY

The main disadvantage of scintigraphy is its non-specificity. To take a common example, an isolated 'hot spot' on a bone scan could be caused by infection, trauma or neoplasia; therefore, correlation with clinical history and other imaging studies is of paramount importance. Conversely, multiple 'hot spots' on the bone scan of an elderly man being staged for prostatic carcinoma are easily diagnosed as skeletal metastases.

Furthermore, given the high sensitivity of bone scans, a normal study in such a patient virtually excludes skeletal metastatic disease. Other disadvantages of scintigraphy relate to the use of ionizing radiation, the cost of equipment, and the extra care required in handling radioactive materials.

MAGNETIC RESONANCE IMAGING

MAGNETIC RESONANCE IMAGING PHYSICS AND TERMINOLOGY

Over the past 20 years, magnetic resonance imaging (MRI) has become accepted as a powerful imaging tool. The following is a brief summary of the physical principles behind MRI.

Magnetic resonance imaging uses the magnetic properties of the hydrogen atom to produce images. The nucleus of the hydrogen atom is a single proton. Being a spinning, charged particle it has magnetic properties and, for the sake of discussion, may be thought of as a small bar magnet with north and south poles (Fig. 1.27). The first step in MRI is the application of a strong, external magnetic field. For this purpose, the patient is placed within a large, powerful magnet. The hydrogen atoms within the patient align in a direction either parallel or antiparallel to the strong external field. A greater proportion aligns in the parallel direction so that the net vector of their alignment, and therefore the net magnetic vector, will be in the direction of the external field (Fig. 1.28). This is known as longitudinal magnetization.

Although aligned in a strong magnetic field, the hydrogen nuclei do not lie motionless. Each nucleus spins around the axis of the magnetic field in a motion known as precession (Fig. 1.29). The frequency of precession is an inherent property of the hydrogen atom in a given magnetic field and is known as the Larmor frequency. The Larmor frequency therefore changes in proportion to magnetic field strength. It is of the order of 10 MHz (megahertz), a frequency in the same part of the electromagnetic spectrum as radio waves.

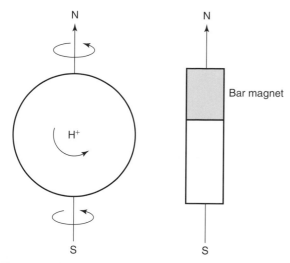

Fig. 1.27 *The spinning hydrogen atom has a small magnetic field analogous to a bar magnet.*

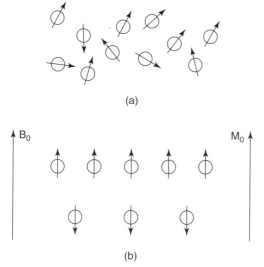

Fig. 1.28 *Effect of application of a strong magnetic field. In (a) the hydrogen atoms are randomly aligned in the normal resting state. In (b) after application of a strong external magnetic field (B_0) the hydrogen atoms align either parallel or antiparallel. Because more align in the parallel direction the net magnetic vector (M_0) is in the direction of the external magnetic field.*

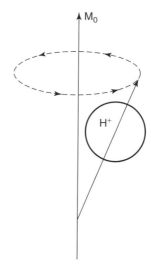

Fig. 1.29 *Precession. The hydrogen atom spins around the line of the magnetic field in a motion known as precession at a frequency called the Larmor frequency.*

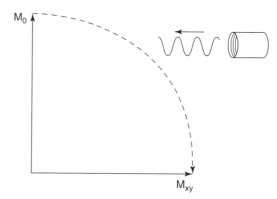

Fig. 1.30 *Application of the radiofrequency (RF) pulse at the Larmor frequency causes the net magnetic vector of the hydrogen atoms (M_0) to rotate on to the x–y plane.*

A second magnetic field is then applied at right angles to the original external field. This second magnetic field is applied at the same frequency as the Larmor frequency and is known as the radiofrequency pulse (RF pulse). A magnetic coil known as the RF coil, applies the RF pulse. The RF pulse causes the net magnetization vector of the hydrogen atoms to turn towards the transverse plane, i.e. a plane at right angles to the direction of the original, strong external field (Fig. 1.30). As such, the RF pulse adds energy to the system. Depending on the strength and duration of the RF pulse the net magnetization vector will rotate away from the longitudinal direction to a varying degree. A 90° pulse rotates the vector into the transverse plane. This is known as transverse magnetization. A 180° pulse rotates the vector to the opposite longitudinal direction. Smaller angles of rotation, known as 'flip angles', of the order of 15–30° are used for gradient-recalled-echo sequences.

The component of the net magnetization vector in the transverse plane induces an electrical current in the RF coil. This current is known as the MR signal and is the basis for formation of an image. Computer analysis of the complex MR signal from the RF receiver coils is used to produce a magnetic resonance image (Fig. 1.31). Note that in viewing MRI images, white or light grey areas are referred to as 'high signal'; dark grey or black areas are referred to as 'low signal'. On certain sequences flowing blood is seen as a black area referred to as a 'flow void'.

The standard MRI unit consists of a number of magnetic coils systems. First is the large magnet itself. This is usually a superconducting magnet that uses liquid helium. Second, a series of gradient coils is used to produce variations to the magnetic field that allow image formation. It is the rapid switching of these gradients that causes the loud noises associated with MRI scanning. Finally are the RF coils. These are applied to or around the area of interest and are used to transmit the RF pulse and to receive the RF signal. The coils come in varying shapes and sizes depending on the part of the body to be examined. Larger coils are required, for example, in imaging the heart or liver, whereas very small extremity coils are used for small parts such as the wrist or ankle.

TISSUE CONTRAST AND IMAGING SEQUENCES

Other imaging modalities rely on a single property of tissue to generate contrast between the various soft-tissue structures; computed tomography depends on the soft-tissue density whereas US depends on tissue echogenicity. Much of the complexity of MRI arises from the fact that the MR signal depends on many varied properties of the tissues and structures being examined. These properties include:

- The number of hydrogen atoms present in tissue (proton density).
- The chemical environment of the hydrogen atoms, e.g. whether in free water or bound by fat.
- Flow: blood vessels or cerebrospinal fluid (CSF).
- Magnetic susceptibility.
- T1 relaxation time (see 'Spin echo' below).
- T2 relaxation time (see 'Spin echo' below).

By altering the duration and amplitude of the RF pulse, as well as the timing and repetition of its application, various imaging sequences use these properties to produce image contrast. Terms used to describe the different types of MR imaging sequences include spin echo, inversion recovery, and gradient recalled echo (gradient echo).

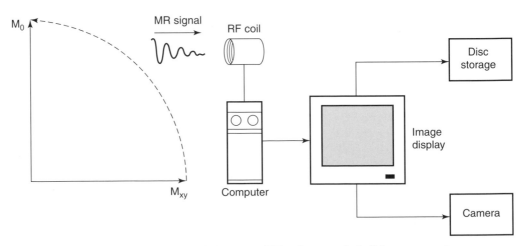

Fig. 1.31 *Production of the MR signal. When the radiofrequency (RF) pulse is switched off the net magnetic vector returns to its original direction emitting a signal that is detected by the RF coil and analysed by computer to produce an image.*

Spin echo

The spin echo sequences include T1-weighted, T2-weighted and proton density. The following paragraph is a brief explanation of the terms T1 and T2.

Following the application of a 90° RF pulse, the net magnetization vector lies in the transverse plane. Also, all of the hydrogen protons are precessing at the same rate – they are said to be 'in phase'. Upon cessation of the RF pulse two things begin to happen. The net magnetization vector will rotate back to the longitudinal direction. This is known as longitudinal relaxation or T1 relaxation. At the same time, the spinning hydrogen atoms will start to precess at slightly varying rates. This dephasing process is known as transverse relaxation or T2 relaxation (decay) and is caused by a number of factors, including minute inhomogeneities in magnetic field strength and interactions with adjacent protons.

The T1 is defined as the time taken for the longitudinal magnetization to resume 63 per cent of its final value. The T2 is defined as the amount of time for the transverse magnetization to decay to 37 per cent of its original value. The rates at which T1 and T2 relaxation occur are inherent properties of the various tissues.

Sequences that primarily use differences in T1 relaxation rates produce T1-weighted images. Tissues with long T1 values are shown as low signal while those with shorter T1 values are displayed as higher signal. The T2-weighted images reflect differences in T2 relaxation rates. Tissues whose protons dephase slowly have a long T2 and are displayed as high signal on T2-weighted images. Tissues with shorter T2 values are shown as lower signal. Both T1- and T2-weighted sequences are performed very commonly in most parts of the body (Fig. 1.32).

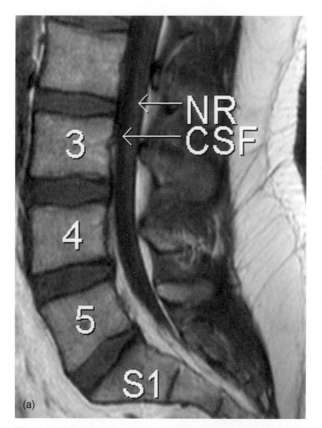
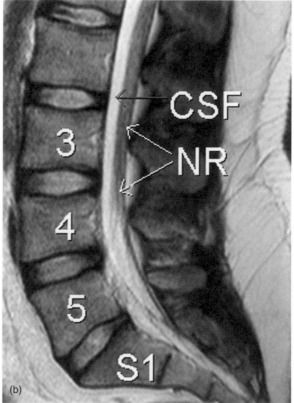

Fig. 1.32 *Magnetic resonance sagittal images of the lower lumbar spine and sacrum. (a) T1-weighted image with dark cerebrospinal fluid (CSF). (b) T2-weighted image with bright CSF and better delineation of nerve roots (NR).*

Proton density images are produced by sequences that accentuate neither T1 nor T2 differences. The signal strength of proton density images (also known as intermediate-weighted) mostly reflects the density of hydrogen atoms (protons) in the different tissues. Proton density images are particularly useful in the skeletal system for the demonstration of small structures as well as articular cartilage.

Gradient recalled echo (gradient echo)

Gradient echo sequences are used in skeletal imaging to display certain structures such as the menisci of the knee. They are also used in the brain to look for blood products in patients with suspected bleeding due to vascular tumours, previous trauma or angiopathy (Fig. 1.33). Gradient echo sequences are also capable of very rapid imaging and are increasingly used for imaging the heart as well as abdominal organs such as the liver.

Inversion recovery

Inversion recovery sequences are used to suppress unwanted signals that may obscure pathology. The two most common inversion recovery sequences are short T1-inversion recovery (STIR), used to suppress fat, and fluid-attenuated inversion recovery (FLAIR), used to suppress water. Fat suppression sequences such as STIR are used for demonstrating pathology in areas containing a lot of fat, such as the orbits and bone marrow. These sequences allow the delineation of bone marrow disorders such as oedema, bruising and infiltration (Fig. 1.34). Fluid-attenuated inversion recovery sequences suppress signal from CSF and are used to image the brain. The FLAIR sequences are particularly useful for diagnosing white matter disorders such as multiple sclerosis.

FUNCTIONAL MRI SEQUENCES

Two commonly used functional MRI sequences (fMRI) are diffusion-weighted imaging (DWI) and perfusion-weighted imaging (PWI). These will be discussed in Chapter 14.

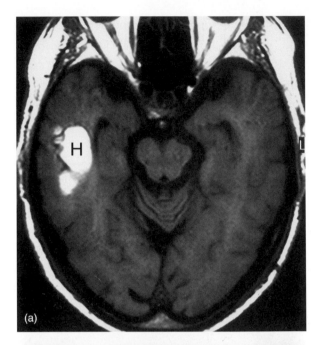

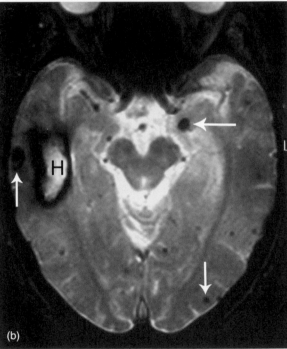

Fig. 1.33 *Gradient echo imaging of the brain. (a) T1-weighted transverse scan showing a haemorrhage (H) in the right temporal lobe of an elderly man. (b) Gradient echo scan shows a low signal rim around the haemorrhage owing to haemosiderin. Further multiple areas of haemosiderin deposition (arrows) not shown on the T1-weighted image are well seen with gradient echo. This appearance is typical of amyloid angiopathy.*

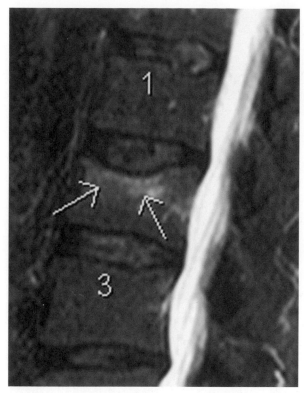

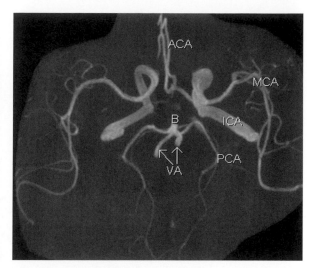

Fig. 1.35 *Magnetic resonance angiography of the brain showing normal arteries: vertebral (VA), basilar (B), posterior cerebral (PCA), internal carotid (ICA), middle cerebral (MCA) and anterior cerebral (ACA).*

Fig. 1.34 *Short T1-inversion recovery (STIR) sagittal image of the lumbar spine shows bone marrow oedema (arrows) in an acute crush fracture of L2.*

Magnetic resonance spectroscopy

Magnetic resonance spectroscopy (MRS) uses different frequencies to identify certain molecules in a selected volume of tissue, known as a voxel. An area of interest is selected by conventional MRI imaging, followed by spectroscopic analysis. Following data analysis, a spectrographic graph of certain metabolites is drawn. Metabolites of interest include lipid, lactate, N-acetyl-aspartate (NAA), choline, creatinine, citrate and myoinositol. Possible uses of MRS include imaging of dementias, differentiation of recurrent cerebral tumour from radiation necrosis or normal postoperative changes, and diagnosis of prostatic carcinoma.

Blood oxygen-level-dependent imaging

Blood oxygen-level-dependent (BOLD) imaging is a non-invasive fMRI technique used for localizing regional brain signal intensity changes in response to task performance. It does not require injection of contrast. Rather, BOLD imaging depends on regional changes in concentration of deoxyhaemoglobin, and is therefore a tool to investigate regional cerebral physiology in response to a variety of stimuli. BOLD fMRI may be used prior to surgery for brain tumour or arteriovenous malformation (AVM), as a prognostic indicator of the degree of postsurgical deficit.

MAGNETIC RESONANCE ANGIOGRAPHY

With varying sequences, flowing blood can be shown as either signal void (black) or increased signal (white). Magnetic resonance angiography (MRA) refers to the use of these sequences to display the anatomy of arteries. Computer reconstruction techniques allow the display of blood vessels in 3D as well as rotation and viewing of these blood vessels from multiple angles (Fig. 1.35). Contrast enhancement with intravenous injection of Gd-DTPA (see 'Contrast medium in MRI', below) is used for MRA of larger areas of the body such as the renal and mesenteric arteries and the arteries to the lower legs.

Magnetic resonance angiography of blood vessels with relatively slow flow rates, such as the deep venous sinuses of the brain or the small vessels of the hand or foot, is also best performed with contrast enhancement. This type of imaging provides a relatively non-invasive alternative to diagnostic angiography. Indications for MRA include:

- Imaging of the carotid arteries for stroke and transient ischaemic attack (TIA).
- Cerebral aneurysm and AVM.
- Imaging of the peripheral vessels for claudication.

Magnetic resonance imaging of veins is also performed; this is known as MR venography (MRV). This is most commonly performed in the brain to outline the major cerebral venous sinuses in cases of suspected venous sinus thrombosis or obstruction.

CONTRAST MATERIAL IN MRI

Gadolinium (Gd) is a paramagnetic substance that causes T1 shortening and therefore increased signal on T1-weighted images. Unbound gadolinium is highly toxic. For this reason, binding agents are required for *in vivo* use. The most common of these is diethylene-triamine pentaacetic acid (DTPA). Gd-DTPA is non-toxic and used in a dose of 0.1 mmol/kg.

The main indications for the use of Gd-DTPA are as follows:

- Brain:
    (i) Inflammation: meningitis, encephalitis;
    (ii) Tumours: primary (Fig. 1.36), metastases;
    (iii) Tumour residuum/recurrence following treatment.
- Spine:
    (i) Postoperative to differentiate fibrosis from recurrent disc protrusion;
    (ii) Infection: discitis, epidural abscess;
    (iii) Tumours: primary, metastases.
- Musculoskeletal system:
    (i) Soft-tissue tumours;
    (ii) Intra-articular Gd-DTPA: MR arthrography.

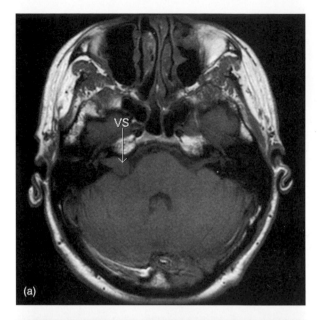

(a)

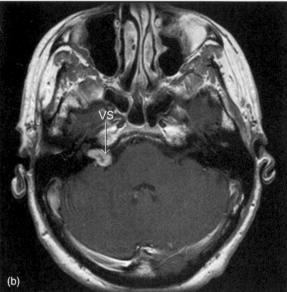

(b)

Fig. 1.36 *Intravenous contrast in magnetic resonance imaging: vestibular schwannoma. (a) A T1-weighted transverse image of the posterior fossa shows a right-sided mass. (b) Following injection of gadolinium the mass shows intense enhancement, typical of vestibular schwannoma (VS). (See also Fig. 15.10, page 237.)*

NEWER DEVELOPMENTS AND APPLICATIONS

Magnetic resonance imaging continues to develop as an imaging modality. Cardiac MR is becoming increasingly accepted in specific applications, including assessment of myocardial mass and viability, congenital heart disease and aortic disorders. Newer high field strength MRI units are becoming more widely available. Most current medical MRI machines have field strengths of 1.5 Tesla. Newer units use field strengths of 3 Tesla or more and '3T imaging' may improve the accuracy and application of MRI in neurological disorders as well as musculoskeletal applications, such as improved visualization of articular cartilage. New contrast materials are also being developed that may increase the specificity of MRI in the characterization of liver tumours.

ADVANTAGES OF MRI

The main advantages of MRI may be summarized as follows:
• Excellent soft-tissue contrast and characterization.
• Lack of artefact from adjacent bones. This makes MRI the imaging modality of choice in areas such as the posterior fossa and pituitary fossa where the quality of CT images may be degraded by artefact.
• Multiplanar capabilities: MRI is able to obtain images in any desired plane.
• Lack of ionizing radiation.

In summary, MRI is the imaging modality of choice for most brain and spine disorders. It has also found wide acceptance in the assessment of musculoskeletal disorders, including internal derangements of joints and staging of musculoskeletal tumours. It has an increasing problem-solving role for various abdominal disorders such as characterization of hepatic, renal and adrenal masses. Cardiac MRI has an accepted role in congenital heart disease and cardiomyopathy and is used increasingly for the assessment of myocardial viability. Magnetic resonance angiography is widely used in the imaging of the cerebral circulation and in some centres is the initial angiographic method of choice for other areas including the renal and peripheral circulations.

LIMITATIONS AND DISADVANTAGES OF MRI

• Cost. The equipment for MRI is very expensive. Running and maintenance costs are also high. Potential benefits to patient care must be carefully weighed against these costs when ordering MRI scans.
• Cardiac pacemakers, metal foreign objects and other hazards (see Chapter 2).
• Claustrophobia.
• Reduced sensitivity for certain substances. MRI is less sensitive than CT in the detection of small amounts of calcification and in the detection of acute haemorrhage. As such, CT is still the imaging modality of choice for the assessment of acute subarachnoid haemorrhage and for acute head injury.

Hazards and precautions in medical imaging

This chapter deals with the hazards and risks associated with the field of medical imaging. It is important for the referring doctor to have a working knowledge of these factors when considering whether to order an imaging investigation. The chapter is divided into the following topics:

1 Contrast media reactions.
2 Radiation hazards.
3 Magnetic resonance imaging (MRI) safety issues.

CONTRAST MEDIA REACTIONS

Iodinated (iodine containing) contrast media were first widely used in radiology in the 1950s. These original contrast media were highly osmolar, with osmolality five to eight times that of blood. These media were also ionic, dissociating in solution into anions and cations. These two properties, ionicity and high osmolality are largely responsible for many of the toxic effects of older contrast media. Newer contrast media gained wide acceptance in the 1980s and continue to be refined to the present day. These newer media are non-ionic and approximately isosmolar with blood with significantly reduced side-effects and adverse reactions.

Most patients injected with iodinated contrast media experience a mild warm feeling plus an odd taste in the mouth. These are normal transient phenomena. Adverse reactions to contrast media may be classified according to aetiology and severity as follows:

• Transient osmotically induced reactions.
• Anaphylactoid reactions: mild, intermediate, severe.
• Contrast media induced nephropathy.

Most adverse reactions such as nausea and vomiting, flushing and arm pain are due to osmotically induced physiological changes. These reactions are minor and transient; their incidence is significantly reduced by the use of nonionic low osmolar media.

ANAPHYLACTOID CONTRAST MEDIA REACTIONS

Immediate generalized reactions are usually classified as anaphylactoid with true anaphylaxis less common. Clinically, these reactions are indistinguishable from anaphylaxis and are classified as mild, intermediate, and severe or life threatening. Mild anaphylactoid reactions include mild urticaria and pruritus. Intermediate reactions include more severe urticaria, hypotension and mild bronchospasm. More severe reactions consist of more severe bronchospasm, laryngeal oedema, pulmonary oedema, unconsciousness, convulsions, pulmonary collapse, and cardiac arrest. The incidences of mild, intermediate and severe reactions with ionic high osmolar contrast media are 15 per cent, 0.22 per cent and 0.04 per cent, respectively. The use of non-ionic low osmolar contrast media results in reduced incidences of 3 per cent, 0.04 per cent and 0.004 per cent, respectively. Fatal reactions are exceedingly rare (1:170 000) with both types of contrast media.

Several predisposing factors are known to increase the risk of adverse reactions to contrast media. A history of asthma increases the risk of reaction to contrast media by a factor of 10 and a history of atopy by a factor of 3. A history of allergy to seafood does not appear to be associated with an increased risk of contrast media reactions. Patients with a definite history of previous anaphylactoid reaction to iodinated contrast media have about a 40 per cent risk of further reactions. Iodinated contrast media are contraindicated in these patients. There is no convincing evidence that pre-treatment with steroids or an antihistamine reduces the risk of contrast media reactions.

In summary, a few points may be made regarding anaphylactoid contrast media reactions:

- All patients should receive a risk assessment before injection of iodinated contrast media.
- Regardless of risk factors, the incidence of most reactions is reduced by the use of nonionic low osmolar contrast media.
- Iodinated contrast media should only be used if they are definitely indicated; their use should never be regarded as routine.
- Reactions are rare and occur unexpectedly.
- All staff working with iodinated contrast materials should be familiar with CPR and emergency procedures should be in place to deal with reactions, including resuscitation equipment and various drugs.

CONTRAST-INDUCED NEPHROPATHY

Contrast-induced nephropathy (CIN) refers to a reduction of renal function induced by iodinated contrast media. Laboratory evidence of CIN consists primarily of an elevation in serum creatinine of over 25 per cent within 3 days of contrast medium injection. The elevation of serum creatinine usually peaks in 3–4 days. Most cases of CIN are self-limiting with resolution in 1–2 weeks. In that time, however, there are problems of prolonged hospitalization and dialysis is required in up to 15 per cent. Therefore, CIN is a significant problem.

The major risk factor for the development of CIN is impaired renal function. Patients with impaired renal function should not receive iodinated contrast media unless absolutely necessary. The risk of CIN increases with the degree of renal impairment and is particularly high in patients with diabetic nephropathy. Other risk factors include old age (>70 years), dehydration, large doses of contrast media and the use of high osmolar media. The risk of developing CIN is reduced if the patient is well hydrated. Various pretreatments have been described such as oral acetylcysteine; however, there is currently no convincing evidence that anything other than hydration is beneficial.

RADIATION HAZARDS

Radiography, scintigraphy and computed tomography (CT) use ionizing radiation. In large doses ionizing radiation is harmful. This has been shown in numerous studies including those on survivors of the atomic bomb attacks in Japan in 1945. The risks of harm from medical radiation are low and are usually expressed as the increased risk of developing cancer as a result of exposure. Public awareness of the possible hazards of medical radiation is growing and it is important for doctors who refer patients for X-rays, nuclear medicine scans or CT scans to have at least a basic understanding of radiation effects and the principles of radiation protection.

RADIATION EFFECTS

Radiation hazards occur as a result of damage to cells caused by radiation. This damage takes many forms including cell death and genetic damage leading to mutations. Actively dividing cells such as are found in the bone marrow, lymph glands and gonads are particularly sensitive. The nature and degree of cell damage vary according to total radiation dose and dose rate, the amount of the body irradiated, and the type of radiation. In general, two types of effects may result from radiation damage: stochastic effects and deterministic effects.

With stochastic effects the probability of the effect, not its severity, is regarded as a function of dose. There is no dose threshold below which a stochastic effect will not theoretically occur. The most commonly discussed stochastic effect is increased cancer risk caused by radiation exposure. Deterministic effects result from cell death and include radiation burns, cataracts and decreased fertility. The severity of deterministic effects varies with dose. A dose threshold may exist below which the effect will not occur.

UNITS OF RADIATION DOSE

Absorbed dose refers to the amount of energy imparted by ionizing radiation in a given mass of matter. The SI unit of absorbed dose is joules per kilogram ($J\,kg^{-1}$) and is referred to as the Gray (Gy): $1\,Gy = 1.0\,J\,kg^{-1}$.

The biological effects of an absorbed radiation dose depend on the type of radiation. The concept of equivalent dose takes into account the fact that some kinds of radiation can produce more damage in tissue than others, even though the absorbed dose may be the same. A dimensionless constant known as the quality factor is used to describe the varying magnitude of biological effects caused by different types of radiation. Photons (X-rays and gamma rays) have a quality factor of 1. Neutrons, protons and alpha particles are much more damaging and have quality factors of 5 to 20. Equivalent dose is calculated by multiplying the absorbed dose by the quality factor. The SI unit of equivalent dose is joules per kilogram and is referred to as the Sievert (Sv): $1 \text{ Sv} = 1.0 \text{ J kg}^{-1}$.

The organs of the body have different susceptibilities to radiation damage. The effective dose is used to compare the risks when different organs receive radiation doses. The effective dose is calculated by multiplying the equivalent dose for each organ by an organ specific weighting factor. Organs and tissues that are more susceptible to radiation damage have higher weighting factors than less susceptible tissues. The effective dose provides a means of calculating the overall risk of radiation effects, especially the risk of cancer. As with equivalent dose, the unit of effective dose is the Sievert. Radiation doses used to compare radiological tests with each other refer to effective dose and are quoted in millisieverts (mSv). Some typical effective doses (mSv) are listed below:

- Posterior–anterior (PA) chest X-ray: 0.02.
- Lumbar spine X-ray: 1.3.
- Intravenous pyelogram (IVP): 2.5.
- Barium enema: 7.0.
- CT head: 2.0.
- CT abdomen: 10.0.
- Bone scan ^{99m}Tc-MDP: 5.2.
- Average natural background radiation: 2.0–3.0 per year.

PROTECTION IN RADIOLOGICAL PRACTICE

The International Commission on Radiological Protection (ICRP) was set up in 1928. It consists of expert delegates from many countries and its recommendations are accepted as worldwide standards. This section is a summary of numerous ICRP publications and recommendations on radiation hazards and protection, as well as recommendations of the National Health and Medical Research Council of Australia.

The aims of radiation protection are to prevent deterministic effects and to limit the probability of stochastic effects. This is done by keeping all justifiable exposure as low as is reasonably achievable (ALARA principle). The ALARA principle includes minimizing radiation doses to individuals as well as minimizing the number of people exposed. No practice is adopted unless its introduction produces a positive net benefit, i.e. a benefit that outweighs its detriment. With these aims and principles in mind the following guidelines are used for radiographic procedures.

Protection of patient

Each radiation exposure is justified on a case-by-case basis. The minimum number of radiographs is taken and minimum fluoroscopic screening time used. The X-ray beam is focused accurately to the area of interest. Only trained personnel are allowed to operate radiographic equipment. Mobile equipment is only used when the patient is unable to come to the radiology department. Modalities that do not use ionizing radiation (ultrasound or MRI) should be used where possible. Quality assurance programmes are carried out in each radiology department, including correct installation, calibration and regular testing of equipment.

Paediatrics

Children are more sensitive to radiation than adults and are at greater risk of developing radiation-induced cancers many decades after the initial exposure. In paediatric radiology, special attention should be paid to minimizing the number of exposures and screening times, and to the use of well-focused beams. The use of gentle restraining devices and/or sedation may reduce the number of repeat exposures required. Gonad shields should be used. If parents are required to be in the room, they should wear lead coats and not be directly exposed to radiation. Scanning parameters for CT should be adjusted for children. Much lower radiation doses are generally required in children than in adults to produce a diagnostically adequate CT scan.

Women of reproductive age

Radiation exposure of the abdomen and pelvis should be minimized. Consider any woman of reproductive age whose period is overdue to be pregnant. Ask all females of reproductive age if they could be pregnant. Post multilingual signs in prominent places asking patients to notify the radiographer of possible pregnancy.

Pregnancy

As organogenesis is unlikely to be occurring in an embryo in the first 4 weeks following the last menstrual period, this is not considered a critical period for radiation exposure. Organogenesis commences soon after the time of the first missed period and continues for the next 3–4 months. During this time the fetus is considered to be maximally radiosensitive. Examination of the abdomen or pelvis should be delayed if possible to a time when fetal sensitivity is reduced, i.e. post-24 weeks gestation or ideally until the baby is born. Where possible, MRI or ultrasound should be used. Exposure to remote areas such as chest, skull and limbs may be undertaken with minimal fetal exposure at any time during pregnancy. Lead aprons draped over the abdomen are more reassuring than of practical value. Nuclear medicine studies are best avoided, if possible, during pregnancy. For nuclear medicine studies in the postpartum period, it is advised that breast-feeding ceases and breast milk discarded for 2 days following the injection of radionuclide.

Protection of staff (including medical students!)

Only necessary staff members are to be present in a room where X-ray procedures are being performed. If TV monitors are placed outside the screening room students may observe procedures at a safe distance. Anyone in the fluoroscopy or CT room at the time of exposure must wear protective clothing such as lead aprons,

thyroid shields and protective glasses. At no time should staff be directly irradiated by the primary beam. Lead gloves must be worn if the hands need to enter the primary beam such as in immobilizing patients or performing stress views. All X-ray rooms should have lead lining in their walls, ceilings and floors.

MAGNETIC RESONANCE IMAGING SAFETY ISSUES

Magnetic resonance imaging involves the use of a strong static magnetic field, rapidly switching magnetic gradient fields and radiofrequency (RF) fields. At the time of writing there is no evidence of direct deleterious biological effects from any of these sources. However, a number of potential hazards associated with MRI do exist. These predominantly relate to the interaction of the magnetic fields with metallic materials and electronic devices.

The field from the MRI unit can be described in terms of two spatial regions. Region 1 refers to the area around the isocentre of the magnetic field within the bore of the magnet. Ferromagnetic objects within region 1 experience rotational forces or torque. Region 2 refers to the field outside the bore of the magnet. The strength of this field decreases with distance from the magnet. Metal objects within region 2 experience rotational and translational forces; objects are pulled toward the magnet. Reports exist of objects such as spanners, oxygen cylinders and drip poles becoming missiles; the hazards to personnel are obvious. The most widely used safety standard is the '5-Gauss line'. This is the line around the magnet in both horizontal and vertical planes beyond which the magnetic field strength is less than 5 Gauss (0.0005 T). Physical barriers and prominent signs should be used to prevent entry within the 5-Gauss line of any person not screened as below and not accompanied by a trained technician.

Ferromagnetic (magnetizable) materials within the patient could potentially be moved by the magnetic field causing tissue damage. Common potential problems are metal fragments in the eye and various medical devices such as intracerebral aneurysm clips. Patients with a past history of penetrating eye injury are at risk for having metal fragments in the eye and should be screened before entering the MRI room with plain films of the orbits. Magnetic resonance imaging-compatible aneurysm clips have been available for many years. The MRI should not be performed until the safety of an individual device has been established. The presence of electrically active implants such as cardiac pacemakers, cochlear implants and neurostimulators is a contraindication to MRI unless the safety of an individual device is proven.

Other causes for concern in MRI include:

• High auditory noise levels. Earplugs should be provided to all patients undergoing MRI examinations.

• Claustrophobia. Although 'open' magnets are available on the market, the majority of MRI machines are in the shape of a tunnel and claustrophobia remains a major issue affecting a significant number of patients. Sedation is therefore a common procedure (used in up to 10 per cent of cases). Adequate monitoring of the sedated patient by properly trained staff using MRI-compatible equipment is mandatory.

• Allergy to injected contrast materials. Although rare, anaphylactoid reactions to gadolinium compounds have been reported.

• RF burns. Rare reports exist of RF burns associated with inductive heating of conducting leads placed against the patient's skin. Where possible MRI-compatible instruments such as pulse oximeters should be used. Care should be taken to separate conducting leads such as ECG leads from the patient's skin.

• Peripheral nerve stimulation. Rapidly switching magnetic fields can stimulate muscles and peripheral nerves. Guidelines are used in MRI to limit the rate of gradient field switching to well below the threshold for nerve stimulation.

• Pregnancy. There is no evidence of any adverse effects of MRI in pregnancy.

Two basic measures involved in reduction and management of risk in MRI are an education programme and suitable screening of staff and patients.

1 Education programme: an education programme covering the risks as outlined above should be given to all medical staff associated with MRI including doctors, nurses, radiographers and other technologists. Other staff who may enter the scanning room such as engineers, cleaners and security staff should be included.

2 Screening of staff and patients: a standard questionnaire should cover any relevant factors such as:
   (i) Previous surgical history;
   (ii) The presence of metal foreign bodies including aneurysm clips, etc.;
   (iii) The presence of cochlear implants and cardiac pacemakers;
   (iv) Any possible occupational exposure to metal fragments and history of penetrating eye injury;
   (v) Any other factors such as previous allergic reaction.

How to read a chest X-ray

The chest X-ray (CXR) remains the most commonly performed radiological investigation. In the acute situation a radiologist's report might not be immediately available and interpretation is up to doctor who has requested the examination. This chapter is an introduction to the principles of CXR interpretation. An overview of the standard CXR projections is followed by a brief outline of normal radiographic anatomy. Some notes on assessment of a few important technical aspects are then provided as well as an outline of a suggested systematic approach. These are followed by the bulk of the chapter, which will outline the common radiographic findings and patterns encountered. Where appropriate, short lists of differential diagnoses are provided.

PROJECTIONS PERFORMED

A standard CXR examination consists of two projections, the posteroanterior (PA) erect plus a lateral view.

THE POSTEROANTERIOR ERECT

The patient stands with his or her anterior chest wall up against the X-ray film. The X-ray tube lies behind the patient so that X-rays pass through in a posterior to anterior (PA) direction.

Reasons for performing the film PA:
- Accurate assessment of cardiac size as a result of minimal magnification.
- Scapulae can be rotated out of the way.

Reasons for performing the film erect:
- Physiological representation of blood vessels of mediastinum and lung. In the supine position mediastinal veins and upper lobe vessels may be distended leading to misinterpretation. In

particular, a normal mediastinum may look abnormally wide on supine CXR.
- Gas passes upwards: pneumothorax is more easily diagnosed, as is free gas beneath the diaphragm.
- Fluid passes downwards; therefore pleural effusion is more easily diagnosed.

LATERAL

Reasons for performing a lateral CXR:
- Further view of lungs, especially those areas obscured on the PA film, e.g. posterior segments of lower lobes, areas behind the hila, and left lower lobe, which lies behind the heart on the PA.
- Further assessment of cardiac configuration.
- Further anatomical localization of lesions.
- More sensitive for pleural effusions.
- Good view of thoracic spine.

In general, the use of two views, PA and lateral, is advocated in the assessment of most chest conditions. Exceptions where a PA film alone would suffice are:
- Infants and children.
- 'Screening' examinations, e.g. for immigration, insurance or diving medicals.
- Follow-up of known conditions seen well on the PA, e.g. pneumonia following antibiotics, metastases following chemotherapy and pneumothorax following drainage.

OTHER PROJECTIONS

Other projections that may be used instead of, or as well as, the two standard views are outlined below.

Anteroposterior/supine X-ray

Anteroposterior (AP) supine films are performed when the patient is too ill to stand. This would include acutely ill or traumatized patients, and patients in intensive care and coronary care units. Note that the mediastinum will appear wider on an AP supine film owing to venous distension and magnification. This may lead to an incorrect diagnosis of widened mediastinum, which may be particularly significant in the setting of chest trauma where aortic injury is suspected.

Expiratory film

A film performed in expiration may be useful for a small pneumothorax and in suspected bronchial obstruction with air trapping e.g. inhaled foreign body in a child.

Decubitus film

A decubitus film refers to a radiograph performed with the patient lying on his or her side. It is used occasionally in patients too ill to stand where pleural effusion or pneumothorax are suspected and not definitely diagnosed on an AP film.

Oblique views

Oblique views may be used to show the ribs or sternum for suspected fracture, or to display other chest wall pathologies.

RADIOGRAPHIC ANATOMY

THE POSTEROANTERIOR VIEW

The trachea is well seen in the midline, as is its division into right and left main bronchi (Fig. 3.1). A thin line on the right margin of the trachea is noted. This is termed the right paratracheal stripe. It is an important

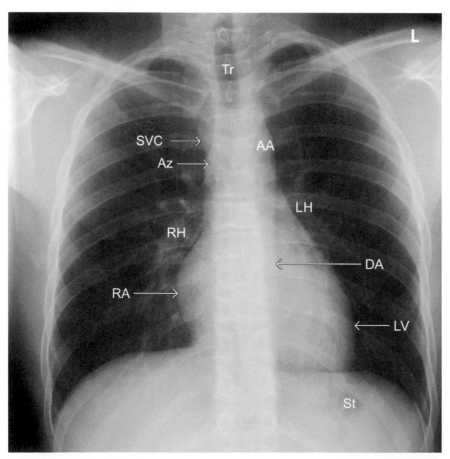

Fig. 3.1 *Normal posteroanterior chest X-ray. Note the following structures: trachea (Tr), superior vena cava (SVC), azygos vein (Az), right hilum (RH), right atrium (RA), aortic arch (AA), left hilum (LH), left ventricle (LV), descending aorta (DA) and stomach (St).*

line to look for on the PA view as it may be lost or thickened in the presence of lymphadenopathy. The right paratracheal stripe is continuous inferiorly with a small convex opacity, which sits in the concavity formed by the junction of the trachea and right main bronchus. The azygos vein, seen 'end-on' as it loops forwards over the right main bronchus to enter the superior vena cava (SVC), forms this opacity. The SVC is often seen as a straight line, continuous inferiorly with the right heart border. The right heart border is formed by the right atrium, outlined by the aerated right middle lobe. The right hilum lies approximately midway between the diaphragm and lung apex. It is formed by the right main bronchus and right pulmonary artery, and their lobar divisions.

The left mediastinal border can be thought of as three convexities. The most superior of these, sometimes termed the aortic knuckle, is formed by the aortic arch. The descending aorta can be traced downwards from this convexity. It forms a line to the left of the spine. This line may be obscured by a posterior mediastinal mass, or by pathology in the left lower lobe. The second convexity is quite variable and is formed by the main pulmonary artery. Posterior to this and extending laterally is the left hilum. It consists of the left main bronchus and left pulmonary artery and their main lobar divisions. The largest and most inferior convexity is the left heart border. The left ventricle forms the left heart border, except in cases where the right ventricle is enlarged. The left atrial appendage lies on the upper left cardiac border; it is not seen unless enlarged.

THE LATERAL VIEW

The lateral view (Fig. 3.2) is usually performed with the patient's arms held out horizontally. The humeral heads may be seen as round opacities projected over the lung apices. They should not be mistaken for abnormal masses. The trachea is seen as an air-filled structure in the upper chest, midway between the anterior and posterior chest walls. The posterior aspect of the aortic arch forms a convexity posterior to the trachea. The trachea can be followed inferiorly to the carina where the right and left main bronchi may be seen end-on as

round lucencies. The left main pulmonary artery forms an opacity posterior and slightly superior to the carina. The right pulmonary artery forms an opacity anterior and slightly inferior to the carina.

On the lateral view, the posterior cardiac border is formed by the left atrium superiorly and the left ventricle inferiorly. The right ventricle forms the anterior cardiac border. The main pulmonary artery forms a convex opacity continuous with the right upper cardiac border.

TECHNICAL ASSESSMENT

Before making a diagnostic assessment it is worthwhile pausing briefly to assess the technical quality of the PA film. The patient should be properly centred on the film with no rotation. Rotation may cause anatomical distortion and apparent increased opacity of one side of the chest, which may lead to incorrect diagnosis of pleural fluid or consolidation (Fig. 3.3). The easiest way to ensure that there is no rotation is to check that the spinous processes of the upper thoracic vertebrae lie midway between the medial ends of the clavicles. The radiograph should include the lung apices and both costophrenic angles.

An inadequate inspiration may lead to overdiagnosis of pulmonary opacity or collapse. With an adequate inspiration the diaphragms should lie at the level of the 5th or 6th ribs anteriorly. A straight trachea should be seen in children.

Any X-ray exposure should be appropriate to the patient being examined. Larger adult patients will need a higher exposure than young children. The film should not be overexposed (too black) or underexposed (too white). With appropriate exposure the lower thoracic vertebral bodies and blood vessels to the left lower lobe should be faintly discernible through the heart.

DIAGNOSTIC ASSESSMENT OF THE CXR

Accurate interpretation of the CXR may be difficult or impossible in the absence of relevant and accurate clinical information. Is the patient febrile or in pain? Is there haemoptysis or shortness of breath? Are there relevant results from other tests such as spirometry or bronchoscopy? Another important factor is the time

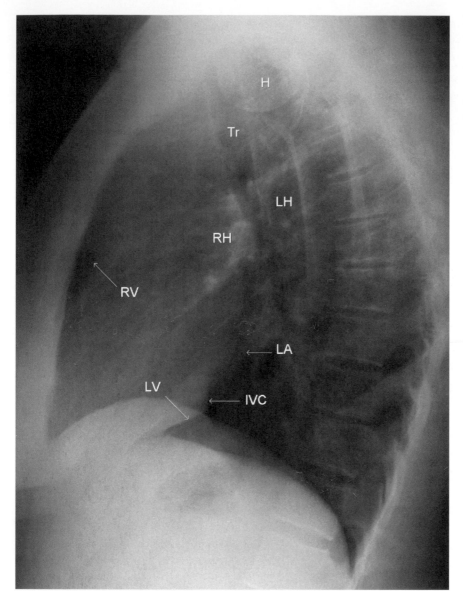

Fig. 3.2 *Normal lateral chest X-ray. Note the following structures: trachea (Tr), humeral head (H), right hilum (RH), left hilum (LH), right ventricle (RV), left atrium (LA), left ventricle (LV) and inferior vena cava (IVC).*

course of any abnormality. Comparison with any previous CXRs is often very useful to assess whether visible abnormalities are acute or chronic.

When starting to look at chest radiographs try to use a system. This will help you avoid missing relevant findings.

Posteroanterior film

1 Heart: position, size, configuration.
2 Assess the pulmonary vascular pattern: compare upper lobe vessels to lower lobe vessels.
3 Mediastinum: trachea, aorta, pulmonary arteries, SVC and azygos vein
4 Right and left hilum.
5 Pleural spaces: Check around the periphery of each lung in the pleural spaces for pneumothorax, pleural effusion, pleural thickening or calcification.
6 Bones and chest wall: ribs, clavicles, scapulae and humeri, sternum on the lateral film, thoracic vertebral bodies.
7 Lungs: lung abnormalities may consist of solitary or multiple nodules/masses or diffuse abnormality that

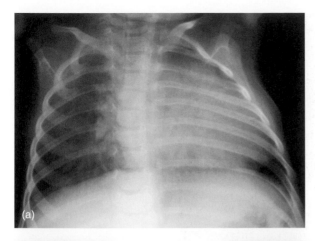

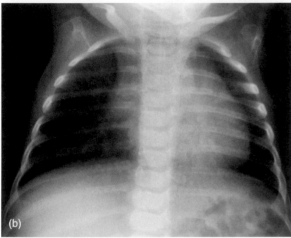

Fig. 3.3 *Effects of rotation. (a) chest X-ray (CXR) of an infant with rotation producing significant anatomical distortion. Note the asymmetry of the ribs and apparent cardiac enlargement. (b) A normally centred CXR shows normal anatomy.*

may be alveolar, interstitial or a combination of both. Divide each lung into thirds, first from top to bottom then from the hilum to the periphery. Look at top, middle and lower thirds, followed by medial, central and lateral thirds. Look particularly at difficult areas where lesions are easily missed:
– Behind the heart;
– Behind each hilum;
– Behind the diaphragms;
– Lung apices.

Check the lung contours for signs of blurring or loss of definition:
– Cardiac borders;
– Mediastinal margins;
– Diaphragms.
8 Other:
– Check below the diaphragm for free gas and to ensure that the stomach bubble is in correct position beneath the left diaphragm;
– In female patients, check that both breast shadows are present and that there has not been a previous mastectomy;
– Check the axillae and lower neck for masses or surgical clips.

Lateral film

1 Heart: size and configuration.
2 Mediastinum: trachea, right and left pulmonary arteries.
3 Lungs
– Retrosternal airspace, between posterior surface of sternum and anterior surface of heart;
– Identify both hemidiaphragms.
– Posterior costophrenic angles: very small pleural effusions are seen with greater sensitivity than on the PA film.
4 Bones
– Sternum and thoracic spine;
– The lower thoracic vertebral bodies should appear blacker than the upper ones. Increased apparent density of the lower vertebral bodies may be the only sign of consolidation in the posterior basal segments of the lower lobes. This area is difficult to see on the PA film because of overlying diaphragm.

ASSESSMENT OF THE HEART

The heart is assessed for position, size and configuration. Other CXR signs such as valvular or pericardial calcification should also be noted.

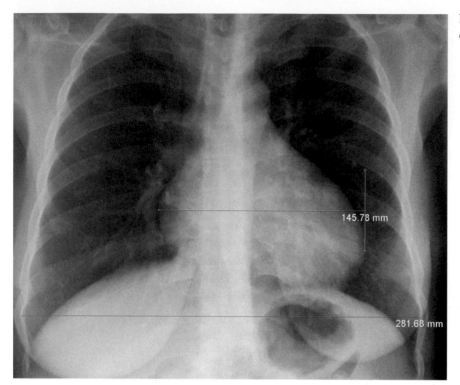

145.78 mm

281.68 mm

Fig. 3.4 *Measurement of cardiothoracic ratio (CTR).*

POSITION

The cardiac apex is directed toward the patient's left chest wall. About two-thirds of the normally positioned heart will lie to the left of midline. Malposition of the heart refers to an abnormally positioned heart, but with normal orientation of chambers and with the apex still pointing to the left. The heart may be malpositioned too far to the left by collapse of the left lung or by a space-occupying process on the right. Conversely, the heart may be pulled to the right by right-sided collapse or pushed to the right by a left-sided space-occupying process. Such space-occupying processes would include tension pneumothorax or a large pleural effusion.

Dextrocardia refers to reversal of the normal orientation of the heart with the cardiac apex directed to the patient's right. In isolated dextrocardia the other organs such as liver and stomach are positioned normally. In situs inversus all of the organs are reversed and the gastric bubble will lie beneath the right diaphragm.

CARDIAC SIZE

The cardiothoracic ratio (CTR) is the ratio between the maximum transverse diameter of the heart and the maximum transverse diameter of the chest. It is usually expressed as the ratio of these measurements in centimetres (Fig. 3.4). A CTR of greater than 0.5 is said to indicate cardiac enlargement although there are a number of variables not least of which is the shape of the patient's chest. The CTR is unreliable as a one-off measurement. Of more significance is an increase in heart size on serial CXRs, or a transverse diameter of greater than 15.5 cm in adult males or 14.5 cm in adult females.

SIGNS OF SPECIFIC CHAMBER ENLARGEMENT

On the PA view the right heart border is formed by the right atrium, outlined by the aerated right middle lung lobe. The left ventricle, except where the right ventricle is enlarged, forms the left heart border. The left atrial appendage lies on the upper left cardiac border; it is not seen unless enlarged.

On the lateral view, the posterior cardiac border is formed by the left atrium superiorly and the left ventricle inferiorly. The right ventricle forms the anterior cardiac border. CXR signs of cardiac chamber enlargement are listed in Table 3.1

Table 3.1 Signs of cardiac chamber enlargement

Cardiac chamber	Radiological signs of enlargement
Right atrium	Bulging right heart border
Left atrium	Prominent left atrial appendage on the left heart border (Fig. 3.5).
	Double outline of the right heart border
	Splayed carina with elevation of the left main bronchus
	Bulge of the upper posterior heart border on the lateral view
Right ventricle	Elevated cardiac apex
	Bulging of anterior upper part of the heart border on the lateral view
Left ventricle	Bulging lower left cardiac border with depressed cardiac apex

PULMONARY VASCULAR PATTERNS

The normal lung vascular pattern has the following features:

- Arteries branching vertically to upper and lower lobes.
- Veins running roughly horizontally towards the lower hila.
- Upper lobe vessels smaller than lower lobe vessels on erect CXR.
- Vessels difficult to see in the peripheral thirds of the lungs.

With pulmonary venous hypertension (Fig. 3.5) blood vessels in the upper lobes are larger than those in the lower lobes on erect CXR. These findings are associated with cardiac failure and mitral valve disease and often accompanied on CXR by pulmonary oedema and pleural effusion.

Pulmonary arterial hypertension is associated with long-standing pulmonary disease, including emphysema, multiple recurrent pulmonary emboli and left to right shunts, such as ventricular septal defect (VSD), atrial septal defect (ASD) and patent ductus arteriosus (PDA). Signs of pulmonary arterial hypertension on CXR include bilateral hilar enlargement due to enlarged proximal pulmonary arteries with rapid decrease in the caliber of peripheral vessels ('pruning').

Pulmonary plethora refers to increased pulmonary blood flow as a result of left to right shunts (VSD, ASD and PDA). On CXR there is increased size and number of pulmonary vessels, with vascular structures seen in the peripheral third of the lung fields. Pulmonary oligaemia refers to reduced pulmonary blood flow and

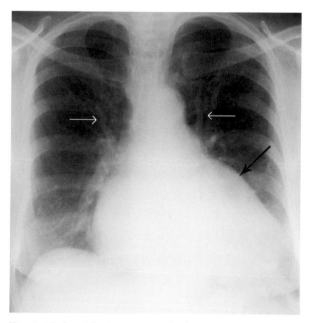

Fig. 3.5 *Left atrial enlargement and pulmonary venous hypertension. The heart is enlarged with prominence of the left atrial appendage producing a bulge of the upper left cardiac border (black arrow). The upper lobe arteries (white arrows) are larger than those in the lower lobe, indicating pulmonary venous hypertension.*

is associated with pulmonary stenosis/atresia, Fallot tetralogy, tricuspid atresia, Ebstein anomaly and severe emphysema. On CXR pulmonary plethora produces general lucency (blackness) of lung fields with decreased size and number of pulmonary vessels and small main pulmonary arteries.

MEDIASTINAL MASSES

Signs on CXR that a central opacity or mass lies within the mediastinum rather than the lung include:

- Continuity with the mediastinal outline.
- Sharp margin.
- Convex margin.
- Absence of air bronchograms.

Logical classification and differential diagnosis of mediastinal masses is based on localization to the anterior, middle or posterior mediastinum. In this regard, the silhouette sign and the lateral film are of most use.

ANTERIOR MEDIASTINAL MASS

Chest X-ray signs of an anterior mediastinal mass (Fig. 3.6):

- Merge with cardiac border.
- Hilar structures can be seen through the mass.
- Masses passing upwards into the neck merge radiologically with the soft tissues of the neck and so are not seen above the clavicles (cervico-thoracic sign); a lesion seen above the clavicles must lie adjacent to aerated lung apices, i.e. posterior and within the thorax.

Differential diagnosis of an anterior mediastinal mass:

- Retrosternal goitre:
  (i) Cervico-thoracic sign, as above, i.e. mass not seen above the clavicles;
  (ii) Displaced trachea.
- Thymic tumour: may be associated with myasthenia gravis.
- Thymic cyst.

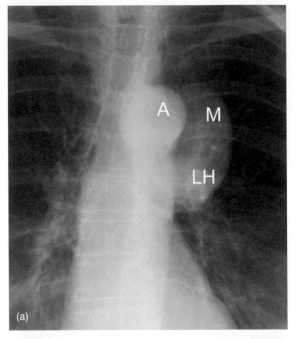

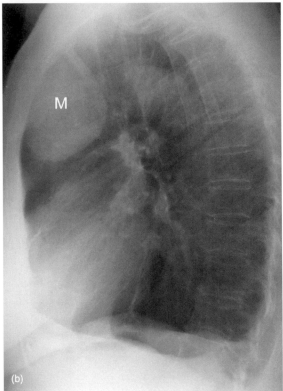

Fig. 3.6 *Anterior mediastinal mass: lymphoma. (a) posteroanterior projection showing the mass (M) and the aorta (A). The left hilum (LH) can be seen through the mass. (b) Lateral projection confirms the anterior position of the mass.*

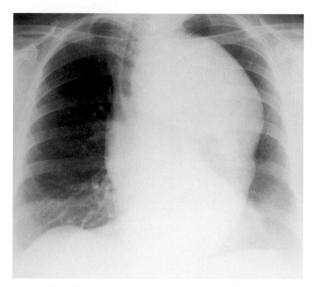

Fig. 3.7 *Middle mediastinal mass: aneurysm of thoracic aorta.*

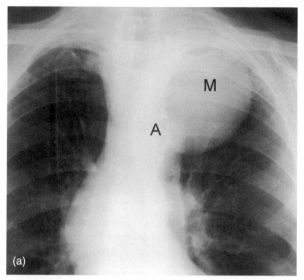

- Lymphadenopathy:
  - (i) Hodgkin disease;
  - (ii) Metastases.
- Aneurysm of ascending aorta.

MIDDLE MEDIASTINAL MASS

A middle mediastinal mass is usually seen on CXR as an opacity that merges with the hilar structures and cardiac borders. Differential diagnosis of a middle mediastinal mass includes:

- Lymphadenopathy:
  - (i) Mediastinal/hilar;
  - (ii) Bronchial carcinoma, less commonly other tumours.
  - (iii) Lymphoma.
- Bronchogenic cyst.
- Aortic aneurysm (Fig. 3.7).

POSTERIOR MEDIASTINAL MASS

The CXR signs of a posterior mediastinal mass:

- Cardiac borders and hila clearly seen.
- Posterior descending aorta obscured.
- May be underlying vertebral changes.

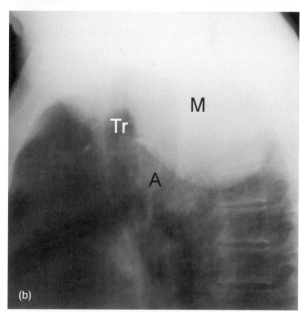

Fig. 3.8 *Posterior mediastinal mass: neurogenic tumour. (a) Posteroanterior projection showing the mass (M) partly obscuring the aorta (A). (b) Lateral view confirms the posterior position of the mass and shows the trachea (Tr) anteriorly.*

Differential diagnosis of a posterior mediastinal mass:

- Hiatus hernia:
  - (i) Located behind the heart;
  - (ii) May contain a fluid level.
- Neurogenic tumour:
  - (i) Well-defined mass in the paravertebral region (Fig. 3.8);

(ii) Erosion or destruction of vertebral bodies/posterior ribs.
- Anterior thoracic meningocele: associated with neurofibromatosis.
- Neurenteric cyst: associated with vertebral abnormalities.
- Oesophageal duplication cyst.
- Paravertebral lymphadenopathy.

HILAR DISORDERS

Each hilar complex, as seen on the PA and lateral chest radiographs, comprises the proximal pulmonary arteries, bronchus, pulmonary veins and lymph nodes. The lymph nodes are not visualized unless enlarged. In assessing hilar enlargement, be it bilateral or unilateral, one must decide whether it is caused by enlargement of the pulmonary arteries or some other cause, such as lymphadenopathy or a mass. If the branching pulmonary arteries are seen to converge towards an apparent mass, this is a good sign of enlarged main pulmonary artery (hilum convergence sign).

Causes of unilateral hilar enlargement:
- Bronchial carcinoma (Fig. 3.9).
- Infective causes:
  (i) Tuberculosis (TB);
  (ii) Mycoplasma.
- Perihilar pneumonia:
  (i) An area of pneumonia lying anterior or posterior to the hilum may cause *apparent* hilar enlargement on the PA film;
  (ii) Usually obvious on the lateral film.
- Other causes of lymphadenopathy (more commonly bilateral):
  (i) Lymphoma;
  (ii) Sarcoidosis.
- Causes of enlargement of a single pulmonary artery:
  (i) Post-stenotic dilatation on the left side due to pulmonary stenosis;
  (ii) Massive unilateral pulmonary embolus;
  (iii) Pulmonary artery aneurysm (often calcified).

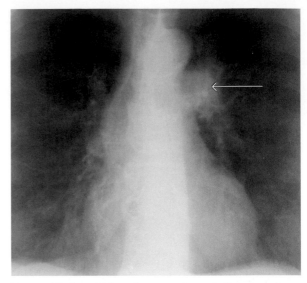

Fig. 3.9 *Unilateral hilar enlargement (arrow): bronchogenic carcinoma.*

Causes of bilateral hilar enlargement:
- Sarcoidosis (Fig. 3.10):
  (i) Symmetrical;
  (ii) Lobulated;
  (iii) Often associated with right paratracheal lymphadenopathy.
- Lymphoma: Often asymmetrical.
- Metastatic malignancy:
  (i) Bronchogenic carcinoma;
  (ii) Non-pulmonary primary, e.g. testis, breast.

SOLITARY PULMONARY NODULE

Factors to assess:
- Size: greater than 3 cm diameter highly suspicious of malignancy.
- Margin: ill-defined margin suggests malignancy.
- Cavitation: malignancy or infection.
- Calcification: rare in malignancy.
- Comparison with previous CXR to assess growth.

Differential diagnosis of solitary pulmonary nodule:
- Bronchogenic carcinoma (Fig. 3.11):
  (i) Evidence of rapid growth on serial CXR examinations;

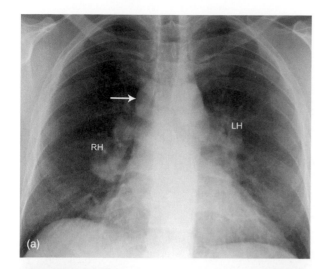

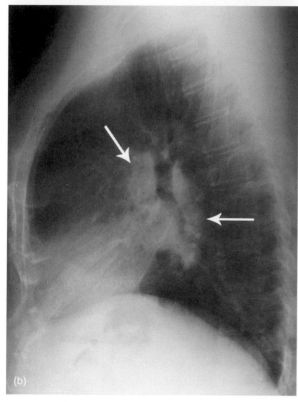

Fig. 3.10 *Bilateral hilar enlargement: sarcoidosis. (a) Posteroanterior view showing enlarged right hilum (RH) and left hilum (LH) due to lymphadenopathy as well as right mediastinal lymphadenopathy (arrow). (b) Lateral view showing lobulated opacity anterior and posterior to the distal trachea indicating bilateral hilar lymphadenopathy (arrows).*

    (ii) Ill-defined margin;
    (iii) Size greater than 3 cm;
    (iv) No calcification;
    (v) For further notes on bronchogenic carcinoma please see Chapter 4.
- Solitary metastasis.
- Granuloma including tuberculoma (see Fig. 4.5):
    (i) Calcification common;
    (ii) Well-defined margin;
    (iii) Usually 0.3–1.0 cm diameter;
    (iv) Unchanged on serial CXR examinations.
- Carcinoid tumour:
    (i) Usually <3 cm diameter;
    (ii) Calcification in one-third;
    (iii) May be associated with peripheral consolidation due to bronchial obstruction.
- Arteriovenous malformation: feeding arteries and draining veins may be seen.

For notes on further investigation of the solitary pulmonary nodule please see Chapter 4.

MULTIPLE PULMONARY NODULES

Differential diagnosis of multiple pulmonary nodules:
- Metastases (Fig. 3.12):
    (i) Usually well defined;
    (ii) Nodules of varying size;
    (iii) More common peripherally and in the lower lobes;
    (iv) Cavitation seen in squamous cell carcinomas, sarcomas and metastases from colonic primaries.
- Abscesses:
    (i) Cavitation: thick, irregular wall;
    (ii) Usually caused by *Staphylococcus aureus*.
- Hydatid cysts: often quite large, i.e. 10 cm or more.
- Wegener's granulomatosis:
    (i) Cavitation of nodules common;
    (ii) Associated paranasal sinus disease;
    (iii) May also produce diffuse airspace shadowing (see below).
- Multiple arteriovenous malformations.

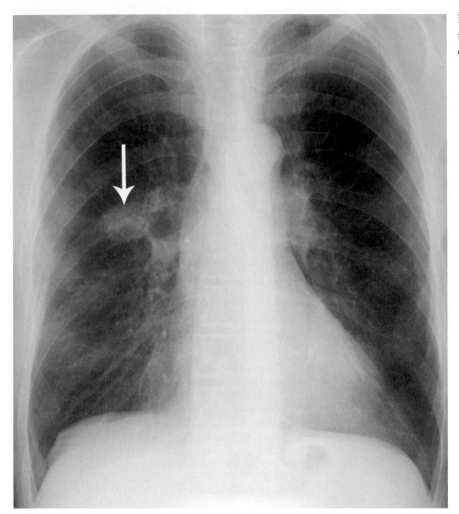

Fig. 3.11 *Solitary pulmonary nodule (arrow): bronchogenic carcinoma.*

DIFFUSE PULMONARY SHADOWING

Anatomically, functionally and radiologically the lungs may be divided into two compartments, the alveoli or airspaces and the interstitium or supporting soft tissues between the airspaces.

The trachea divides into right and left bronchi. Each bronchus divides into lobar and segmental bronchi, and by repeated branching into smaller bronchi and bronchioles. The branching bronchi and bronchioles, accompanying arteries, veins and lymphatics, plus supporting connective tissue form the interstitium of the lung. The most distal small bronchioles are the terminal bronchioles. The lung distal to each terminal bronchiole is termed the lung acinus. The lung acinus consists of multiple generations of tiny respiratory bronchioles and alveolar ducts. The alveoli or airspaces arise from the respiratory bronchioles and alveolar ducts.

Disease processes may involve the alveoli or the interstitium, or both. One of the most important factors in narrowing the differential diagnosis of diffuse pulmonary shadowing is the ability to differentiate alveolar from interstitial shadowing.

ALVEOLAR PROCESSES

Alveolar shadowing may be caused by oedema fluid, inflammatory fluid, blood and protein or tumour cells. All of these abnormalities have the same soft-tissue

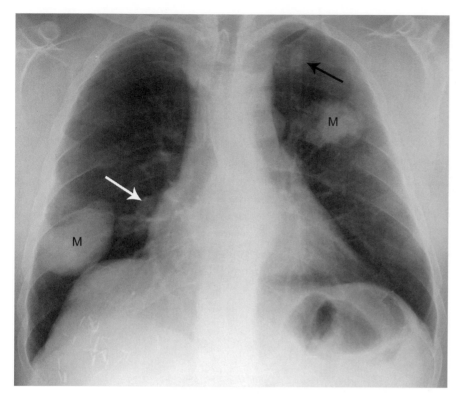

Fig. 3.12 *Multiple pulmonary metastases from colorectal carcinoma. Note two obvious masses (M) plus more subtle masses behind the right heart (white arrow) and partly obscured by the left first rib (black arrow). Surgical staples in the right upper abdomen indicate previous partial hepatectomy for metastatic disease.*

density on X-ray. Abnormalities may be acute or chronic. Acute changes are seen with common infections, oedema and haemorrhage, while chronic changes are seen with atypical infections, proteinosis and tumour. Because appearances are non-specific, definitive diagnosis is usually only made where the CXR findings are correlated with the clinical signs and symptoms.

Signs of alveolar shadowing:

- Opacity tends to appear rapidly after the onset of symptoms.
- Fluffy, ill-defined areas of opacification.
- Areas of consolidation tend to coalesce.
- Air bronchograms (Fig. 3.13): air-filled bronchi can be seen as they are outlined by surrounding consolidated lung; air bronchograms are not seen in pleural or mediastinal processes.

Three patterns of distribution of alveolar shadowing tend to occur:

1 Segmental or lobar distribution.
2 Bilateral opacification spreading from the hilar regions into the lungs with relative sparing of the

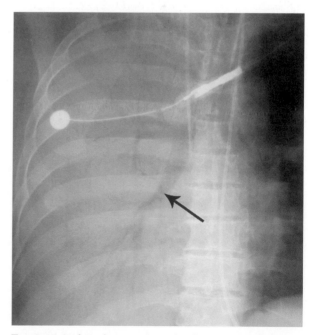

Fig. 3.13 *Air bronchograms (arrow) indicating extensive alveolar opacification.*

peripheral lungs, sometimes referred to as a 'bat wing' distribution.

3 Bilateral opacification involving the peripheral lungs with relative sparing of the central regions, sometimes referred to as 'reversed bat wing' distribution.

Differential diagnosis lists based on distribution of changes plus whether changes are acute or chronic may be developed as below.

Segmental/lobar alveolar pattern:

- Pneumonia (see below).
- Segmental/lobar collapse (see below).
- Pulmonary infarct.
- Alveolar cell carcinoma.
- Contusion (associated with rib fractures, pneumothorax, and other signs of trauma).

Acute bilateral central 'bat wing' pattern (Fig. 3.14):

- Pulmonary oedema:
  - (i)　Cardiac failure;
  - (ii)　Adult respiratory distress syndrome (ARDS);
  - (iii)　Fluid overload;
  - (iv)　Drowning and other causes of aspiration;
  - (v)　Head injury or other causes of raised intracranial pressure;
  - (vi)　Drugs and poisons (e.g. snake venom, heroin overdose);
  - (vii)　Hypoproteinaemia (e.g. liver disease);
  - (viii)　Blood transfusion reaction.
- Pneumonia: *Pneumocystis carinii* (acquired immune-deficiency syndrome); TB; viral pneumonias; *Mycoplasma*.

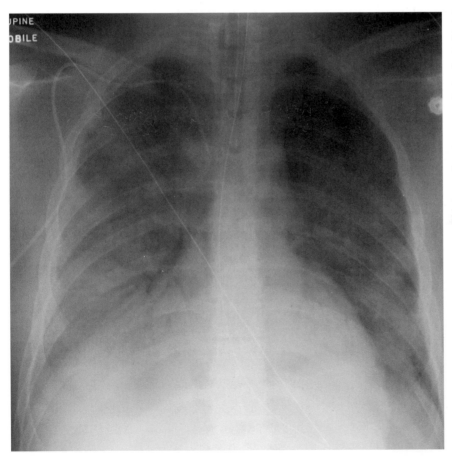

Fig. 3.14 *'Bat's wing' pattern: pulmonary oedema. Extensive bilateral airspace opacification with well-defined air bronchograms in the right lung. Opacification on the left shows the typical parahilar distribution known as the 'bat wing' pattern with relative sparing of the lung periphery.*

- Pulmonary haemorrhage: Goodpasture's syndrome; anticoagulants; bleeding diathesis: haemophilia, disseminated intravascular coagulation (DIC).

Chronic bilateral central 'bat wing' pattern:

- Atypical pneumonia: TB, fungi.
- Lymphoma/leukaemia.
- Sarcoidosis: interstitial form much more common.
- Pulmonary alveolar proteinosis.
- Alveolar cell carcinoma: localized form more common.

Reversed 'bat wing' pattern (Fig. 3.15):

- Loeffler's syndrome: transient pulmonary infiltrates associated with blood eosinophilia.
- Eosinophilic pneumonias.

- Wegener's granulomatosis.
- Fat embolism: occurs 1–2 days after major trauma, particularly with fractures of the large bones of the lower limbs.

INTERSTITIAL PROCESSES

Three types of pattern are seen in interstitial processes: linear, nodular and honeycomb pattern. These may occur separately or together in the same patient with considerable overlap in appearances often encountered.

1 Linear pattern: this consists of a network of fine lines running through the lungs. Lines are caused by thickened connective tissue septae and may be further classified as:
   – Kerley A lines: long, thin lines in the upper lobes;

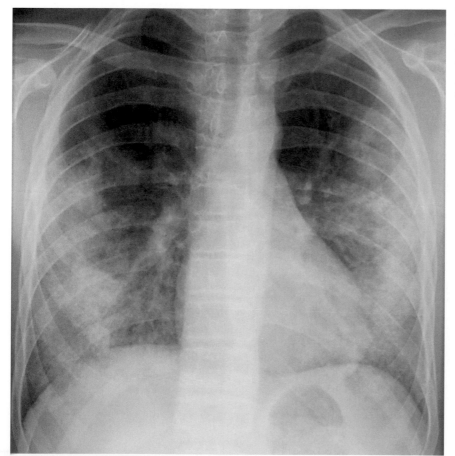

Fig. 3.15 *'Reversed bat's wing' pattern: Wegener's granulomatosis. Note the presence of bilateral airspace opacity in a predominantly peripheral distribution with relative sparing of the central parahilar regions.*

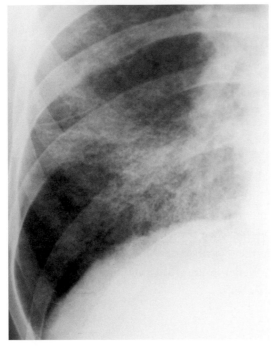

Fig. 3.16 *Interstitial nodules: sarcoidosis. Note the presence of multiple small nodular opacities throughout the right lower lobe.*

– Kerley B lines: short, thin lines predominantly in the lower zones extending 1–2 cm horizontally inwards from the lung surface.

2 Nodular pattern (Fig. 3.16): nodules caused by interstitial disease are small (1–5 mm), well defined and not associated with air bronchograms. They tend to be very numerous and are distributed evenly throughout the lungs.

3 Honeycomb pattern (Fig. 3.17): the honeycomb pattern represents the end-stage of many of the interstitial processes listed below. It may also be seen with tuberous sclerosis, amyloidosis, neurofibromatosis and cystic fibrosis. The honeycomb pattern implies extensive destruction of pulmonary tissue. Cysts that range in size from tiny up to 2 cm in diameter replace the lung parenchyma. These cysts have very thin walls. Normal pulmonary vasculature cannot be seen. Pneumothorax is a frequent complication of honeycomb lung.

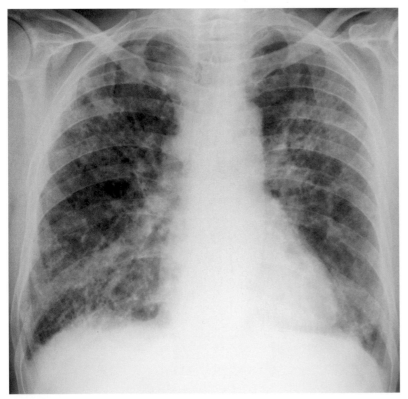

Fig. 3.17 *Honeycomb lung. Note coarse interstitial opacity throughout both lungs with 'shaggy' appearance of the cardiac borders and hemidiaphragms.*

The list of interstitial disease processes is extensive. As with alveolar processes, CXR appearances are non-specific. Short differential diagnosis lists of the more common disorders have been developed and are based on whether CXR findings are acute, subacute or chronic. Chronic disorders may be further subdivided based on their distribution in the lungs, i.e. whether upper or lower zones are predominantly involved.

Acute interstitial shadowing

- Interstitial oedema:
    (i) Kerley B lines (Fig. 3.18);
    (ii) Associated with cardiac enlargement and pleural effusions;
    (iii) May progress to, or be associated with, an alveolar pattern.
- Acute interstitial pneumonia: usually viral.

Subacute interstitial shadowing

In patients with a history of carcinoma, lymphangitis carcinomatosa may cause localized or diffuse interstitial shadowing. Lymphangitis carcinomatosa is caused by direct malignant infiltration and obstruction of the lymphatic pathways in the pulmonary interstitium. It produces prominent linear and nodular shadowing with Kerley B lines, often associated with mediastinal/hilar lymphadenopathy.

Chronic, upper zones

- Tuberculosis:
    (i) Upper lobe fibrosis with loss of volume (Fig. 3.19);
    (ii) Associated calcification in cavities;
    (iii) Acute miliary form gives a widespread fine nodular pattern;
- Sarcoidosis:
    (i) Nodular form dominates;
    (ii) Often associated with hilar lymphadenopathy, though pulmonary involvement alone occurs in 25 per cent of cases.
- Silicosis:
    (i) Nodular and linear pattern;
    (ii) Associated with hilar lymph node calcification and enlargement;

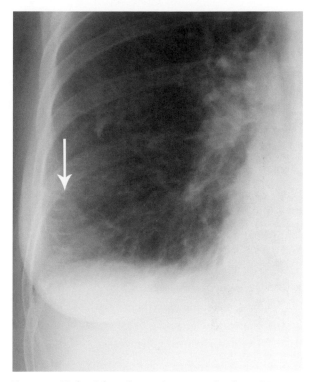

Fig. 3.18 *Kerley B lines (arrows): interstitial oedema. Note the typical appearance of short linear opacities extending into the lung from the peripheral surface.*

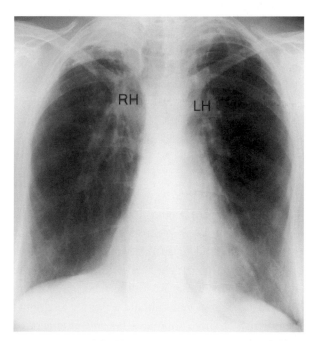

Fig. 3.19 *Upper lobe fibrosis. Note elevation of right and left hila (RH and LH, respectively).*

(iii) May be associated with large confluent masses, i.e. progressive massive fibrosis (PMF).
- Extrinsic allergic alveolitis.
- Bronchopulmonary aspergillosis.
- Histiocytosis-X.

Chronic, lower zones

- Fibrosing alveolitis.
- Asbestosis: may be associated with pleural plaques and calcification particularly of the diaphragmatic pleura.
- Rheumatoid disease:
  (i) Associated with pleural effusions;
  (ii) Rheumatoid nodules.
- Other connective tissue disorders:
  (i) Systematic lupus erythematosis (SLE);
  (ii) Systemic sclerosis;
  (iii) Dermatomyositis/ polymyositis.

LOBAR PULMONARY CONSOLIDATION

'Pulmonary consolidation' refers to filling of the pulmonary alveoli with fluid (pus, blood, and oedema), protein, or cells. The radiographic signs of alveolar opacification are described above. Consolidation of a pulmonary lobe or segment (Fig. 3.20) is usually caused by pneumonia, with other less common causes such as pulmonary infarct or contusion usually differentiated on the basis of clinical history. Several radiographic signs may be helpful in localizing areas of pulmonary consolidation.

The silhouette sign

Remember that in Chapter 1 it was stated that an object would be seen with conventional radiography if its borders lie beside tissue of different density. This especially applies in the chest where diaphragms, heart and mediastinal outlines are well seen because they lie adjacent to aerated lung. Should a part of lung lying against any of these structures become non-aerated owing to collapse, consolidation or the presence of a

Table 3.2 Examples of the silhouette sign

Part of lung that is non-aerated	Border that is obscured
Right middle lobe (Fig. 1.3)	Right heart border
Left lingula (Fig. 3.20)	Left heart border
Right lower lobe (Fig. 1.3)	Right diaphragm
Left lower lobe (Fig. 3.21)	Left diaphragm Descending aorta
Right upper lobe (Fig. 3.22)	Right border of ascending aorta Right mediastinal margin
Left upper lobe	Aortic knuckle* Upper left cardiac border

* Note that in severe collapse of the left upper lobe, the apical segment of the left lower lobe may be pulled upwards and forwards enough such that aerated lung lies beside the aortic knuckle. The aortic knuckle will therefore be seen in this situation.

mass, the outline of that structure will no longer be seen. This is known as the 'silhouette' sign and is one of the most important principles in chest radiography (Table 3.2).

Consolidation adjacent to fissures

Straight margins occur in the lungs at the pulmonary fissures. If an area of consolidation or collapse has a straight margin, that margin must abut a fissure and this can help in localization (Table 3.3).

Increased density of lower thoracic spine

On the lateral view the thoracic vertebral bodies should show a gradual apparent decrease in density as one peruses from top to bottom (see Fig. 3.2, page 34). Opacification in the right or left lower lobes may produce an apparent increase in density of the lower thoracic vertebral bodies. This may be the most obvious radiographic sign of lower lobe pneumonia (Fig. 3.21b), particularly small areas of consolidation obscured by the heart on the PA view.

Table 3.3 Location of pulmonary consolidation or collapse according to fissure abutment

Lobe of lung	Cause of straight margin
Right upper lobe (Figs 3.22 & 3.23)	Horizontal fissure inferiorly on posteroanterior (PA) film Oblique fissure posteriorly on lateral film
Right middle lobe (Fig. 3.24)	Horizontal fissure superiorly on PA film Oblique fissure posteriorly on lateral film
Right lower lobe (Fig. 3.25)	Oblique fissure anteriorly on lateral film Collapse causes rotation and visualization of the oblique fissure on the PA film
Left upper lobe (Fig. 3.26)	Oblique fissure posteriorly on lateral film
Left lower lobe (Fig. 3.27)	Oblique fissure anteriorly on lateral film Collapse causes rotation and visualization of the oblique fissure on the PA film

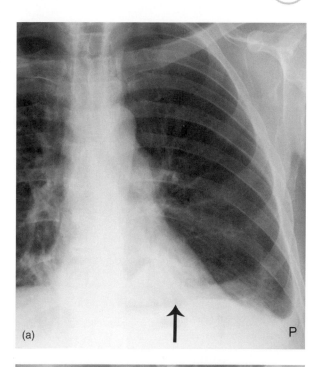

(a)

P

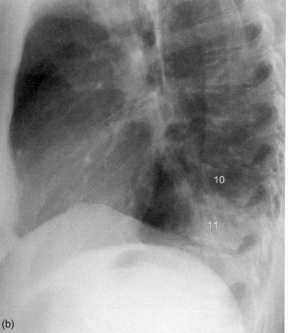

(b)

Fig. 3.21 *Left lower lobe consolidation: pneumonia. (a) On the posteroanterior view consolidation of the left lower lobe produces opacity behind the left heart (arrow). There is also a small pleural effusion (P). (b) Consolidation in either lower lobe may produce apparent increase in density of the lower thoracic vertebral bodies. In this case T11 is of greater apparent density than T10 because of consolidation in the left lower lobe.*

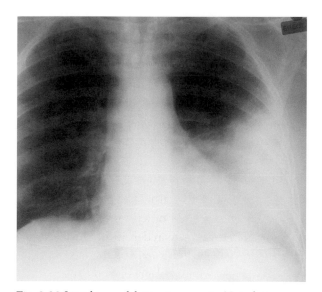

Fig. 3.20 *Lingula consolidation: pneumonia. Note that consolidation in the lingula obscures the left cardiac border.*

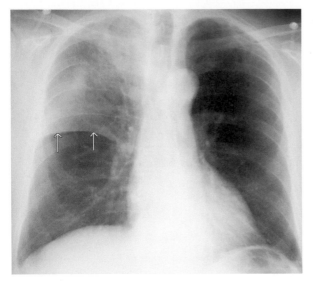

Fig. 3.22 *Right upper lobe consolidation: pneumonia. Note opacification of the right upper lobe bordered inferiorly by the horizontal fissure (arrows).*

PULMONARY COLLAPSE

Pulmonary collapse most commonly takes the form of linear or disc-like areas of focal collapse. These are referred to as linear or discoid atelectasis. Causes of linear atelectasis include:

- Following thoracic or abdominal surgery.
- Inflammatory or other painful pathology beneath the diaphragm, e.g. pancreatitis, acute cholecystitis.
- Pulmonary embolus.
- Following resolution of pneumonia.

More extensive collapse may involve pulmonary segments or lobes. Causes of pulmonary lobar collapse include:

- Bronchial obstruction:
  - (i) Tumour;
  - (ii) Foreign body;
  - (iii) Mucous plug, e.g. asthma.
- Passive collapse owing to external pressure on the lung:
  - (i) Pneumothorax;
  - (ii) Pleural effusion or haemothorax;
  - (iii) Diaphragmatic hernia (neonate).

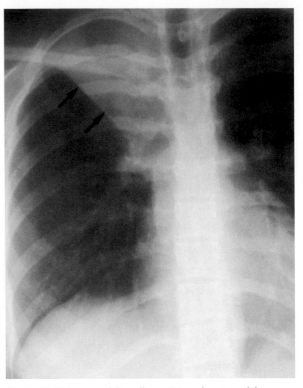

Fig. 3.23 *Right upper lobe collapse. Note elevation of the horizontal fissure (arrows).*

- Scarring or fibrosis:
  - (i) TB (upper lobes);
  - (ii) Radiation pneumonitis (post-radiotherapy).

GENERAL SIGNS OF LOBAR COLLAPSE

The most important initial sign of lobar collapse is decreased volume of the affected lung. Other signs include:

- Displacement of pulmonary fissures.
- Local increase in density due to non-aerated lung.
- Elevation of hemidiaphragm.
- Displacement of hila.
- Displacement of mediastinum.
- Compensatory overinflation of adjacent lobes.

SPECIFIC SIGNS OF LOBAR COLLAPSE

Right upper lobe (Fig. 3.23):

- Collapses upwards and anteriorly.
- Decreased volume of right lung.
- Elevation of horizontal fissure.

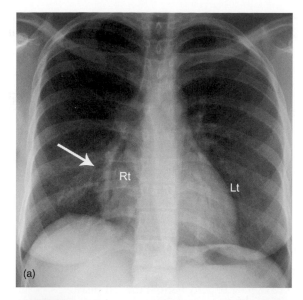

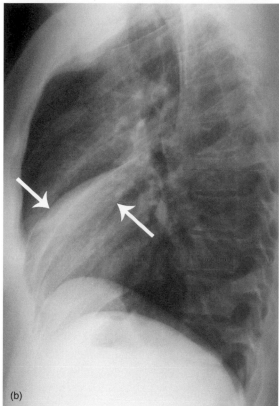

Fig. 3.24 *Right middle lobe collapse. (a) posteroanterior view shows loss of volume on the right with opacity (arrow) obscuring the right heart border (Rt). Compare this with the left heart border (Lt), which is clearly seen. (b) Lateral view shows the typical triangular-shaped opacity produced by collapsed right middle lobe (arrows).*

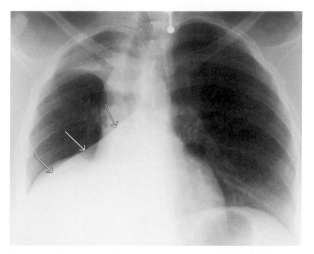

Fig. 3.25 *Right lower lobe collapse. Triangular opacity behind the right heart (arrows) with loss of definition of the right diaphragm. The right heart border is still seen. Note that in this case the right upper lobe is also collapsed.*

- Increased density of right upper zone.
- Loss of definition of right mediastinal margins.
- Elevation of right hilum.
- Tracheal deviation to the right.

Right middle lobe (Fig. 3.24)

- Increased density in right midzone with loss of definition of the right cardiac border.
- Lateral film: triangular opacity projected over the heart.

Right lower lobe (Fig. 3.25)

- Collapses downwards and posteriorly.
- Decreased volume of right lung.
- Triangular opacity at the right base medially.
- Loss of definition of the right hemidiaphragm.
- Heart border not obscured.
- Elevation of right hemidiaphragm.
- Depression of right hilum.
- Non-visualization of the right lower lobe artery.
- Lateral film: increased apparent density of lower thoracic vertebral bodies.

Left upper lobe (Fig. 3.26):

- Collapses upwards and anteriorly.
- Decreased volume of left lung.

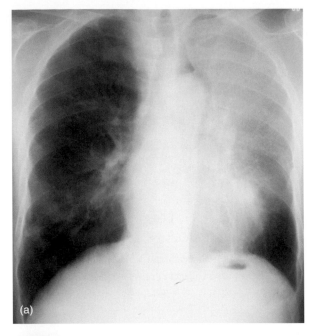

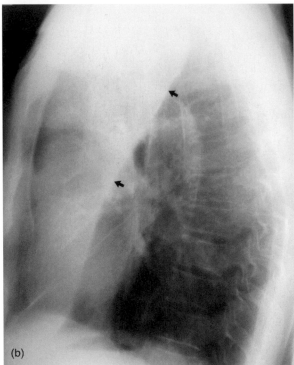

Fig. 3.26 *Left upper lobe collapse. (a) Posteroanterior view shows loss of volume on the left and opacity in the left upper zone. The aortic arch can be seen because of elevation of the aerated left lower lobe. (b) Lateral view shows the typical pattern of left upper lobe collapse with the oblique fissure pulled upwards and anteriorly (arrows).*

- Increased density of left upper zone.
- Loss of definition of left upper cardiac border and left mediastinal margin; in severe left upper lobe collapse the aortic knuckle may be well outlined by elevated apical segment of the left lower lobe.
- Elevation of left hilum.
- Tracheal deviation to the left.
- Lateral film: increased opacity anteriorly, which has a well-defined posterior margin because of the oblique fissure.

Left lower lobe (Fig. 3.27):

- Collapses downwards and posteriorly.
- Decreased volume of left lung.
- Triangular opacity behind the left heart.
- Loss of definition of the left hemidiaphragm.
- Left heart border not obscured.
- Elevation of left hemidiaphragm.
- Depression of left hilum.
- Non-visualization of left lower lobe artery.
- Lateral film: increased apparent density of lower thoracic vertebral bodies.

PLEURAL DISORDERS

Pleural disorders include accumulation of fluid in the pleural spaces (pleural effusion), air leaks (pneumothorax and pneumomediastinum), and pleural soft-tissue thickening and plaque formation.

PLEURAL EFFUSION

The X-ray appearances of pleural effusion are not related to the nature of the fluid, which may include transudate, exudates, blood, pus or lymph (chylothorax).

Signs of pleural effusion on erect CXR (Fig. 3.28, page 54) include homogeneous dense opacity at the base of the lung, with a concave upper surface higher laterally than medially, producing a meniscus. Small pleural effusions produce blunting of the normal sharp angle between the lateral curve of the diaphragm and the inner chest wall, referred to as blunting of the

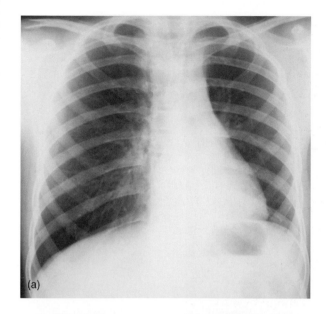

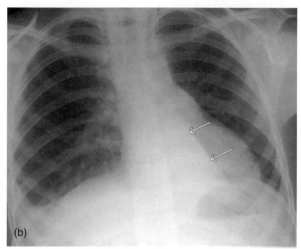

Fig. 3.27 *Left lower lobe collapse: two separate examples. (a) Note loss of volume on the left, opacity behind the left heart and loss of definition of the medial part of the left diaphragm. (b) A more classical, though less commonly seen pattern of left lower lobe collapse with a sharply defined triangular opacity behind the left heart (arrows).*

costophrenic angle. The lateral film is more sensitive to the presence of small pleural effusions than the PA view. It is estimated that about 300 mL of fluid is required to show costophrenic angle blunting on the PA, whereas only 100 mL is required to produce this sign (posteriorly) on the lateral view. Large pleural effusions displace the mediastinum towards the contralateral side.

Variations to the 'normal' appearance of pleural effusion include:
- Loculations that may resemble pleural masses.
- Fluid in fissures that may mimic pulmonary masses.
- Subpulmonic effusion: fluid trapped beneath the lung produces opacity parallel to the diaphragm with a convex upper margin.

Signs of pleural fluid on supine CXR (Fig. 3.29, page 55) opacity over lung apex (pleural cap) and increased opacity of the hemithorax through which lung structures can still be seen. There is often loss of definition of the hemidiaphragm and blunting of the costophrenic angle. The opacity of pleural effusion may be differentiated from pulmonary consolidation by the absence of air bronchograms.

Causes of pleural effusion

- Cardiac failure:
  (i) Bilateral;
  (ii) Right larger than left.
- Malignancy:
  (i) Bronchogenic carcinoma;
  (ii) Metastatic;
  (iii) Mesothelioma.
- Infection:
  (i) Bacterial pneumonia;
  (ii) Tuberculosis;
  (iii) Mycoplasma;
  (iv) Empyema;
  (v) Subphrenic abscess.
- Pulmonary embolus with infarct.
- Pancreatitis: effusion is usually left-sided.
- Trauma: associated with rib fractures.
- Connective tissue disorders:
  (i) Rheumatoid arthritis;
  (ii) SLE.
- Liver failure.
- Renal failure.
- Meig's syndrome: associated with ovarian fibroma.

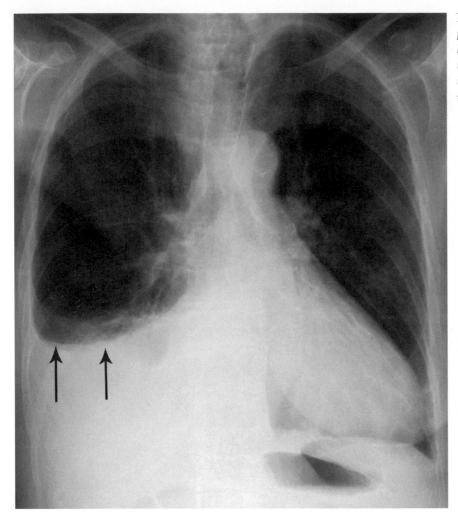

Fig. 3.28 *Pleural effusion producing a fluid level at the right base (arrows). The outer edge of the fluid tracks a small distance up the chest wall producing a typical meniscus shape.*

PNEUMOTHORAX

Pneumothorax is usually well seen on a normal inspiratory PA film. The diagnosis of small pneumothorax may be easier on an expiratory film. This is because of the reduced volume of the lung in expiration, which makes the pneumothorax look relatively larger. Whether the film is performed in inspiration or expiration, the sign to look for is the lung edge outlined by air in the pleural space (Fig. 3.30).

Tension pneumothorax occurs with continued air leak from the lung into the pleural space. This results in increased pressure in the pleural space with expansion of the hemithorax and further compression and collapse of the lung. The CXR signs of tension pneumothorax include marked collapse and distortion of the lung and increased volume of hemithorax with displacement of the mediastinum, depressed diaphragm and increased space between the ribs (Fig. 3.31).

Supine AP CXR may have to be performed in intensive care unit (ICU) patients or following severe trauma. Pleural air lies anteromedially and beneath the lung so that the usual appearance, as described for an erect PA film, is not seen. Signs of pneumothorax on a supine CXR include:

- Mediastinal structures including heart border, inferior vena cava (IVC) and SVC are sharply outlined by adjacent free pleural air.
- Upper abdomen appears lucent because of overlying air.
- Deep lateral costophrenic angle (Fig. 3.32, page 56).

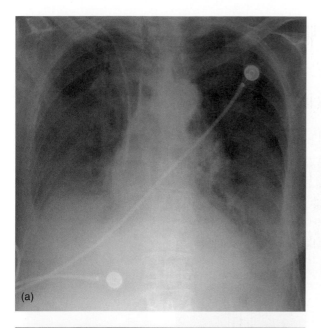

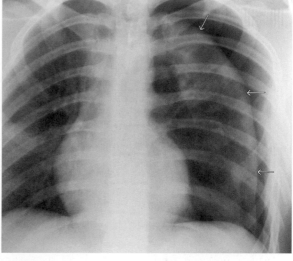

Fig. 3.30 *Pneumothorax. The edge of the partly collapsed lung (arrows) is outlined by the pneumothorax.*

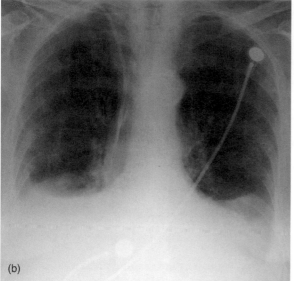

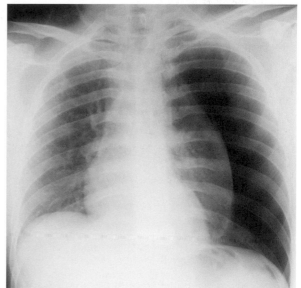

Fig. 3.29 *Pleural effusions on chest X-ray (CXR). (a) Supine CXR: pleural effusions produce vague opacity over both lower zones with poor definition of each hemidiaphragm. Lack of air bronchograms and visualization of pulmonary structures helps differentiate pleural effusions from pulmonary consolidation. (b) Erect CXR confirms the diagnosis of bilateral pleural effusions.*

Fig. 3.31 *Tension pneumothorax. Signs of tension include expansion of the left hemithorax, increased space between the left ribs, shift of the mediastinal structures to the right and severe collapse of the left lung.*

Causes of pneumothorax

- Spontaneous:
  (i) Tall, thin males;
  (ii) Smokers.

- Iatrogenic:
  (i) Following percutaneous lung biopsy;
  (ii) Ventilation;
  (iii) Central venous line line insertion;
  (iv) Trauma: associated with rib fractures.

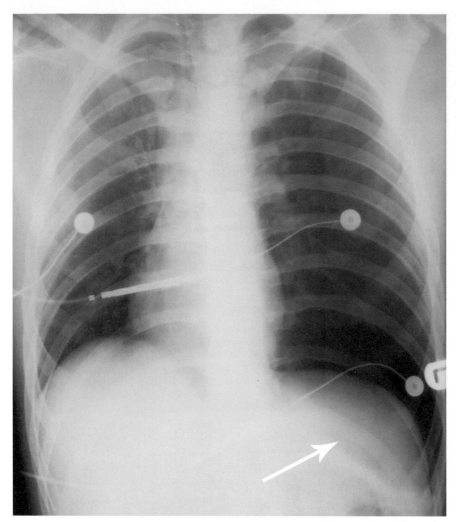

Fig. 3.32 *Supine pneumothorax. Pneumothorax in a supine patient shows as an area of lucency over the lower left hemithorax and upper left abdomen (arrow). Note also increased volume on the left indicating tension. (See also Fig. 16.3, page 245)*

- Emphysema.
- Malignancy: high incidence in osteogenic sarcoma metastases.
- Honeycomb lung.
- Cystic fibrosis.

PNEUMOMEDIASTINUM

Pneumomediastinum refers to air leak into the soft tissues of the mediastinum. Radiographic signs of pneumomediastinum result from air outlining the normal mediastinal structures. These signs include a strip of air outlining the left side of the mediastinum, air around the aorta, pulmonary arteries and pericardium, and subcutaneous air extending upwards into the soft tissues of the neck (Fig. 3.33).

Causes of pneumomediastinum

- Spontaneous: following severe coughing or strenuous exercise.
- Asthma.
- Foreign body aspiration in neonates.
- Chest trauma.
- Oesophageal perforation: tumour, severe vomiting, and endoscopy.

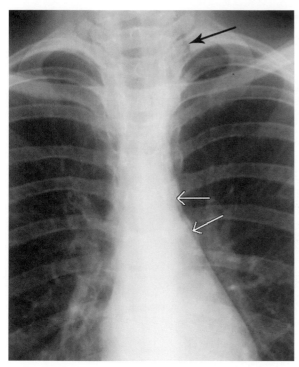

Fig. 3.33 *Pneumomediastinum. A thin layer of air is seen parallel to the left mediastinal margin (white arrows). Air is also seen tracking into the soft tissues of the neck (black arrow).*

PLEURAL THICKENING

Pleural thickening may occur in a variety of circumstances as follows:

- Secondary to trauma:
  - (i) Associated with healed rib fractures;
  - (ii) Dense layer of soft tissue, often calcified.
- Following empyema:
  - (i) More common over the lung bases;
  - (ii) Often calcified.
- Tuberculosis.
- Asbestos exposure:
  - (i) Irregular pleural thickening and pleural plaques (Fig. 3.34);
  - (ii) Calcification common, especially of diaphragmatic surface of pleura;
  - (iii) Note that pleural disease is not asbestosis; the term 'asbestosis' refers to the interstitial lung disease secondary to asbestos exposure.

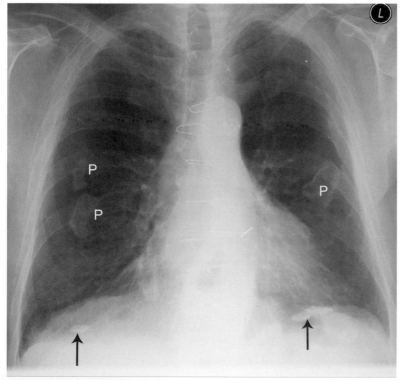

Fig. 3.34 *Pleural plaques: asbestos exposure. Multiple plaques (P) are seen as well-defined though irregular opacities projected over the lungs. Note also linear regions of pleural calcification (arrows).*

- Mesothelioma:
    - (i) Diffuse or localized pleural mass;
    - (ii) Rib destruction uncommon;
    - (iii) Large pleural effusions common;
    - (iv) Pleural plaques elsewhere in 50 per cent.

- Pancoast tumour:
    - (i) Primary apical lung neoplasm;
    - (ii) Rib destruction with irregular pleural thickening.
- Pleural metastases: often obscured by associated pleural effusion.

Respiratory system

Common symptoms caused by respiratory disease include cough, production of sputum, haemoptysis, dyspnoea and chest pain. These may be accompanied by systemic manifestations including fever, weight loss and night sweats. As always, accurate history plus findings on physical examination, in particular auscultation of the chest, are vital in directing further investigation and management. History and examination may be supplemented by relatively simple tests such as white cell count, erythrocyte sedimentation rate (ESR), and sputum analysis for culture or cytology. A variety of pulmonary function tests may be performed. These include measurements of static lung volumes and airways resistance with spirometry, measurements of gas exchange such as carbon monoxide (CO) diffusing capacity and arterial blood gas, and exercise testing.

More sophisticated and invasive tests include:
- Flexible fibreoptic bronchoscopy:
  - (i) Endobronchial biopsy;
  - (ii) Transbronchial biopsy;
  - (iii) Bronchoalveolar lavage.
- Percutaneous transthoracic needle biopsy under computed tomography (CT) guidance.
- Mediastinoscopy.
- Open (surgical) lung biopsy.
- Video-assisted thorascopic surgery (VATS): minimally invasive surgical technique for biopsy of lung, mediastinum, pleura or chest wall.

A complete discussion of these methods is beyond the scope of this book.

Virtually all symptoms and clinical situations related to the respiratory system will be investigated by chest X-ray (CXR). Interpretation of CXRs has been outlined in Chapter 3. In this chapter the roles of the other main imaging modalities in respiratory disease are outlined and followed by examples of imaging findings in the more common respiratory conditions.

IMAGING INVESTIGATION OF THE RESPIRATORY SYSTEM

COMPUTED TOMOGRAPHY

Computed tomography is the investigation of choice for the following:
- Mediastinal mass:
  - (i) Accurate localization;
  - (ii) Characterization of internal contents of mass (fat, air, fluid and calcification);
  - (iii) Displacement/invasion of adjacent structures such as aorta, heart, trachea, oesophagus, vertebral column, chest wall.
- Hilar mass:
  - (i) Greater sensitivity than plain films for the presence of hilar lymphadenopathy.
  - (ii) Greater specificity in differentiating lymphadenopathy or hilar mass from enlarged pulmonary arteries.
- Staging of bronchogenic carcinoma:
  - (i) Greater sensitivity than plain films for the presence of mediastinal or hilar lymphadenopathy (Fig. 4.1);
  - (ii) Greater sensitivity for complications such as chest wall or mediastinal invasion, and cavitation.
- Detection of pulmonary metastases:
  - (i) CT has greater sensitivity than plain films for the detection of small pulmonary lesions, including metastases;

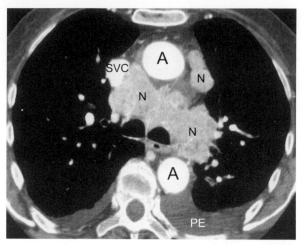

Fig. 4.1 *Mediastinal lymphadenopathy caused by bronchogenic carcinoma: computed tomography. Note enlarged mediastinal lymph nodes (N), superior vena cava (SVC), aorta (A) and pleural effusions (PE).*

  (ii) This is particularly so in areas of the lung seen poorly on CXR, including the apices, posterior segments of the lower lobes, and medial areas that are obscured by the hila.
- Characterization of a pulmonary mass seen on CXR:
  (i) More accurate than plain films for the presence of calcification;
  (ii) Other factors also well assessed by CT include cavitation and relation of a mass to the chest wall or mediastinum;
  (iii) Intravenous contrast material may help to identify aberrant vessels and arteriovenous malformations.
- Demonstration of mediastinal vasculature:
  (i) Thoracic aortic aneurysm;
  (ii) Aortic dissection;
  (iii) Superior vena cava (SVC) compression/invasion by tumour;
  (iv) Vascular anomalies that may cause abnormalities on CXR, e.g. azygos continuation of inferior vena cava (IVC), partial anomalous pulmonary venous drainage.
- Trauma:
  (i) Exclusion of mediastinal haematoma in a haemodynamically stable patient with a widened mediastinum on CXR following chest trauma.
  (ii) CT angiogram to assess aorta (see below).
- Characterization of pleural disease:
  (i) CT gives excellent delineation of pleural abnormalities that may produce confusing appearances on CXR;
  (ii) Pleural masses, fluid collections, calcifications and tumours such as mesothelioma are well shown, as are complications such as rib destruction, mediastinal invasion and lymphadenopathy.
- Guidance of percutaneous biopsy and drainage procedures: CT-guided biopsy is especially useful for peripheral lesions not amenable to bronchoscopic biopsy.

HIGH-RESOLUTION COMPUTED TOMOGRAPHY

High-resolution computed tomography (HRCT) is a technique used in the assessment of disorders of the lungs. Conventional CT of the chest uses sections 3–10 mm thick. The high-resolution technique uses much thinner sections of around 1 mm. The thinner sections show the lung in much greater detail. Intravenous contrast material is not used and the mediastinal and chest wall structures are less well seen than with conventional chest CT. High-resolution CT is useful for the following:
- Bronchiectasis (Fig. 4.2):
  (i) HRCT is the investigation of choice in the assessment of bronchiectasis;
  (ii) As well as showing dilated bronchi, HRCT accurately shows the anatomical distribution of changes, in addition to complications such as scarring, collapse, consolidation and mucous plugging.
- Interstitial lung disease:
  (i) HRCT is more sensitive and specific than plain films in the diagnosis of many interstitial lung diseases;

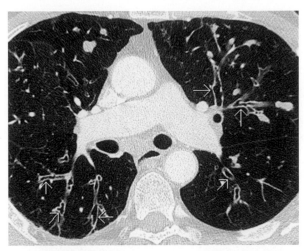

Fig. 4.2 *Bronchiectasis: high-resolution computed tomography. Dilated thick walled bronchi (arrows). Compare this appearance with the normal lungs in Fig. 1.10a.*

(ii) Sarcoidosis, idiopathic interstitial pneumonias, lymphangitis carcinomatosa and histiocytosis-X are examples of disorders that have specific appearances on HRCT, often obviating the need for biopsy in these patients;

(iii) Where biopsy is felt necessary, HRCT may aid in guiding the operator to the most favourable biopsy site.

- Atypical infections:
  (i) HRCT provides diagnosis of many atypical infections earlier and with greater specificity than plain CXR;
  (ii) Examples include: *Pneumocystis carinii,* aspergillosis and *Mycobacterium avium intracellulare* – infections that occur in immunocompromised patients, including those with AIDS;
  (iii) As well as diagnosis, HRCT may be useful for monitoring disease progress and response to therapy.

- Normal CXR in symptomatic patients: HRCT has a definite role in the assessment of patients with an apparently normal CXR, despite the clinical indications of respiratory disease, including dyspnoea, chest pain, haemoptysis and abnormal pulmonary function tests.

COMPUTED TOMOGRAPHY PULMONARY ANGIOGRAPHY (SEE CHAPTER 5)

SCINTIGRAPHY

A number of examples exist of the use of scintigraphy in the assessment of disorders of the respiratory system.

- Pulmonary embolism: ventilation/perfusion lung scan (see Chapter 5).
- Early infection:
  (i) Gallium-67 (^{67}Ga);
  (ii) The most common example in clinical use would be in the detection of early *Pneumocystis carinii* infection in acquired immune-deficiency syndrome (AIDS) patients;
  (iii) Increased lung uptake of ^{67}Ga may be seen prior to the appearance of CXR changes.
- Positron-emission tomography (PET) with fluorodeoxyglucose (FDG):
  (i) Characterization of a solitary pulmonary nodule – increased uptake in neoplastic masses;
  (ii) Staging of bronchogenic carcinoma;
  (iii) Differentiation of recurrent bronchogenic carcinoma from postoperative or postradiation changes. Such differentiation may be difficult or impossible with CXR and CT.

ULTRASOUND

Ultrasound (US) is useful for the confirmation of pleural effusion suspected on CXR. It can readily differentiate pleural fluid from other causes of pleural opacity such as pleural thickening or mass. It is particularly useful for guidance of aspiration and drainage of small pleural fluid collections.

ANGIOGRAPHY AND INTERVENTIONAL RADIOLOGY

Angiography of bronchial arteries followed by embolization may be useful in the setting of massive haemoptysis.

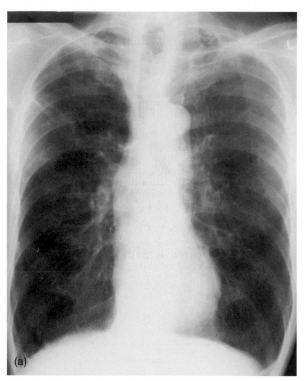

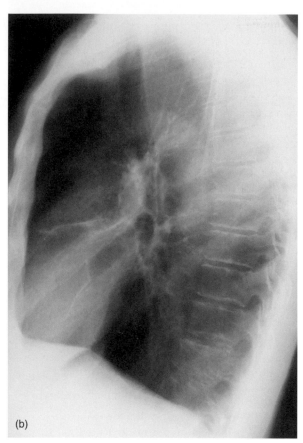

Fig. 4.3 *Emphysema. (a) Posteroanterior radiograph showing over-expansion of both lungs. (b) Lateral radiograph showing flattening of the hemidiaphragms and increased size of retrosternal airspace posterior to the sternum.*

COMMON PULMONARY DISORDERS

EMPHYSEMA

Emphysema refers to enlarged airspaces secondary to destruction of the alveolar walls. Centrilobular emphysema is the most common form. It occurs in smokers and predominantly affects the upper lobes. Panlobular emphysema is seen in association with α-1 antitrypsin deficiency. It tends to affect predominantly the lower lobes. Chest X-ray signs of emphysema (Fig. 4.3) include:

• Overexpanded lungs.
• Flat diaphragms lying below the 6th rib anteriorly.
• Increased retrosternal airspace on lateral film.
• Decreased vascular markings in lung fields.

• Increased anteroposterior diameter of the chest, with in some cases kyphosis and anterior bowing of the sternum.
• Bulla formation: bullae are seen as thin-walled air-containing cavities.
• Pulmonary arterial hypertension: prominent main pulmonary arteries.

High-resolution CT may be used to accurately assess the severity and distribution of emphysema, quantify the percentage of residual healthy lung, and identify conditions that would exclude surgical treatment, such as bronchogenic carcinoma.

ASTHMA

Between acute attacks, the CXR of an asthma sufferer is often normal. 'Baseline changes' that may be seen

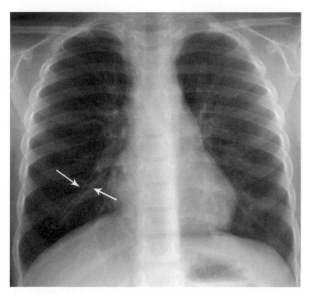

Fig. 4.4 *Asthma. Note prominent thickening of bronchial walls in the central lungs (arrows).*

include overexpanded lungs, thickening of bronchial walls – most marked in the parahilar regions – and focal scarring from previous infections (Fig. 4.4). During acute asthma attacks the lungs are overinflated because of air trapping. Lobar or segmental atelectasis caused by mucous plugging is common. It is important to differentiate atelectasis from consolidation to avoid unnecessary use of antibiotics. Other complications of asthma that may be diagnosed on CXR include pneumonia, pneumomediastinum and pneumothorax, and secondary aspergillosis.

PNEUMONIA

Organisms that commonly cause pneumonia include *Streptococcus pneumoniae*, *Haemophilus influenzae*, *Klebsiella pneumoniae* and *Mycoplasma pneumoniae*. Early subtle areas of alveolar shadowing progress to dense lobar consolidation. See Chapter 3 for notes on patterns of lobar consolidation. Expansion of a lobe with bulging pulmonary fissures may be seen with *Klebsiella*. Necrosis and cavitation may complicate severe cases of lobar pneumonia. Small pleural effusions commonly accompany pneumonia. More aggressive organisms such as *Staphylococcus aureus* and *Pseudomonas* can cause more extensive consolidation. This may involve multiple lobes, with cavitation leading to abscess formation.

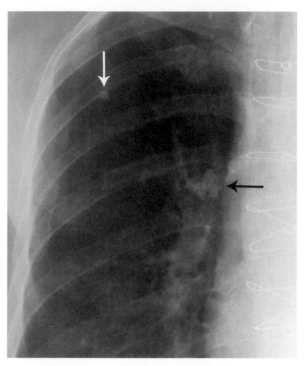

Fig. 4.5 *Tuberculosis: healed primary. Calcified granuloma in right upper lobe (white arrow) and calcified mediastinal lymph nodes (black arrow).*

Other complications include empyema and bronchopleural fistula.

For further information on pulmonary infections in children, see Chapter 16.

TUBERCULOSIS

Primary tuberculosis

Primary tuberculosis (TB) is usually asymptomatic. The healed pulmonary lesion of primary TB may be seen on CXR as a small calcified peripheral pulmonary nodule with calcified hilar lymph node (Fig. 4.5).

Post-primary pulmonary tuberculosis (reactivation TB)

Post-primary TB has a predilection for the apical and posterior segments of the upper lobes, plus the apical segments of the lower lobes. Variable CXR appearances may include ill-defined areas of alveolar consolidation and thick-walled, irregular cavities (Fig. 4.6).

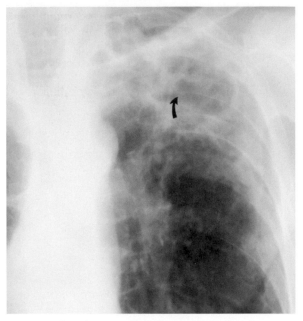

Fig. 4.6 *Tuberculosis: post-primary. Opacity in the left upper lobe with cavitation (arrow).*

Haemoptysis, aspergilloma, tuberculous empyema and broncho-pleural fistula may complicate cavitation. Subsequent fibrosis may cause volume loss in the upper lobes. Fibrosis and calcification usually indicate disease inactivity and healing, but one should never diagnose inactive TB on a single CXR: serial films are essential to prove inactivity.

Miliary tuberculosis

Miliary TB occurs because of haematogenous dissemination, which may occur at any time following primary infection. On CXR, miliary TB appears as tiny densities of approximately 2 mm diameter spread evenly through both lungs.

SOLITARY PULMONARY NODULE

The definition of a solitary pulmonary nodule is a spherical lung opacity seen on CXR without associated findings such as pulmonary collapse or lymphadenopathy. Characterization of a solitary pulmonary nodule is often a diagnostic challenge. Features on CXR that tend to indicate malignancy include a diameter of greater than 3.0 cm and an ill-defined margin (see Fig. 3.11, page 42).

Two findings on CXR that are sufficiently predictive of a benign aetiology to preclude further investigation are calcification and lack of growth over 2 years. Comparison with previous X-rays is therefore essential, if these are available. These features are seen in a minority of solitary pulmonary nodules and most require further imaging investigations, particularly where there are underlying risk factors for lung cancer. These include cigarette smoking, exposure to asbestos, and a history of lung cancer in a first-degree relative. The two most commonly used investigations are CT and FDG-PET.

Computed tomography

Detection of even small amounts of calcification or fat on CT virtually excludes bronchogenic carcinoma. Calcification may be seen in granuloma (usually small well-defined opacity) or bronchial carcinoid. Contrast enhancement tends to indicate malignancy rather than granuloma.

Fluorodeoxyglucose positron-emission tomography

This may be useful to characterize solitary pulmonary nodules where other imaging is unhelpful. Neoplastic masses show increased uptake of FDG. However, FDG-PET is unable to accurately characterize lesions less than 1 cm diameter and false positive findings may occur in active inflammatory lesions.

Biopsy

Lesions that have positive findings for malignancy on CT or FDG-PET will require biopsy. Lesions that remain indeterminate may also require biopsy or follow-up with further imaging after a certain period of time, depending on risk factors and other findings. Biopsy may be performed via bronchoscopy, percutaneously with CT guidance, with VATS, or by open surgical biopsy and resection.

STAGING OF BRONCHOGENIC CARCINOMA (LUNG CANCER)

Bronchogenic carcinoma is classified into small cell lung cancer (SCLC) and non-small cell lung cancer

(NSCLC). The TNM system is widely used to stage bronchogenic carcinoma. In this system the 'T' refers to features of the primary tumour and includes features such as tumour size and evidence of chest wall or mediastinal invasion. The 'N' refers to lymph node involvement and the 'M' to distant metastasis. Small cell lung cancer accounts for about 15 per cent of new cases of bronchogenic carcinoma and is more aggressive than NSCLC. It is often staged using a two-stage system, where patients are classified as having limited or extensive disease. Limited disease implies tumour confined to one hemithorax and to regional lymph nodes. Extensive disease describes anything beyond this, either to contralateral hemithorax or distant metastasis.

Chest X-ray

The majority of bronchogenic carcinomas are initially diagnosed on CXR. The usual appearance is a pulmonary mass (see Fig. 3.11, page 42). This may be quite small, and may be an incidental finding on a CXR performed for other reasons, such as pre-anaesthetic or as part of a routine medical check-up.

Complications of bronchogenic carcinoma that may produce a more complex appearance on CXR include:

- Segmental/lobar collapse (Fig. 4.7).
- Persistent areas of consolidation.
- Hilar lymphadenopathy.
- Mediastinal lymphadenopathy.
- Pleural effusion.
- Invasion of adjacent structures: mediastinum, chest wall (Fig. 4.8).
- Metastases: lungs, bones.

Computed tomography

Computed tomography is the major imaging modality of choice for the staging of bronchogenic carcinoma. It is more accurate than CXR for the diagnosis of mediastinal lymphadenopathy, hilar lymphadenopathy, mediastinal invasion and chest wall invasion. The CT examination should include the adrenal glands (a common site of metastases from NSCLC). It may also be used for primary diagnosis where the CXR is negative

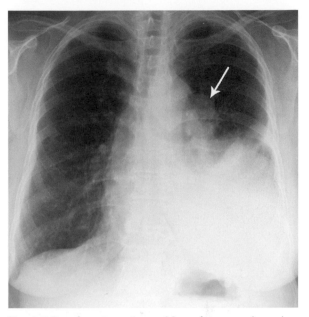

Fig. 4.7 *Bronchogenic carcinoma. Note a large mass (arrow) adjacent to the left hilum. Loss of volume and irregular opacity at the left base are caused by a combination of left lower lobe collapse and pleural effusion.*

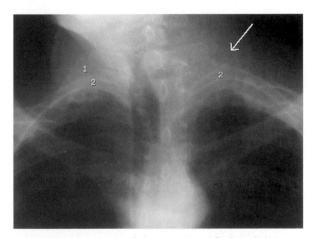

Fig. 4.8 *Pancoast tumour left apex. Note right first rib (1), bilateral second ribs (2), absent left first rib (arrow) due to destruction by tumour.*

and the presence of a tumour is suspected on clinical grounds, e.g. haemoptysis, positive sputum cytology or paraneoplastic syndrome.

Biopsy

Diagnosis of cell type is important, first to confirm the diagnosis of bronchogenic carcinoma, and second to

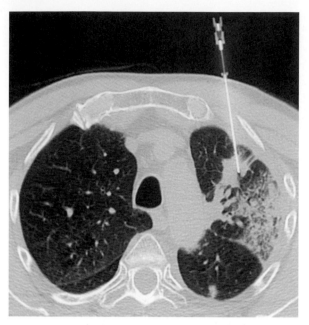

Fig. 4.9 *Computed tomography-guided lung biopsy.*

classify the tumour. Tumour cells may be obtained from sputum cytology or from aspiration of pleural fluid. More commonly, some form of invasive biopsy will be required. Centrally located tumours may be amenable to diagnosis with bronchoscopy. Most peripheral tumours can be accessed by CT-guided biopsy (Fig. 4.9). Exceptions to this are very small masses, or tumours in difficult locations such as deep to the scapula. These may require open biopsy or VATS.

Fluorodeoxyglucose positron-emission tomography

Recent studies have shown PET with FDG to be useful in staging of bronchogenic carcinoma. It has been found that FDG-PET is highly sensitive to areas of increased metabolic activity and shows neoplastic tissue as areas of increased activity ('hot spots'). It provides views of the whole body and, therefore, will show the primary tumour, lymph node involvement and metastases to distant sites. In particular, it has a high negative predictive value, indicating that a negative PET scan can obviate the need for other imaging or more invasive studies.

HAEMOPTYSIS

Haemoptysis refers to the expectoration of blood from the tracheobronchial tree or lung. The commonest cause of haemoptysis is erosion of bronchial mucosa in smokers with chronic bronchitis. The next most common cause is bronchogenic carcinoma. Haemoptysis may also be encountered with pulmonary infections, including TB. The initial imaging investigation of haemoptysis is CXR followed by other investigations such as CT, bronchoscopy or biopsy, as required.

Massive haemoptysis is defined as expectoration of more than 300 mL of blood per 24 hours. Causes include erosion of bronchial arteries in bronchiectasis and arteriovenous malformation. Urgent CXR is followed by angiography. Selective catheterization of the bronchial arteries with identification of a bleeding site may be followed by embolization. If this is not curative, surgical removal of the affected segment or lobe may be required.

IDIOPATHIC PULMONARY FIBROSIS

The term idiopathic interstitial pneumonia refers to a group of diffuse lung diseases that share many features despite being separate disease entities. Diseases classified under this term include usual interstitial pneumonia (UIP), non-specific interstitial pneumonia (NSIP), desquamative interstitial pneumonia (DIP), acute interstitial pneumonia (AIP), lymphoid interstitial pneumonia (LIP) and cryptogenic organizing pneumonia (COP). The commonest form of idiopathic interstitial pneumonia is UIP and this is also known as idiopathic pulmonary fibrosis.

Idiopathic pulmonary fibrosis is a chronic lung disorder characterized by diffuse interstitial inflammation and fibrosis. Peak incidence is at 50–60 years of age. Patients present with insidious onset of dyspnoea with exertion. Diagnosis relies on abnormal pulmonary function tests with evidence of restriction and impaired gas exchange, exclusion of other causes of interstitial lung disease, such as connective tissue disorders and drug toxicity, and typical findings on HRCT.

The CXR signs of idiopathic pulmonary fibrosis include an interstitial linear pattern, predominantly at

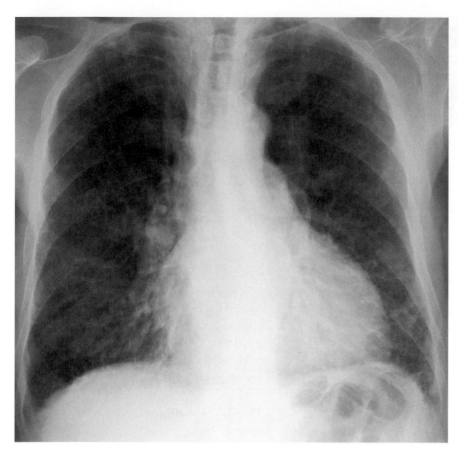

Fig. 4.10 *Pulmonary fibrosis of unknown cause in a patient with a long history of shortness of breath. Note extensive linear opacity throughout both lungs with irregularity of the heart borders and hemidiaphragms.*

the lung bases (Fig. 4.10). This produces an irregular 'shaggy' heart border. As the disease progresses there is loss of lung volume and development of the honey-comb lung pattern.

The HRCT findings include a peripheral linear pattern involving predominantly the lower lobes. There is often also diffuse density known as a 'ground-glass' pattern. These changes progress over time to a honey-comb pattern that may be seen on HRCT as coarse irregular linear opacity with cyst-like air spaces.

CHEST TRAUMA

Severely traumatized patients are unable to stand. For this reason, the CXR in the setting of acute trauma is often performed with the patient in the supine position. This leads to a number of problems with interpretation:

- The mediastinum appears widened because of normal distension of venous structures.

- Pleural fluid may be more difficult to diagnose in the absence of a fluid level.
- Pneumothorax may be more difficult to diagnose.

If possible therefore, an erect CXR should be performed.

Findings to look for on the CXR of a trauma patient include pneumothorax, haemothorax, haemopneumo-thorax, pulmonary contusion, mediastinal haematoma, ruptured diaphragm, and skeletal injuries including fractures of ribs, sternum and scapula.

Pneumothorax

Tension pneumothorax is indicated by depression of the diaphragm and contralateral mediastinal shift (see Fig. 3.31). Haemopneumothorax shows as a straight fluid level (Fig. 4.11). Traumatic pneumothorax is often associated with pneumomediastinum and sub-cutaneous emphysema of the chest wall and neck.

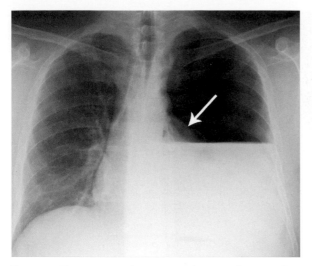

Fig. 4.11 *Haemopneumothorax. Note that a combination of air and fluid in the pleural space produces a straight line without the typical meniscus of a pleural effusion. Compare this appearance with Fig. 3.28. In this case there is also evidence of tension with increased volume on the left and marked collapse and distortion of the left lung (arrow).*

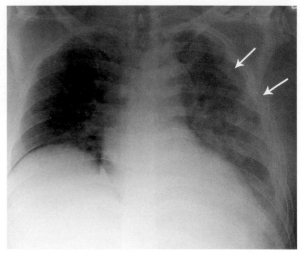

Fig. 4.12 *Haemothorax producing opacification of the left hemithorax. Note multiple rib fractures (arrows).*

Pneumomediastinum is seen on CXR as vertical lucencies in the paratracheal tissues with air outlining the mediastinal pleura, especially on the left (see Fig. 3.33). Subcutaneous emphysema is seen as patchy lucency in the soft tissues of the chest wall and neck. It may produce a striped appearance in the pectoralis muscles with air dissecting between muscle fibre bundles. Severe pneumomediastinum in association with tension pneumothorax may indicate a tear in a major bronchus.

Haemothorax

Haemothorax may give the appearance of a classical pleural effusion. More commonly it is seen as more loculated pleural-based opacity, often in association with other findings such as rib fractures and pulmonary contusion (Fig. 4.12). A large haemothorax may cause contralateral mediastinal shift. As mentioned above, haemopneumothorax shows as a straight fluid level on an erect CXR.

Pulmonary contusion

Pulmonary contusion may be solitary or multiple. Contusion shows on CXR as a focal area of alveolar shadowing that appears within hours of the trauma and usually clears after 4 days. Contusion is usually, though not always, associated with rib fractures.

Ruptured diaphragm

The CXR signs of ruptured diaphragm include herniation of abdominal structures into the chest, apparent elevation of the hemidiaphragm and contralateral mediastinal shift.

Aortic rupture

Full-thickness aortic rupture is usually fatal. Approximately 20 per cent of aortic ruptures are not full thickness (i.e. the adventitia is intact). Untreated, there is a high mortality rate with delayed complete rupture occurring up to 4 months following trauma. Only around 5 per cent of incomplete ruptures develop a false aneurysm associated with a normal life span. Note that incomplete aortic rupture implies an intact adventitia. Therefore, mediastinal haematoma arises from other blood vessels such as the intercostal or internal mammary arteries or veins. The mediastinal haematoma is associated with, not caused by, the aortic injury. The CXR signs of aortic injury result from the associated mediastinal haematoma. It is therefore important to recognize signs of mediastinal haematoma on CXR and

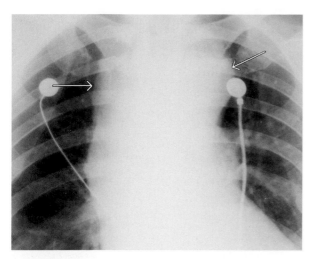

Fig. 4.13 *Aortic injury. Note that there is widening of the mediastinum (arrows) with loss of definition of mediastinal structures owing to mediastinal haematoma.*

CT. Twenty per cent of patients with mediastinal haematoma on CXR or CT will have an aortic injury. Absence of mediastinal haematoma is a reliable predictor of an intact aorta.

The CXR signs of aortic rupture (Fig. 4.13):

- Widened mediastinum that may be difficult to assess on a supine film.
- Obscured aortic knuckle and other mediastinal structures.
- Displacement of trachea and nasogastric tube to the right.
- Depression of left main bronchus.
- Left haemothorax giving pleural opacification, including depression of the apex of the left lung.

Incomplete rupture of the aorta is confirmed by CT angiogram, aortogram or transoesophageal echocardiogram (TEE) with most tears occurring at the aortic isthmus, just distal to the left subclavian artery. Choice of modality is dependent on local expertise and availability. With the wide availability of multidetector CT, CT angiogram is now most commonly employed. Where definite CXR signs of mediastinal haematoma are present, or where the CXR is equivocal, chest CT including CT angiogram should be performed. Aortogram or TEE may be used as problem-solving tools in difficult or equivocal cases.

Rib fractures

Oblique views looking for subtle rib fractures are not advised in the acute situation. Associated soft-tissue injuries and complications are more important. Fractures of the upper three ribs indicate a high level of trauma, though there is no proven increase in the incidence of great vessel damage. Fractures of the lower three ribs have an association with upper abdominal injury (liver, spleen and kidney).

A flail segment refers to segmental fractures of three or more ribs. This produces paradoxical movement of a segment of the chest wall with respiration. This is often very difficult to appreciate clinically and as such flail segment is usually a radiological diagnosis. Flail segment has a high incidence of associated injuries, such as pneumothorax, subcutaneous emphysema and haemothorax, and adequate pain management is crucial to prevent lobar collapse and pneumonia.

Other fractures

Sternal fractures usually involve the body of the sternum, rarely the manubrium. They are only seen on a lateral view. Sternal fracture has a high association with myocardial and pulmonary contusion and airway rupture. Dislocation of the sternoclavicular joint is an uncommon injury, usually caused by a direct blow. This joint is notoriously difficult to see on plain films and CT is the investigation of choice where this injury is suspected. Computed tomography will show the medial end of the clavicle lying in an abnormally posterior position. Fractures of the clavicle, scapula and humerus may also be seen in association with chest trauma.

SARCOIDOSIS

Sarcoidosis is a disease of unknown aetiology characterized by the widespread formation of non-caseating granulomas (see Figs 3.10 and 3.16). The chest is the commonest site with hilar and mediastinal lymphadenopathy and lung changes. Lymphadenopathy alone occurs in 50 per cent of cases, lymphadenopathy plus lung changes in 25 per cent of cases and lung changes alone in 15 per cent of cases. Hilar lymphadenopathy is usually symmetrical and lobulated, and associated with right paratracheal lymphadenopathy. The lung changes of sarcoidosis consist of small interstitial nodules 2–5 mm diameter spread through both lungs, predominantly in the midzones. Healing may lead to bilateral upper zone fibrosis.

Extrathoracic sites of involvement with sarcoidosis include:

- Liver and spleen.
- Peripheral lymph nodes.
- CNS: granulomatous meningitis.
- Eyes: uveitis.
- Bone.
- Salivary glands: bilateral parotid gland enlargement.
- Skin: erythema nodosum.

CYSTIC FIBROSIS (MUCOVISCIDOSIS)

Cystic fibrosis is an autosomal recessive condition with dysfunction of exocrine glands and reduced mucociliary function. Pancreatic insufficiency leads to steatorrhoea and malabsorption. Meconium ileus may be seen in infants (see Chapter 16), with recurrent pancreatitis and meconium ileus equivalent occurring in older patients. Pulmonary symptoms include recurrent infections and chronic cough.

The CXR changes include overinflated lungs with thickening of bronchial walls and dilated bronchi

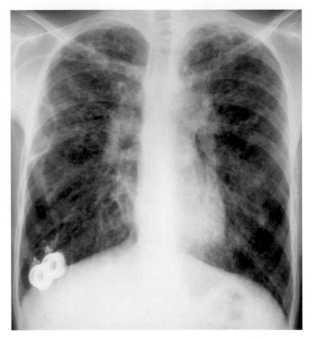

Fig. 4.14 *Cystic fibrosis. The lungs are overexpanded with extensive linear densities owing to bronchial wall thickening and mucous plugs. A right-sided central venous catheter is also present.*

(Fig. 4.14). Localized areas of collapse and finger-like opacities caused by mucoid impaction in dilated bronchi may occur. There is a high incidence of pneumonia-producing focal areas of consolidation. Pulmonary arterial hypertension may produce large pulmonary arteries.

Cardiovascular system

With advances in computed tomography (CT) and magnetic resonance imaging (MRI), imaging of the heart and blood vessels is undergoing a major revolution. This chapter begins with an overview of current cardiac imaging, with the current roles of various imaging modalities outlined. This section is followed by discussion of imaging investigation of the more common diseases of arteries and veins, including aortic dissection, abdominal aortic aneurysm, peripheral vascular disease, pulmonary embolism and deep venous thrombosis, venous insufficiency and hypertension. The chapter concludes with a brief discussion of interventional radiology of the peripheral vascular system.

IMAGING INVESTIGATION OF CARDIAC DISEASE

CHEST X-RAY

The most common use of plain films in cardiac disease is in the assessment of cardiac failure and its treatment. Plain films should be perused for cardiac position and size, specific cardiac chamber enlargement, and changes to the pulmonary vascular pattern (see Chapter 3). Cardiac valve calcification may also be visualized on chest X-ray (CXR). Calcification of the mitral valve annulus is common in elderly patients. It may be associated with mitral regurgitation. Calcification of the mitral valve leaflets may occur in rheumatic heart disease or mitral valve prolapse. Mitral valve leaflet or annulus calcification is seen on the lateral CXR inferior to a line from the carina to the anterior costophrenic angle, and on the posteroanterior (PA) CXR inferior to a line from the right cardiophrenic angle to the left hilum. Aortic valve calcification is seen on the lateral

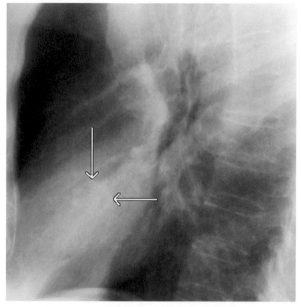

Fig. 5.1 *Aortic valve calcification. Lateral chest X-ray shows curvilinear calcification in the aortic valve (arrows) in a patient with aortic stenosis.*

CXR lying above and anterior to a line from the carina to the anterior costophrenic angle (Fig. 5.1). It is usually associated with severe aortic stenosis.

ECHOCARDIOGRAPHY

Echocardiography is a highly sophisticated and accurate tool for investigation of a wide range of cardiac disorders. Direct visualization of cardiac anatomy is accompanied by Doppler analysis of flow rates through valves and septal defects. Colour Doppler helps in the identification of septal defects and quantification of gradients across stenotic valves. In difficult cases, echocardiography may be further enhanced by the injection of ultrasound (US) contrast agents. A common application of this is to visualize small intracardiac shunts such as atrial septal defect.

A significant limitation of echocardiography is the difficulty of imaging through the anterior chest wall. This is particularly true in large patients and in patients with emphysema in whom the heart may be largely obscured by overexpanded lung. These problems have been overcome with the use of transoesophageal probes, giving transoesophageal echocardiography (TEE). The most useful applications of TEE include acute aortic dissection, endocarditis, and congenital heart disease and paraprosthetic leaks.

Indications for echocardiography include:

- Quantification of cardiac function:
    - (i) Systolic function: measurement of ejection fraction;
    - (ii) Quantification of stroke volume and cardiac output;
    - (iii) Measurement of chamber volumes and wall thicknesses;
    - (iv) Diastolic function: measurement of left ventricular 'relaxation'.
- Congenital heart disease.
- Diagnosis and quantification of valvular dysfunction.
- Stress echocardiography: diagnosis of regional wall motion abnormalities induced by exercise as a sign of coronary artery disease.
- Miscellaneous: cardiac masses, pericardial effusion, aortic dissection (TEE).

SCINTIGRAPHY

Myocardial perfusion and viability

Myocardial perfusion scintigraphy is performed with thallium-201 (^{201}Tl), ^{99m}Tc-sestamibi, or ^{99m}Tc-tetrofosmin. Fluorodeoxyglucose positron-emission tomography (FDG-PET) may also be used to assess myocardial viability. Indications for myocardial perfusion imaging include:

- Acute chest pain with normal or inconclusive electrocardiogram (ECG).
- Abnormal stress ECG in patients at low or intermediate risk of coronary artery disease (high-risk patients should have coronary angiography).

- To determine haemodynamic significance of coronary artery disease.
- To assess cardiac risk prior to major surgery.

Multiple gated acquisition scan

Multiple gated acquisition (MUGA) scan, also known as gated blood pool imaging, is performed with ^{99m}Tc-labelled red blood cells. It is used to quantify cardiac systolic function by calculation of ejection fraction and may also provide information about areas of myocardial infarction by regional wall motion analysis. The MUGA scan has been largely replaced by echocardiography.

CORONARY ANGIOGRAPHY

Coronary angiography is performed by placement of preshaped catheters into the origins of the coronary arteries and injection of contrast material. Catheters are inserted via femoral artery puncture or, less commonly, via the brachial artery. Coronary angiography is the investigation of choice for diagnosis and quantification of coronary stenosis. It is combined with therapeutic interventions including angioplasty and stent deployment. The limitations of coronary angiography are discussed below.

COMPUTED TOMOGRAPHY

Modern 16- and 64-slice scanners are able to image the heart, including the performance of CT coronary angiography (Fig. 5.2). The current roles of cardiac CT include:

- Calculation of coronary artery calcium score.
- CT angiography (CTA) of coronary arteries in patients at intermediate risk for coronary artery disease (see below).
- CTA for assessment of coronary artery bypass grafts and stent patency.
- Mapping of the anatomy of the left atrium and pulmonary veins prior to radiofrequency catheter ablation for atrial fibrillation.

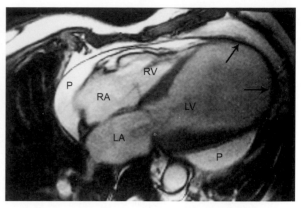

Fig. 5.3 *Left-ventricular aneurysm: transverse magnetic resonance imaging scan showing a 'four-chamber' view of the heart. Note the following structures: right atrium (RA), right ventricle (RV), left atrium (LA), left ventricle (LV) and pericardial effusion (P). The apex of the left ventricle has a markedly thinned wall and is dilated (arrows).*

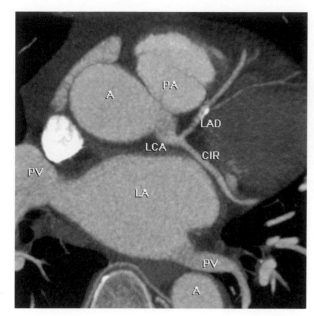

Fig. 5.2 *Computed tomography angiogram of the coronary arteries. Note the following structures: aorta (A), pulmonary artery (PA), pulmonary veins (PV), left atrium (LA), left coronary artery (LCA), left anterior descending artery (LAD) and circumflex artery (CIR).*

MAGNETIC RESONANCE IMAGING

Technical advances in MRI have led to increased application of this modality in the investigation of cardiac disease. The term 'cardiac MR' (CMR) is used widely. The obvious advantages of MRI include: no ionizing radiation, no iodinated contrast media, good soft-tissue differentiation, multiplanar imaging and no interference from bone or air. Disadvantages include: relatively long scan times, general anaesthetic required for infants and young children, and various contraindications including cardiac pacemakers.

Current applications of CMR include:
• Cardiac function: calculation of ejection fraction, myocardial mass, and regional wall motion where echocardiography is difficult or equivocal.
• Congenital heart disease: complementary to echocardiography.
• Cardiac anatomy: cardiomyopathy, left-ventricular aneurysm (Fig. 5.3), etc., where echocardiography is difficult or equivocal.

• Myocardial viability: increasing role; may replace scintigraphy in the future.
• Infarct scan: contrast material accumulates in infarcted myocardium, allowing direct visualization on a delayed scan.
• Great vessel disease: aortic dissection, coarctation.
• Miscellaneous: cardiac masses; pericardial disease.

CONGESTIVE HEART FAILURE

Dyspnoea may have a variety of causes including cardiac and respiratory diseases as well as anaemia and anxiety states. Certain features in the history may be helpful, such as whether dyspnoea is acute or chronic, worse at night, or accentuated by lying down (orthopnoea). Initial tests include full blood count, ECG and CXR followed by pulmonary function tests where a respiratory cause such as emphysema or asthma is suspected.

Congestive heart failure is the commonest cardiac cause of dyspnoea. It may be caused by systolic or diastolic dysfunction, or a combination of the two. Systolic dysfunction may be thought of as failure of ventricular contraction, while diastolic dysfunction refers to failure of ventricular relaxation between contractions. With systolic dysfunction the amount of blood pumped out of

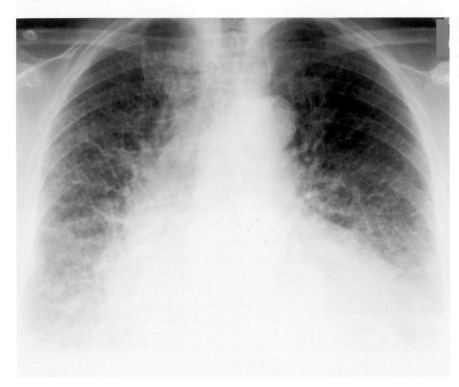

Fig. 5.4 *Acute cardiac failure: cardiac enlargement, interstitial and alveolar oedema, bilateral pleural effusions.*

the ventricles in systole is reduced. In diastolic dysfunction there is failure of relaxation of the ventricular walls, leading to reduced filling of the ventricular chambers. The commonest underlying cause of cardiac failure is ischaemic heart disease. Other causes include valvular heart disease, hypertension, hypertrophic cardiomyopathy, infiltrative disorders, such as amyloidosis, pericardial effusion or thickening, or congenital heart disease.

Imaging is performed to confirm that congestive cardiac failure is the cause of dyspnoea, to quantify and classify cardiac dysfunction, and to search for underlying causes. Chest X-ray and echocardiography are the usual imaging tests employed for the assessment of congestive heart failure.

CHEST X-RAY

The CXR signs of cardiac failure include cardiac enlargement, pulmonary vascular redistribution, and pulmonary oedema (Fig. 5.4).
- Cardiac enlargement:
  - (i) Cardiothoracic ratio is unreliable as a one-off measurement;
  - (ii) Of more significance is an increase in heart size on serial CXRs, or a transverse diameter of greater than 15.5 cm in adult males or 14.5 cm in adult females.
- Pulmonary vascular redistribution: upper lobe blood vessels larger than those in the lower lobes (see Fig. 3.5, page 37).
- Interstitial oedema: reticular (linear) pattern with Kerley B lines (see Fig. 3.18, page 47).
- Alveolar oedema: fluffy, ill-defined areas of alveolar opacity in a bilateral central or 'bat wing' distribution.
- Pleural effusions: the pleural effusions associated with congestive heart failure tend to be larger on the right.

ECHOCARDIOGRAPHY

Echocardiography may be used to calculate cardiac chamber size and wall thickness, and to diagnose the presence of valvular dysfunction and pericardial effusion. Systolic dysfunction may be diagnosed and quantified by calculation of left-ventricular ejection fraction.

Ejection fraction is a measurement of the amount of blood ejected from the left ventricle with systolic contraction. To calculate ejection fraction, the maximum cross-sectional area of the left ventricle is calculated at the end of diastole (D) and then at the end of systole (S). Ejection fraction, expressed as a percentage is calculated by the formula $D - S/D \times 100$. Normal values for ejection fraction are 70 ± 7 per cent for males and 65 ± 10 per cent for females. Other measurements such as stroke volume and cardiac output may also be calculated with echocardiography. Somewhat more complex measurements may also be done to assess diastolic dysfunction.

ISCHAEMIC HEART DISEASE

OVERVIEW OF CORONARY ARTERY DISEASE

Coronary artery disease (CAD) is the leading cause of death worldwide. The rates of mortality and disability due to CAD are increasing in industrialized and developing countries. This is a diffuse disease of the coronary arteries characterized by atheromatous plaques. Plaques may cause stenosis of coronary arteries, producing limitation of blood flow to the myocardium. It is also well recognized, however, that the external membranes of coronary arteries can expand in the presence of atherosclerotic plaque. As such, significant coronary atherosclerosis may be present without narrowing of the vessel lumen.

Rupture of atherosclerotic plaques with subsequent arterial thrombosis leads to acute cardiac events (acute cardiac syndrome) such as unstable angina, myocardial infarction and sudden death. Instability and rupture of atherosclerotic plaque is mediated by inflammatory factors, and may occur with stenosing or non-stenosing plaque. Coronary artery disease with multiple arterial stenoses may present clinically with chronic cardiac disease, most commonly cardiac failure. This is caused by pump failure due to ischaemic myocardium. This may be accompanied by chronic stable angina.

The roles of imaging in CAD include:
- Screening for CAD.
- Diagnosis and quantification of CAD in acute cardiac events.
- Planning of revascularization procedures, including coronary artery bypass graft, and interventional procedures, such as angioplasty and coronary artery stent placement.
- Assessment of myocardial viability.
- Assessment of cardiac function.

SCREENING FOR CORONARY ARTERY DISEASE

The traditional approach to prevention of CAD has been identification and reduction of risk factors such as hypertension, tobacco smoking, lack of physical activity, obesity, diabetes and dyslipidaemias. Despite this, over half of acute clinical events are not explained by these well-known risk factors. Furthermore, a large percentage of patients with high risk factors will not suffer a cardiac event. Coronary angiography has been the standard method for assessing CAD. The major limitation of coronary angiography is that it only provides an image of the vessel lumen. Therefore, only atherosclerotic plaques that cause significant narrowing of the lumen of the artery are diagnosed with coronary angiography.

Screening tests may be performed to identify clinically silent CAD, to calculate the risk of future acute cardiac events and to identify those patients that may benefit from revascularization procedures. These screening tests are designed to detect abnormalities such as ECG changes or regional ventricular wall motion abnormalities in response to exercise or pharmacologically induced myocardial stress. Methods of exercise stress testing include:
- Stress ECG: ST segment depression induced by exercise.
- Stress echocardiogram: segmental wall motion abnormalities induced by exercise.
- Myocardial perfusion scintigraphy with ^{201}Tl or ^{99m}Tc-sestamibi.

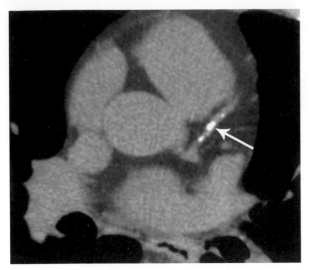

Fig. 5.5 *Computed tomography coronary calcium scoring. Note calcification in the left anterior descending artery (arrow) in a man with atherosclerosis of the coronary arteries.*

An abnormal exercise test has a high predictive value for the presence of obstructive CAD.

Another method of screening for the presence of CAD is coronary calcium detection and scoring by CT. Multidetector row CT is highly sensitive to the presence of coronary artery calcification (Fig. 5.5). The amount of coronary artery calcification increases with the overall burden of coronary atherosclerotic disease. Computer software programs are able to provide a coronary calcium score that represents a reasonable measure of the amount of atherosclerotic plaque. Calcium scores adjusted for age and gender, in combination with other known risk factors, can help to predict the risk of future cardiac events, though precise correlation is yet to be established. A calcium score of zero is a strong indicator of a very low risk of subsequent cardiac events. Calcium scoring may also be useful for monitoring CAD in patients undergoing interventions for risk factor reduction.

Computed tomography coronary angiography has a developing role in the diagnosis of CAD; 16- and 64-multislice CT scanners allow accurate depiction of the coronary arteries. As well as imaging the vessel lumen, CT is able to image non-stenotic plaque in the vessel wall. Current research is directed at characterizing plaque based on measurement of CT density; this may further increase the accuracy of risk assessment with this technique.

ACUTE CHEST PAIN

As outlined above, sudden rupture of an atherosclerotic plaque with subsequent arterial thrombosis and occlusion may lead to acute cardiac events such as sudden death, myocardial infarction, and acute unstable angina. The classical symptoms of acute angina are chest pain and tightness radiating to the left arm. Other causes of acute chest pain include aortic dissection, pulmonary embolism, gastro-oesophageal reflux, muscle spasm, and a variety of respiratory causes. Initial workup for a cardiac cause includes ECG and serum markers such as CK-MB (creatine kinase isoenzyme MB) and cardiac treponins. Initial imaging assessment in the acute situation consists of a CXR to look for evidence of cardiac failure and to diagnose a non-cardiac cause of chest pain such as pneumonia or pneumothorax. This will be followed by coronary angiography, as well as interventional procedures aimed at restoring coronary blood flow. These include coronary artery angioplasty and stent deployment.

MYOCARDIAL VIABILITY AND CARDIAC FUNCTION

Further imaging in the setting of CAD and ischaemic heart disease consists of tests of myocardial viability, including thallium scintigraphy to assess the amount of viable versus non-viable myocardium, and echocardiography to quantify cardiac function.

The thallium exercise test is used to differentiate viable from non-viable myocardium and hence identify those patients who would benefit from coronary revascularization procedures such as angioplasty or bypass graft. Myocardial perfusion scintigraphy is performed with ^{201}Tl or ^{99m}Tc-sestamibi. Fluorodeoxyglucose-PET may also be used to assess myocardial viability. Following injection of radiopharmaceutical, the heart is put under stress through exercise or with various pharmacological agents such as dobutamine or dipyridamole. Images are

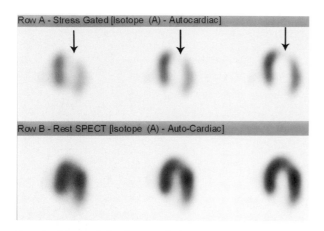

Row A - Stress Gated [Isotope (A) - Autocardiac]

Row B - Rest SPECT [Isotope (A) - Auto-Cardiac]

Fig. 5.6 *Myocardial ischaemia: thallium scintigraphy. The top three images are of the left ventricle after exercise and below these are corresponding images after a rest period. Note the presence of a region of reduced myocardial uptake of thallium with exercise (arrows). There is normal distribution of activity at rest indicating reversible ischaemia rather than established infarction.*

acquired with the heart under stress and then repeated after a period of rest. Areas of ischaemia or infarction show as areas of decreased or no uptake, i.e. 'cold' spots. Reversible ischaemia is seen as a 'cold' spot on exercise that returns to normal after 4 hours of rest (Fig. 5.6). An infarct is seen as a 'cold' spot on exercise unchanged after 4 hours of rest.

Echocardiography is a more accurate non-invasive method for the quantification of left ventricular ejection fraction. It will also diagnose complications of myocardial infarction such as papillary muscle rupture, ventricular septal defect, left-ventricular aneurysm and pericardial effusion.

Increasingly cardiac MRI is being used to assess myocardial viability and cardiac function in patients with CAD. Cardiac MR is able to provide a quantitative assessment of ventricular wall motion and assess myocardial perfusion, at rest and with pharmacologically induced stress.

SUMMARY OF IMAGING IN CORONARY ARTERY DISEASE

The Framingham risk score is a well-recognized tool used to provide a global risk assessment for future 'hard'

cardiac events, including myocardial infarction and sudden death. Based on gender and age, cholesterol and HDL levels, systolic blood pressure and tobacco use, individuals are categorized as low, intermediate or high risk. Low-risk individuals have no risk factors and comprise about 35 per cent of those tested. Low-risk asymptomatic patients require no imaging. High-risk individuals have established atheromatous disease and/or multiple risk factors and comprise about 25 per cent of those tested. High-risk or symptomatic patients should be assessed with coronary catheter angiography and tests of myocardial viability. The choice of the particular test will hinge on a number of factors, including local expertise and availability, as well as the individual circumstances of the patient. Intermediate risk individuals comprise about 40 per cent of those tested and include those with one or more risk factor outside the normal range or a positive family history of CAD. Intermediate risk individuals will increasingly be assessed by non-invasive means, including stress tests and CTA. Computed tomography angiography is less invasive than coronary catheterization and is able to detect most haemodynamically significant plaques. Perhaps most importantly, CTA of the coronary arteries has a very high negative predictive value. As such, it may be able to reduce the number of normal or negative catheter studies.

AORTIC DISSECTION

Aortic dissection occurs when a tear in the surface of the intima allows flow of blood into the aortic wall. This creates a false lumen with re-entry of blood into the true lumen more distally. Dissection may involve the aorta alone or may cause occlusion of major arterial branches. Aortic dissection usually presents with acute chest pain, often described as a 'tearing' sensation. The pain may be anterior, or posterior between the scapulae. It may radiate more distally as the dissection progresses. Aortic dissections are classified by the Stanford system into type A and B. Type A refers to all dissections involving the ascending aorta, with the

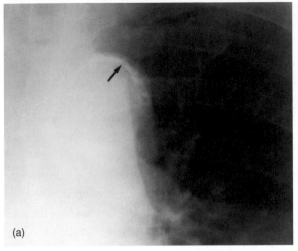 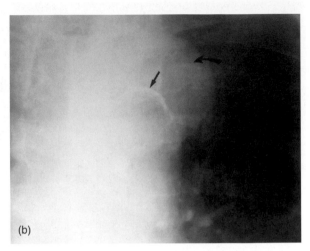

(a)　　　　　　　　　　　　　　　　　　(b)

Fig. 5.7 *Aortic dissection on chest X-ray (CXR). (a) A CXR obtained fortuitously about 10 days prior to dissection shows curvilinear intimal calcification in the aortic arch (arrow). (b) At the time of dissection the intimal calcification (straight arrow) is displaced centrally by blood in the wall of the aorta (curved arrow).*

re-entry site anywhere distally down to and sometimes beyond the aortic bifurcation. Type B dissections are confined to the descending aorta distal to the origin of the left subclavian artery.

A CXR is performed in the initial assessment of the patient with chest pain. In the context of suspected aortic dissection, CXR is mainly to exclude other causes of chest pain before more definitive investigation. Most of the CXR signs that may be seen with aortic dissection such as pleural effusion are non-specific and may be seen in a range of other conditions. Alterations to the contour of the aortic arch and displacement of intimal calcification may be more specific but are only occasionally seen, and even then with some difficulty (Fig. 5.7).

Computed tomography of the chest including CTA of the aorta is the investigation of choice for suspected aortic dissection (Fig. 5.8). The roles of CT in the evaluation of suspected aortic dissection are:

- To confirm the diagnosis.
- Classify the dissection as type A or B.
- Identify involvement of arterial branches, including the coronary arteries.
- Delineation of bleeding: mediastinal haematoma, pleural or pericardial effusion.

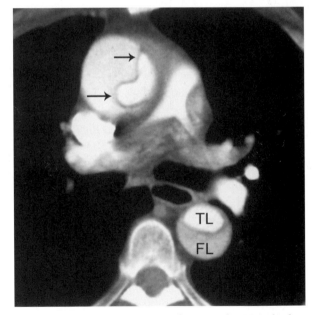

Fig. 5.8 *Aortic dissection: computed tomography. Note the thin intimal flap in the ascending aorta (arrows). In the descending aorta the flap is seen separating the true lumen (TL) from the false lumen (FL).*

Depending on local availability and expertise, TEE or MRI may be used to confirm the diagnosis in difficult or equivocal cases. The TEE must be performed and interpreted by experienced operators. As well as

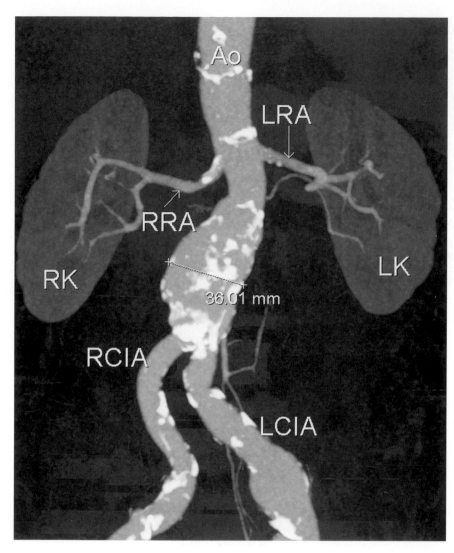

Fig. 5.9 *Abdominal aortic aneurysm: CT. A reconstructed image from a CT angiogram shows the following structures: aorta (Ao), left and right renal arteries (LRA, RRA), left and right kidneys (LK, RK), left and right common iliac arteries (LCIA, RCIA).*

the dissection, TEE will diagnose complications such as aortic insufficiency and pericardial fluid. Angiography may be required for better definition prior to surgery, although less so with the advent of TEE and MRI.

ABDOMINAL AORTIC ANEURYSM

Abdominal aortic aneurysm (AAA) may present clinically as a pulsatile abdominal mass or less commonly with leakage causing acute abdominal pain. It may also be seen as an incidental finding on abdomen X-ray (AXR) or X-ray of the lumbar spine. Plain-film signs of AAA

may include a soft-tissue mass with curvilinear calcification (see Fig. 6.3, page 94).

Computed tomography is the investigation of first choice for measurement, definition of anatomy and diagnosis of complications such as leakage. Multislice CT with multiplanar and three-dimensional (3D) reconstructions is particularly useful for AAA assessment as the whole of the aorta may be scanned during peak contrast enhancement giving excellent definition. Precise CT measurements of aneurysm diameter, length and distance from renal arteries are essential to planning of treatment with percutaneous stent placement (Fig. 5.9). Leakage of AAA may be seen on CT as soft tissue surrounding the aneurysm (Fig. 5.10).

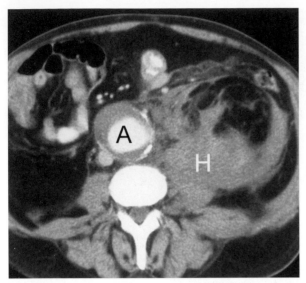

Fig. 5.10 *Leaking abdominal aortic aneurysm: computed tomography (CT). This was obtained in a patient with acute onset of abdominal pain and shows an aortic aneurysm (A) and a large left retroperitoneal haematoma (H).*

Computed tomography may also be performed after stent deployment or surgical repair for diagnosis of problems such as infection, blockage and leakage, or less common complications such as aortoduodenal fistula and retroperitoneal fibrosis.

Ultrasound may be used where CT is unavailable or for follow-up measurement of a known asymptomatic aneurysm.

PERIPHERAL VASCULAR DISEASE

The commonest clinical presentation of the patient with peripheral vascular disease is claudication. Claudication is characterized by muscle pain and weakness reproducibly produced by a set amount of exercise and relieved by rest. Patients with severe arterial disease may have pain at rest or tissue changes such as ischaemic ulcers and gangrene. Non-arterial causes of claudication such as spinal stenosis and chronic venous occlusion may be seen in 25 per cent of cases. The presence of peripheral vascular disease in patients with claudication may be confirmed with noninvasive physiological tests.

These tests include ankle–brachial index (ABI), pulse volume recordings and segmental pressures including measurements performed at rest and following exercise. The presence of a normal ABI at rest and following exercise usually excludes significant peripheral arterial disease and in such cases no further arterial imaging is required.

The noninvasive vascular laboratory combines physiological tests with Doppler US imaging to determine those patients requiring angiography and possible further treatment (either surgery or interventional radiology). Signs of arterial stenosis on Doppler US include visible narrowing of the artery seen on two-dimensional (2D) US and colour images associated with a focal zone of increased flow velocity and an altered arterial wave pattern distally. Doppler US is particularly useful to differentiate focal stenosis from diffuse disease and occlusion. Other arterial abnormalities such as aneurysm, pseudoaneurysm and arteriovenous malformation (AVM) are well seen and Doppler US is also useful for postoperative graft surveillance.

Therapy is required if physiological testing with or without Doppler US reveals the presence of significant peripheral arterial disease in a patient with claudication. In these cases a complete accurate assessment of the arterial system from the aorta to the foot arteries is required. This may consist of catheter angiography, though is being increasingly performed with CTA and MR angiography (MRA).

CATHETER ANGIOGRAPHY

Catheter angiography refers to the placement of selective arterial catheters and injection of contrast material to outline arterial anatomy. Most catheters are placed via femoral artery puncture and less commonly via the brachial or axillary artery. Catheter insertion is performed by the Seldinger technique as follows:

• The artery is punctured with a needle;
• A wire is threaded through the needle into the artery;
• The needle is removed leaving the wire in the artery;
• A catheter is inserted over the wire into the artery.

Various preshaped catheters are available allowing selective catheterization of most major arteries.

Post-procedure care following catheter angiography consists of bed rest for a few hours with observation of the puncture site for bleeding and swelling. The complication rate of modern angiography is very low. Most complications relate to the arterial puncture as follows:

- Haematoma at the puncture site.
- False aneurysm formation.
- Arterial dissection.
- Embolism caused by dislodgement of atheromatous plaques.

Other possible complications relate to the use of iodinated contrast material (allergy and contrast induced nephropathy: see Chapter 2).

With the increasing use of less invasive diagnostic methods such as Doppler ultrasound, CTA and MRA, catheter angiography is less commonly performed for purely diagnostic purposes. Catheter angiography is now more usually performed in association with interventional techniques such as angioplasty, arterial stent placement and thrombolysis.

COMPUTED TOMOGRAPHY ANGIOGRAPHY AND MAGNETIC RESONANCE ANGIOGRAPHY

Computed tomography angiography (CTA) and MRA are being used increasingly for planning of therapy for peripheral vascular disease. With CTA and MRA it is possible to obtain highly accurate images of the peripheral vascular system without arterial puncture. Magnetic resonance angiography generally uses sequences which show flowing blood as high signal (bright white) and stationary tissues as low signal (dark). Increasingly for peripheral studies, contrast material (gadolinium) is used to enhance blood vessels and reduce scanning times. Problems with MRA include long examination times, inability to image patients with pacemakers, and artefacts from surgical clips and metallic stents. Conversely, CTA with multidetector CT has very short examination times, uses less radiation than catheter angiography, and

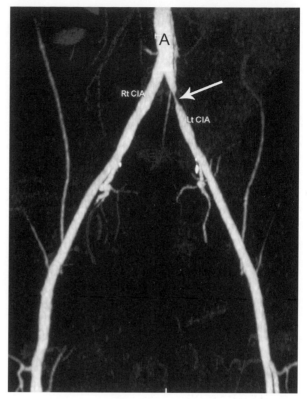

Fig. 5.11 *Stenosis of left common iliac artery (CIA) (arrow): computed tomography angiogram.*

is usually not significantly degraded by stents and surgical clips. Choice of modality to some extent is governed by local expertise and availability; however, CTA has fewer problems and is more widely used for assessment of peripheral vascular disease (Fig. 5.11).

PULMONARY EMBOLISM

Pulmonary embolism (PE) is one of the commonest preventable causes of death in hospital inpatients. It is a common cause of morbidity and mortality in postoperative patients, as well as in patients with other risk factors such as prolonged bed rest, malignancy and cardiac failure. Symptoms include pleuritic chest pain, shortness of breath, cough and haemoptysis, though a large number of pulmonary emboli are clinically silent. Clinical signs such as hypotension, tachycardia, reduced oxygen saturation and ECG changes (S1, Q3, T3) are non-specific and often absent. As such, the clinical diagnosis of pulmonary embolism is problematic and must be confirmed with imaging studies. These include CXR, CT pulmonary angiography (CTPA), ventilation/perfusion nuclear lung scan (V/Q scan), and pulmonary angiography. Pulmonary angiography with selective catheterization of the pulmonary arteries, although considered the gold standard for the imaging diagnosis of PE, is only rarely performed and then only in specialized centres. It will not be considered further.

The initial imaging investigation in all patients is CXR. Signs of PE on CXR include pleural effusion, localized area of consolidation contacting a pleural surface or a localized area of collapse. These signs are quite non-specific and the main role of CXR in this context is to diagnose other causes for the patient's symptoms such as pneumonia. A CXR may also assist in the interpretation of a V/Q scan.

COMPUTED TOMOGRAPHY PULMONARY ANGIOGRAPHY

Helical and multislice CT allow imaging of the thorax in a single breath hold and imaging of the entire pulmonary vascular bed during optimum peak contrast enhancement. Pulmonary emboli are seen on CTPA as filling defects within contrast-filled blood vessels (Fig. 5.12). Compared with scintigraphy (see below) CTPA has a very low percentage of intermediate or equivocal results. It may also help make alternative diagnoses such as pneumonia, aortic dissection, etc. In most cases, CTPA is now the investigation of choice for confirming the diagnosis of PE. The major disadvantages of CTPA are the need for intravenous injection of iodinated contrast material and radiation dose. Scintigraphy is indicated if the patient has a history of previous allergic reaction to intravenous contrast material. Scintigraphy is also indicated in young women as the absorbed radiation dose to the breasts from CTPA is quite high, increasing the risk of developing a subsequent breast cancer. Alternatively, if scintigraphy is not available or is non-diagnostic, CTPA may be performed using breast shields to reduce the breast radiation dose.

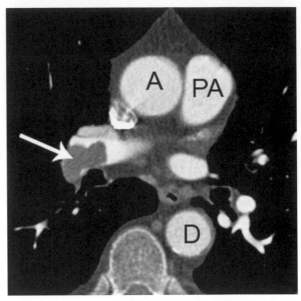

Fig. 5.12 *Pulmonary embolism: computed tomography pulmonary angiography. Pulmonary embolus seen as a low density filling defect in the right pulmonary artery (arrow). Note also ascending aorta (A), descending aorta (D) and main pulmonary artery (PA).*

SCINTIGRAPHY: V/Q SCAN

In V/Q scans, a ventilation phase is first performed with the patient breathing a ^{99m}Tc-labelled aerosol. Six images are performed using anterior, posterior and oblique projections. This is followed by the perfusion phase in which images are obtained using an intravenous injection of ^{99m}Tc-labelled macroalbumin aggregates (MAA). These aggregates have a mean diameter of 30–60 μm and are trapped in the pulmonary microvasculature on first pass through the lungs. The same six projections are performed and the perfusion phase compared with the ventilation phase. The diagnostic hallmark of PE is one or more regions of ventilation/perfusion mismatch (i.e. a region of lung where perfusion is reduced or absent and ventilation is preserved; Fig. 5.13). After correlation with an accompanying CXR, lung scans are graded as low, intermediate or high probability of PE. A high-probability scan is an accurate predictor of PE, while a low probability scan accurately excludes the diagnosis. Unfortunately, a large proportion of patients (up to

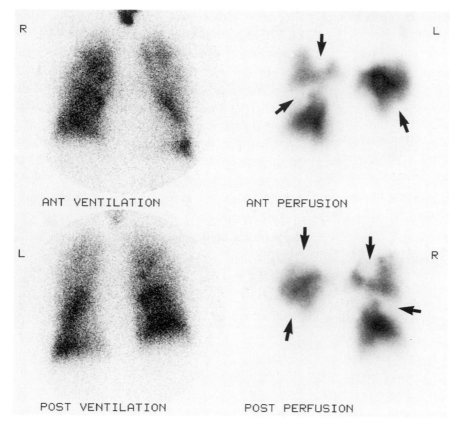

ANT VENTILATION ANT PERFUSION

POST VENTILATION POST PERFUSION

Fig. 5.13 *Pulmonary embolism: V/Q scan. Pulmonary emboli seen as defects on the perfusion phase (arrows) not matched on the ventilation phase.*

75 per cent in some series) have an intermediate probability scan.

RATIONAL USE OF IMAGING IN THE DIAGNOSIS OF PULMONARY EMBOLISM

A number of factors have contributed to the overuse of CTPA. These include:

- The wide availability of multislice CT scanners.
- The high level of accuracy of CTPA.
- The ability of CTPA to make alternative diagnoses.
- The popularization of the concept of the 'triple rule-out': contrast-enhanced CT in patients with chest pain to rule out pulmonary embolism, coronary artery disease and aortic dissection.
- Wide public awareness of PE with popular press coverage of cases of PE following long-haul air travel.

This overuse of CTPA is not only expensive but also has major implications with respect to radiation dose. The rate of negative studies can be reduced by assignment of pretest probability of pulmonary embolism in a patient presenting with suggestive history and clinical findings by the use of a logical clinical assessment system and a D-dimer assay. D-dimer is a plasma constituent present when fibrin is released from active thrombus. It has a sensitivity of over 95 per cent, though is highly non-specific. It therefore has a very high negative predictive value. The most widely used clinical model is the Simplified Wells Scoring System in which points are assigned as follows:

- Leg pain, swelling and tenderness suggestive of deep venous thrombosis (DVT): 3.0.
- Heart rate >100 beats per minute: 1.5.
- Immobilization for ⩾3 consecutive days: 1.5.
- Surgery in the previous 4 weeks: 1.5.
- Previous confirmed DVT or PE: 1.0.
- Haemoptysis: 1.0.
- Malignancy: 1.0.
- PE more likely as or more likely than alternate diagnosis: 3.0.

Pretest probability is assigned depending on the points score as follows:

- <2.0:   low.
- 2.0–6.0:   moderate.
- <6.0:   high.

The diagnosis of PE is reliably excluded if the clinical pretest probability is low and the D-dimer assay is negative. In such patients, imaging with CTPA or scintigraphy is not indicated. Imaging is indicated where the clinical pretest probability is moderate or high or where the D-dimer assay is positive.

DEEP VENOUS THROMBOSIS

Deep venous thrombosis of the leg presents clinically with local pain and tenderness accompanied by swelling. Acute provoking causes of DVT include recent hospitalization and immobilization, trauma or surgery, particularly surgery to the lower limb or major abdominal surgery. Chronic predisposing factors may also be present such as malignancy, obesity, history of previous DVT or factor V Leiden. Sequelae of DVT include pulmonary embolism, recurrent DVT and post-thrombotic syndrome, in which venous incompetence and stasis cause chronic leg pain and swelling and venous ulcers.

Doppler US is the investigation of choice for DVT. It is non-invasive and painless, relatively inexpensive and highly reliable for the assessment of the deep venous system from the lower calf to the inferior vena cava (IVC) (Fig. 5.14). Ultrasound may also detect conditions that can mimic DVT, such as ruptured Baker's cyst.

Signs of DVT on US examination include:

- Visible thrombus within the vein.
- Non-compressibility of the vein.
- Failure of venous distension with Valsalva's manoeuvre.
- Lack of normal venous Doppler signal.
- Loss of flow on colour images.

UPPER LIMB DEEP VENOUS THROMBOSIS

Upper limb DVT usually presents clinically with acute onset of upper limb swelling. It may be seen in association with central venous catheters including PICC (peripherally inserted central catheter) lines or it may be a complication of trauma. In young adult patients, especially body-builders, upper limb DVT may occur secondary to compression of the subclavian vein where it crosses the first rib. Many cases are idiopathic. The differential diagnosis of the acutely swollen arm includes lymphatic obstruction, cellulitis or a functional venous obstruction caused by compression of central veins by a mass.

Imaging diagnosis of the cause of an acutely swollen upper limb is aimed primarily at excluding upper limb DVT. Doppler US is the first investigation of choice with the signs of upper limb DVT the same as listed above for the leg. If this is negative, a contrast-enhanced CT is indicated to provide further assessment of the large central veins including the superior vena cava (SVC). Venography and thrombolysis may be indicated for acute thrombosis of the larger more central veins, such as the axillary or subclavian veins. In cases of SVC compression by tumour or lymph node mass, stent deployment may provide palliation.

VENOUS INSUFFICIENCY

For the patient with varicose veins for whom surgery is contemplated, US with Doppler is the imaging investigation of choice for assessment. The competence of a leg vein, deep or superficial, is determined with Doppler US using calf compression and release. A competent vein will show no or minor reflux (reversal of flow) on release of calf compression. Incompetence is defined as reflux of greater than 0.5 s duration. The following information may be obtained with Doppler US:

- Patency and competence of the deep venous system from the common femoral vein to the lower calf.
- Competence and diameter of saphenofemoral junction.
- Competence and diameter of long saphenous vein.
- Duplications, tributaries and varices arising from the long saphenous vein.

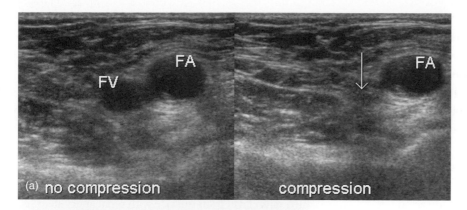

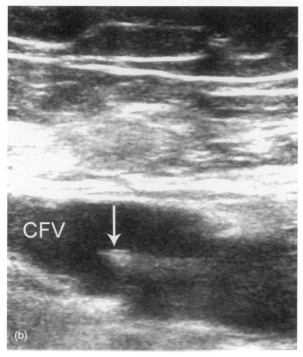

Fig. 5.14 *Deep venous thrombosis (DVT): duplex ultrasound (US). (a) Normal deep veins: duplex US. The US images obtained just below the inguinal ligament in the transverse plane show the common femoral artery (FA) and vein (FV). The common femoral vein can be compressed with gentle pressure (arrow), excluding the presence of DVT. (b) DVT: thrombus is seen as echogenic material (arrow) projecting into the common femoral vein (CFV).*

- Competence and diameter of the saphenopopliteal junction.
- Document location of saphenopopliteal junction.
- Anatomical variants of the saphenopopliteal junction.
- Course and connections of superficial varicose veins.
- Incompetent perforator veins connecting deep system with superficial system and their position in relation to anatomical landmarks such as groin crease, knee crease and medial malleolus.

To assist further with surgical planning marks may be placed on the skin over incompetent perforating veins preoperatively. For clarity, a diagram of the venous system based on the US examination is usually provided.

HYPERTENSION

The vast majority of hypertensive patients have essential hypertension. The clinical challenge is to identify the small percentage of patients with secondary hypertension and to delineate any treatable lesions. All hypertensive patients should have a CXR for the diagnosis of cardiovascular complications (cardiac enlargement, aortic valve calcification or cardiac failure) and to establish a baseline for monitoring of future changes or complications such as aortic dissection. Further imaging investigation of hypertension is indicated in the following:

- Children and young adults less than 40 years old.
- Hypertension that is severe or malignant in nature.
- Failure of antihypertensive medication.
- Certain clinical signs such as a bruit heard over the renal arteries or clinical evidence of endocrine disorders.

The more common causes of secondary hypertension include renal artery stenosis, chronic renal failure and endocrine disorders such as phaeochromocytoma, Conn syndrome (primary hyperaldosteronism) and Cushing syndrome. For notes on imaging of adrenal gland disorders please see Chapter 9.

Initial screening for renal artery stenosis may be performed with Doppler US or scintigraphy. Doppler US is non-invasive with no radiation required and should be the initial investigation of choice where local expertise is available. Renal artery stenosis is indicated by an increase in blood flow velocity. A major limitation of US is the difficulty of imaging renal arteries because of overlying bowel gas and obesity. Scintigraphy with ^{99m}Tc-DTPA (diethylenetriamine pentaacetic acid) may be used where US is technically inadequate. The use of an angiotensin-converting enzyme (ACE) inhibitor such as intravenous captopril increases the accuracy of the study. Renal artery stenosis is indicated by reduced perfusion and delayed function on the affected side. Computed tomography angiography or MRA may be used for further relatively non-invasive imaging where the above screening tests are equivocal.

Where the screening tests are positive, renal angiography and interventional radiology are indicated. Most patients with renal artery stenosis are treated with interventional radiology. This consists of renal artery percutaneous transluminal angioplasty (PTA) and stent insertion. The goals of treatment with interventional radiology are: normal blood pressure, or hypertension that can be controlled medically, plus improved renal function.

In some specialist centres, renal vein renin assays may be performed prior to treatment of renal artery stenosis. In this technique, catheters are inserted through the femoral vein and positioned in the renal veins. Blood samples are taken from each renal vein to assess renin levels, with a positive study indicated by a relatively high renin level from the side with renal artery stenosis. A positive renal vein renin assay indicates a favourable outcome from surgery or interventional radiology.

INTERVENTIONAL RADIOLOGY OF THE PERIPHERAL VASCULAR SYSTEM

VENOUS ACCESS

Indications for access to the central venous system include chemotherapy, antibiotic therapy, hyperalimentation, and haemodialysis. Various radiologically guided methods of venous access are used. The type of access depends largely on the period of time that access is required. The most commonly used devices are:

- Percutaneously inserted central venous catheters (PICC lines).
- Tunnelled catheters.
- Implanted ports.

These techniques use a combination of US and fluoroscopic guidance. Ultrasound is used to obtain initial venous access. It is able to localize the vein, confirm its patency and diagnose relevant variants, such as the internal jugular vein lying medial to the internal carotid artery. Fluoroscopic guidance is used to confirm the final position of the catheter. In general, a central venous catheter should be positioned with its tip at the junction of the SVC and right atrium. PICC lines are usually inserted with local anaesthetic; the other methods usually require sedation and in some cases including children, general anaesthetic. All venous access techniques must be performed with strict sterility.

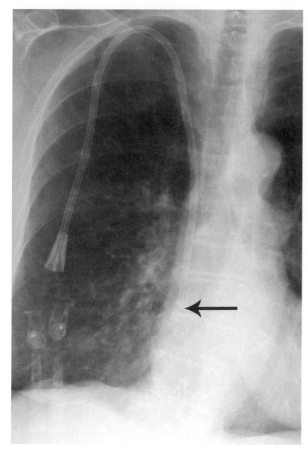

Fig. 5.15 *Tunnelled central venous port. The tip of the catheter is well positioned at the junction of the superior vena cava and right atrium (arrow).*

PICC lines are used for short to intermediate term central venous access. They are inserted via a peripheral arm vein. PICC lines may be inserted without imaging guidance via the median cubital vein, which is palpable at the elbow. The main disadvantage of this technique is that the elbow cannot be flexed, limiting use of the arm. With US guidance PICC lines may be inserted above the elbow into the basilic or brachial vein. Patients generally prefer this method as they are able to use their arm.

Tunnelled catheters are used for intermediate term access (Fig. 5.15). The internal jugular vein is usually the preferred route for insertion. A subcutaneous tunnel is made with blunt dissection from a skin incision in the upper chest wall to the venous access site. The venous catheter is pulled through this subcutaneous tunnel with a tunnelling device and inserted into the internal jugular vein. The catheter is held at the skin insertion site with a purse-string suture.

Implantation ports are used for longer term (3 months or more) intermittent access. They are particularly suitable for cyclical chemotherapy. Access ports are made of steel, titanium or plastic. A subcutaneous pocket is fashioned in the chest wall for the port. Venous access is via the internal jugular or subclavian vein. After placement, the skin is sutured over the port.

Complications of venous access may include the following:

- Infection (rate of infection expressed as the number of infections per 10 000 catheter days):
    - (i) PICC lines: 4–11;
    - (ii) Tunnelled catheters: 14;
    - (iii) Implantation ports: 6.
- Catheter blockage caused by thrombosis and fibrin sheath formation: 3–10 per cent.
- Venous thrombosis (upper limb DVT): 1–2 per cent.
- Other complications such as catheter malposition and kinking are rare with careful placement.

PERCUTANEOUS TRANSLUMINAL ANGIOPLASTY

The usual indication for PTA is a short-segment arterial stenosis with associated clinical evidence of limb ischaemia. It is performed via arterial puncture. Depending on the location of the stenosis the femoral, brachial, axillary or popliteal arteries may be punctured. A wire is passed across the arterial stenosis. A balloon catheter is passed over the wire and the balloon dilated to expand the stenosed arterial segment. Pressure readings proximal and distal to the stenosis pre- and post-dilatation may be performed. A post-dilatation angiogram is also performed to assess the result (Fig. 5.16). Post-procedure care consists of haemostasis and bed rest as for angiography. Patients may be maintained on low-dose aspirin or heparin following a complicated procedure. Complications are

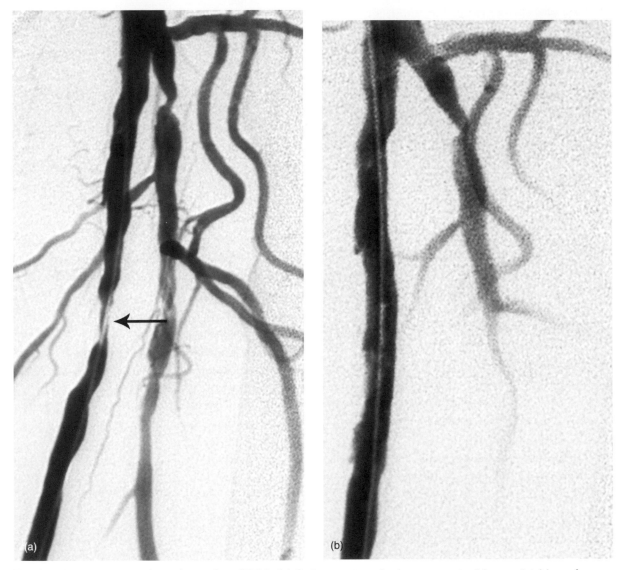

Fig. 5.16 *Percutaneous transluminal angioplasty (PTA). (a) Catheter angiography shows a stenosis of the superficial femoral artery in the upper thigh (arrow). (b) Following PTA the stenosis is no longer seen.*

uncommon and include arterial occlusion, arterial rupture and haemorrhage, and distal embolization.

ARTERIAL STENT PLACEMENT

Arterial stents are of two types: balloon-expandable (Palmaz) and self-expanding (Wallstent). Self-expanding stents consist of stainless steel spring filaments woven into a flexible self-expanding band. Both types of stent are deployed via arterial puncture. With improvements in design and ease of deployment, arterial stents are commonly used by interventional radiologists in the management of stenotic and occlusive arterial disease.

Particular indications for stent deployment include:

- Severe or heavily calcified iliac artery stenosis/occlusion.
- Acute failure of PTA caused by recoil of the vessel wall.
- PTA complicated by arterial dissection.
- Late failure of PTA caused by recurrent stenosis.

THROMBOLYSIS

Indications for thrombolysis include:

- Acute, or acute on chronic arterial ischaemia.
- Arterial thrombosis complicating PTA.
- Surgical graft thrombosis.
- Acute upper limb DVT.

Thrombolysis is performed via arterial puncture or venous puncture for upper limb DVT. A catheter is positioned in or just proximal to the thrombosis followed by infusion of a thrombolytic agent such as urokinase or tissue plasminogen activator (tPA). Regular follow-up angiograms or venograms are performed to ensure dissolution of thrombus with repositioning of the catheter as required. A PTA or arterial stent deployment may be performed for any underlying stenosis. The patient is maintained on anticoagulation following successful thrombolysis.

Contraindications to thrombolysis include bleeding diathesis, active or recent bleeding from any source, and recent surgery, pregnancy, or significant trauma. Complications of thrombolysis may include haematoma formation at the arterial puncture site, distal embolization of partly lysed thrombus and systemic bleeding, including cerebral haemorrhage, haematuria and epistaxis.

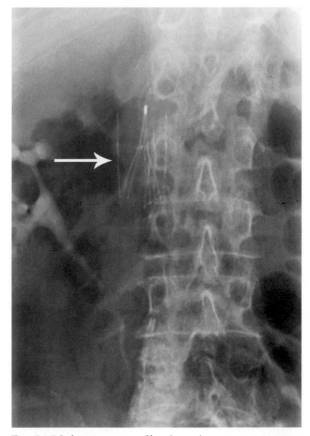

Fig. 5.17 *Inferior vena cava filter (arrow).*

INFERIOR VENA CAVA FILTRATION

In certain situations, self-expanding metal filters may be deployed in the IVC to prevent pulmonary embolus (Fig. 5.17). The technique of IVC filter insertion consists of venous puncture, either common femoral or internal jugular vein. An inferior cavogram is performed to check IVC patency, exclude anatomical anomalies, measure IVC diameter and document the position of the renal veins. The filter is then deployed via a catheter.

Indications for IVC filtration include:

- PE or DVT, where anticoagulation therapy is contraindicated.
- Recurrent PE despite anticoagulation.
- During surgery in high-risk patients.

Permanent or removable filters may be used. Removable filters are particularly useful in younger patients who

may be at risk of PE for a short time-period, such as during recovery from surgery.

Complications of IVC filtration are rare and may include femoral vein or IVC thrombosis, perforation of the IVC and filter migration.

VASCULAR EMBOLIZATION

This covers a wide range of topics and indications. Uses of vascular embolization includes:

- Control of bleeding.
  - (i) Trauma: penetrating injuries; pelvic trauma;
  - (ii) Arteriovenous malformations and aneurysms;
  - (iii) Severe epistaxis.
- Management of tumour.
  - (i) Palliative: embolic agents labelled with cytotoxic agents, radioactive isotopes or monoclonal antibodies;

(ii) Definitive treatment for tumours of vascular origin, e.g. aneurysmal bone cyst;

(iii) Preoperative to decrease vascularity or deliver chemotherapy.

- Systemic arteriovenous malformation: definitive treatment, preoperative, palliative.

For vascular embolization the embolic material is delivered through an arterial catheter. This could be either a standard diagnostic angiographic catheter or one of a number of specialized catheters now available. These include microcatheters, which can be coaxially placed through a larger guiding catheter to gain far more distal access in small arteries. Embolic materials include:

- Metal coils with or without thrombogenic fibres attached.
- Particles such as polyvinyl alcohol particles.
- Glue: superglue acrylates.

- Detachable balloons: latex or silicon.
- Gelfoam pledgets.
- Chemotherapeutic agents.
- Absolute alcohol.

The type of material used depends on the site and blood flow characteristics, whether a permanent or temporary occlusion is required and the type of catheter in use. Personal preference is also important. The procedures usually require good imaging facilities, especially digital subtraction angiography, to monitor the progress of embolization and to diagnose complications.

Complications of vascular embolization may include:

- Inadvertent embolization of normal structures.
- Pain.
- Postembolization syndrome: fever, malaise, and leukocytosis 3–5 days post-embolization.

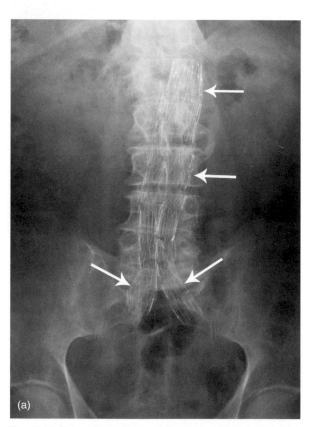

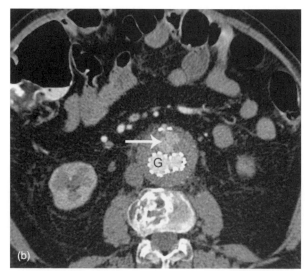

Fig. 5.18 *Covered stent (arrows) for aortic aneurysm. (a) Abdomen X-ray shows the position of the stent graft (arrows). (b) Computed tomography with intravenous contrast injection shows the stent graft (G) within the aortic aneurysm. Note the presence of contrast enhancement in the aneurysm sac anterior to the graft indicating an endoleak (arrow).*

ENDOVASCULAR ABDOMINAL AORTIC ANEURYSM REPAIR

Endoluminal devices consisting of combining metallic stents with graft material may be used to treat aneurysms of the abdominal aorta. These devices are inserted percutaneously via an endovascular approach, removing the need for open surgery. Two types are available, these being stented grafts and covered stents. Stented grafts consist of grafts attached to the internal wall of the aorta by proximal and distal stents. Covered stents consist of graft material stented throughout its entire length. These are used more commonly and consist of an inverted 'Y'-shaped graft with the lower limbs of the 'Y' projecting into the common iliac arteries (Fig. 5.18(a)). The aim of endovascular AAA repair is to prevent aneurysm rupture by excluding the aneurysm sac from blood flow and arterial pressure. Complications of endovascular AAA repair include graft migration, kinking and distortion, and endoleak. Endoleak refers to blood flow in the aneurysm sac outside the graft. Post-procedure imaging consists of AXR to confirm graft position and structural integrity plus contrast enhanced CT to exclude endoleak (Fig. 5.18(b)).

6

How to read an abdomen X-ray

With the widespread use of ultrasound (US) and computed tomography (CT) in the imaging of abdominal disorders, the abdomen X-ray (AXR) is less commonly performed in modern practice. However, the AXR is still an important initial investigation for a number of disorders. It is important for the student to be able to recognize radiographic signs of intestinal obstruction, perforation of the gastrointestinal tract and foreign bodies resulting from penetrating injuries or ingestion (Fig. 6.1). Furthermore, it should be possible to differentiate mechanical intestinal obstruction from generalized paralytic ileus. In some cases, a specific cause of intestinal obstruction may be recognized on AXR. These include caecal or sigmoid volvulus, obstructed inguinal or femoral hernia, and gallstone ileus. An AXR may suggest a specific diagnosis in other causes of acute abdomen though in most acute inflammatory disorders findings are non-specific.

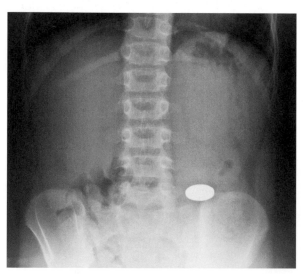

Fig. 6.1 *Abdomen X-ray of a young child showing a swallowed coin.*

THE STANDARD ABDOMINAL SERIES

The standard plain-film abdominal series consists of three films as follows:
1 Supine anteroposterior (AP) abdomen: standard projection used in all cases.
2 Erect AP abdomen. The erect abdomen film is used to look for fluid levels and free gas. It is therefore used for cases of possible intestinal obstruction or perforation. If the patient is too ill for the erect position, a decubitus film may be a useful substitute.
3 Erect chest. An erect chest X-ray (CXR) should be a part of a routine abdominal series for the following reasons:
   – Free gas beneath the diaphragms;
   – Chest complications of abdominal conditions such as pleural effusion in pancreatitis;
   – Chest conditions presenting with abdominal pain such as lower lobe pneumonia.

METHOD OF ASSESSMENT

Owing to a number of variable factors, including body habitus, distribution of bowel gas and the size of individual organs, such as the liver, the 'normal' AXR may show a wide range of appearances. For this reason, a methodical approach is important and the following check-list of 'things to look for' should be used (Fig. 6.2).
1 Hollow organs:
   – Stomach;
   – Small bowel: generally contains no visible gas, although a few non-dilated gas-filled loops may be seen in elderly patients as a normal finding;

- Large bowel;
- Bladder: seen as a round, soft-tissue 'mass' arising from the pelvic floor.
2 Solid organs: liver, spleen, kidneys, uterus.
3 Margins: diaphragm, psoas muscle outline, flank stripe, otherwise known as the properitoneal fat line
4 Bones: lower ribs, spine, pelvis, hips and sacroiliac joints.
5 Calcifications (Fig. 6.3):
  - Aorta;
  - Other arteries: a calcified splenic artery in the elderly is seen as tortuous calcification in the left upper abdomen;
  - Phleboliths: small, round calcifications within pelvic veins; common even in young patients; do not confuse with ureteric calculi;

- Lymph nodes: lymph node calcification caused by previous infection is common in the right iliac fossa and the pelvis;
- Costal cartilages commonly calcify in older patients.

SOME SPECIFIC FINDINGS ON ABDOMEN X-RAY

SMALL BOWEL OBSTRUCTION

Small bowel obstruction may present with a variety of symptoms ranging from mild abdominal pain to acute abdomen with vomiting, constipation, and abdominal distension. The most common cause (about 60 per cent)

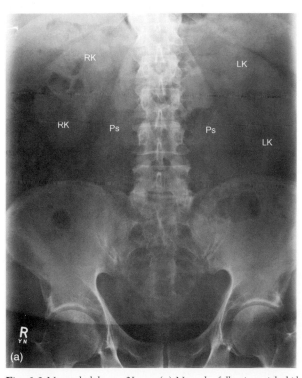

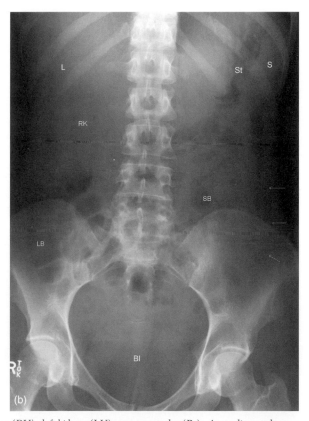

Fig. 6.2 *Normal abdomen X-ray. (a) Note the following: right kidney (RK), left kidney (LK), psoas muscles (Ps). According to the principles explained in Chapter 1 the margins of the kidneys and psoas muscles are outlined by retroperitoneal fat. (b) Note the following: liver (L), right kidney (RK), stomach (St), spleen (S), small bowel (SB), large bowel (LB), bladder (Bl), and properitoneal fat stripe (arrows).*

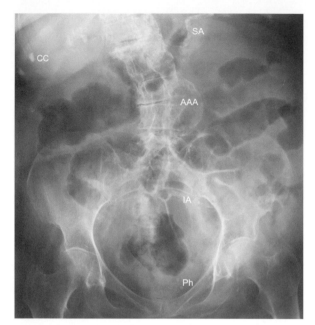

Fig. 6.3 *Abdominal calcifications. Some examples of the types of calcifications that may be seen on abdomen X-ray. These include extensive vascular calcification in the splenic artery (SA), aortic aneurysm (AAA), and iliac arteries (IA). Note also calcified costal cartilages (CC) adjacent to the anterior ends of lower ribs and phleboliths (Ph), small calculi that are a common normal finding in the veins of the pelvis.*

is adhesions and a history of previous abdominal or pelvic surgery should be sought. Less common causes include obstructed hernia, tumour, and rare conditions such as gallstone ileus.

Radiographic signs of small bowel obstruction (Fig. 6.4) include:

- Dilated small bowel loops, which have the following features:
  - (i) Tend to be central;
  - (ii) Numerous;
  - (iii) 2.5–5.0 cm diameter;
  - (iv) Have a small radius of curvature;
  - (v) Valvulae conniventes, seen as thin white lines that are numerous, close together and extend right across the bowel;
  - (vi) Do not contain solid faeces.
- Multiple fluid levels on the erect AXR.
- 'String of beads' sign on the erect AXR caused by small gas pockets trapped between valvulae conniventes.
- Absent or little air in the large bowel.
- Occasionally the specific cause of small bowel obstruction may be detected on AXR; some examples are given below.

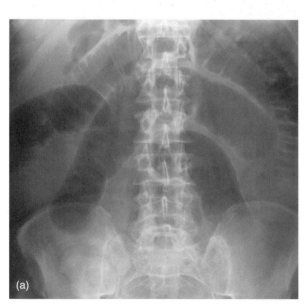

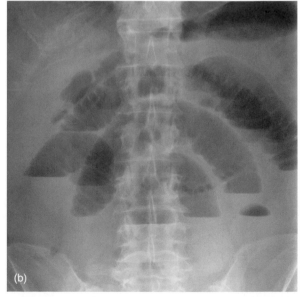

Fig. 6.4 *Small bowel obstruction. (a) Supine view showing multiple loops of small bowel. Note the features of small bowel loops as described in the text. (b) Erect view showing multiple relatively short fluid levels.*

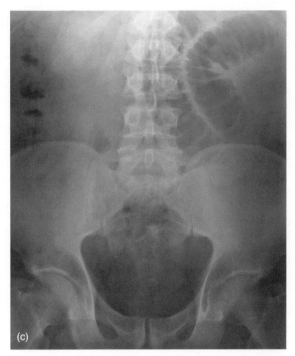

Fig. 6.4 (c) A further example of small bowel obstruction. This is a proximal obstruction with only a few dilated jejunal loops seen in the left upper abdomen.

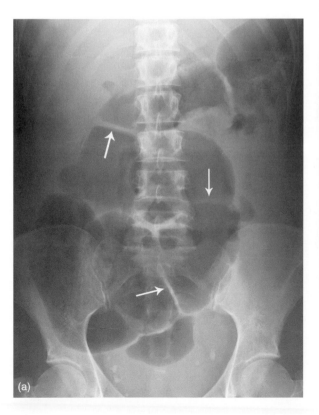

LARGE BOWEL OBSTRUCTION

Large bowel obstruction usually presents with abdominal distension and constipation with varying degrees of abdominal pain. The most common cause (70 per cent) is colorectal carcinoma. Other causes of large bowel obstruction include acute diverticulitis and stricture, obstructed hernia, volvulus, inflammatory bowel disease and extrinsic compression due to pelvic mass.

Radiographic signs of large bowel obstruction (Fig. 6.5) include:

- Dilated large bowel loops which have the following features:
  (i) Tend to be peripheral;
  (ii) Few in number;
  (iii) Large: above 5.0 cm diameter;
  (iv) Wide radius of curvature;
  (v) Haustra, seen as thick white lines that are widely separated, and may or may not extend right across the bowel (compare these features

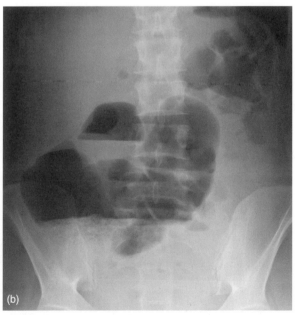

Fig. 6.5 *Large bowel obstruction. (a) Supine view showing multiple dilated loops of large bowel. These extend as far as the splenic flexure where subsequent investigation showed an obstructing tumour. Note the thick haustral folds (arrows) and compare with the valvulae conniventes shown in Fig. 6.4. (b) Erect view showing fluid levels.*

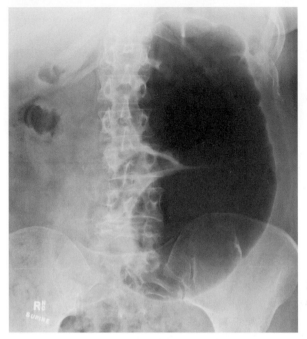

Fig. 6.6 *Caecal volvulus. Massively distended caecum passing across to the left. This is differentiated from sigmoid volvulus by its shape, plus the absence of large bowel dilatation.*

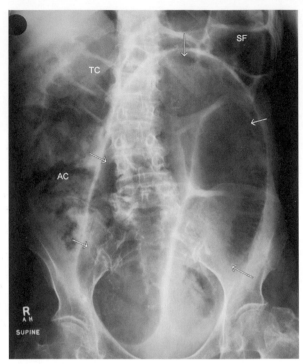

Fig. 6.7 *Sigmoid volvulus. Note the typical inverted 'U' appearance of sigmoid volvulus (arrows). Note also dilatation of ascending colon (AC), transverse colon (TC) and splenic flexure (SF). Note the characteristic overlap of dilated left colon and sigmoid loop below the splenic flexure.*

with those of the small bowel valvulae conniventes described above);

(vi) Contain solid faeces.

- Small bowel may also be dilated if the ileocaecal valve is 'incompetent'.

CAECAL VOLVULUS

Caecal volvulus refers to twisting and obstruction of the caecum. Caecal volvulus occurs most commonly in patients aged 20–40 years and is associated with an abnormally long mesentery and malrotation. Radiographic signs of caecal volvulus include:

- Markedly dilated caecum containing one or two haustral markings (Fig. 6.6).
- The dilated caecum may lie in the right iliac fossa or left upper quadrant.
- Attached gas-filled appendix.
- Small bowel dilatation.
- Collapse of left half of colon.

SIGMOID VOLVULUS

Sigmoid volvulus refers to twisting of the sigmoid colon around its mesenteric axis with obstruction and marked dilatation. It occurs in elderly and psychiatrically disturbed patients. Unlike caecal volvulus, the proximal large bowel is dilated. Radiographic signs of sigmoid volvulus include:

- Massively distended sigmoid loop in the shape of an inverted 'U', which can extend above T10 and overlap the lower border of the liver (Fig. 6.7).
- Usually has no haustral markings.
- The outer walls and adjacent inner walls of the 'U' form three white lines that converge towards the left side of the pelvis.
- Overlap of the dilated descending colon: 'left flank overlap' sign (good differentiating feature from caecal volvulus in which the remainder of the large bowel is not dilated).

STRANGULATED HERNIA

The term hernia refers to abnormal protrusion of intra-abdominal contents, usually peritoneal fat and bowel loops. Inguinal hernia accounts for about 80 per cent of abdominal wall hernias. Femoral hernia is more common in females. Other types of external hernia include umbilical hernia and hernia related to previous surgery, either incisional or parastomal. Most hernias present with an inguinal or abdominal wall mass that increases in size when the patient stands. Occasionally, hernias may become strangulated and present with localized pain and intestinal obstruction.

Radiographic signs of strangulated hernia include:
- Gas-containing soft-tissue mass in the inguinal region (Fig. 6.8).
- May have a fluid level on the erect view.
- Gas in the bowel wall within the hernia indicates incarceration and bowel wall infarction.

GALLSTONE ILEUS

Gallstone ileus refers to small bowel obstruction secondary to gallstone impaction. It usually occurs in a setting of chronic cholecystitis where a large gallstone erodes through the inflamed gallbladder wall to enter the duodenum. This gallstone then becomes impacted in the distal small bowel causing small bowel obstruction.

Radiographic signs of gallstone ileus include:
- Small bowel obstruction.
- Gas in the biliary tree seen as a branching pattern of gas density in the right upper quadrant (Fig. 6.9).
- Calcified gallstone lying in an abnormal position is occasionally seen.

LOCALIZED ILEUS

Localized ileus refers to dilated loops of bowel ('sentinel loops'), usually small bowel, overlying a local inflammation. Sentinel loops may be seen in the following sites:
- Right upper quadrant: acute cholecystitis.
- Left upper quadrant: acute pancreatitis.
- Lower right abdomen: acute appendicitis.

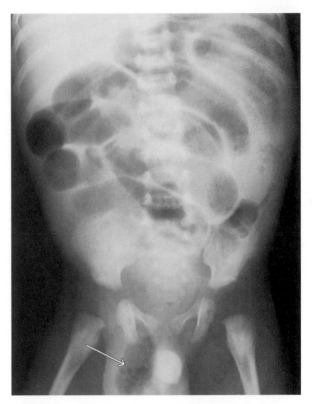

Fig. 6.8 *Strangulated hernia. Multiple dilated small bowel loops indicating intestinal obstruction are seen in an infant with abdominal distension. Note that in infants small and large bowel loops tend to be rather featureless making differentiation of small bowel from large bowel difficult. The most reliable differentiating feature is the position, with small bowel loops tending to lie more centrally. Note the obstructed right inguinal hernia (arrow).*

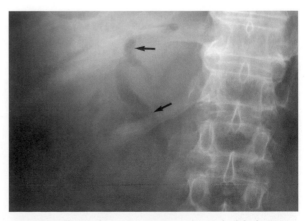

Fig. 6.9 *Gallstone ileus. Gas is seen outlining the bile ducts (arrows).*

GENERALIZED ILEUS

Generalized ileus refers to non-specific dilatation of small and large bowel, which may occur postoperatively or with peritonitis (Fig. 6.10(a)). Scattered irregular fluid levels are seen on the erect X-ray (Fig. 6.10(b)).

PERFORATION OF THE GASTROINTESTINAL TRACT

Perforation of the gastrointestinal tract (GIT) may be caused by peptic ulceration, inflammation including acute diverticulitis and appendicitis, and blunt or penetrating injury, including iatrogenic trauma. Perforation of the stomach, small intestine and most of the colon produces free gas in the peritoneal cavity. Perforation of the duodenum and posterior rectum will result in free retroperitoneal gas.

Radiographic signs of free gas:

- Erect CXR: gas beneath diaphragm (Fig. 6.11).
- Supine abdomen: gas outlines anatomical structures such as the liver, falciform ligament and spleen; bowel walls are seen as white lines outlined by gas on both sides, i.e. inside and outside the bowel lumen (Fig. 6.12).
- Free gas is also identified on erect abdomen film.
- If the patient is too ill to stand then either decubitus or shoot-through lateral films can be performed.

RENAL CALCULUS

As outlined in Chapter 9, CT is now the investigation of choice for the investigation of renal colic and the diagnosis of renal tract calculi. An AXR may be used after primary diagnosis to confirm spontaneous passage of a calculus or to direct further management. It may

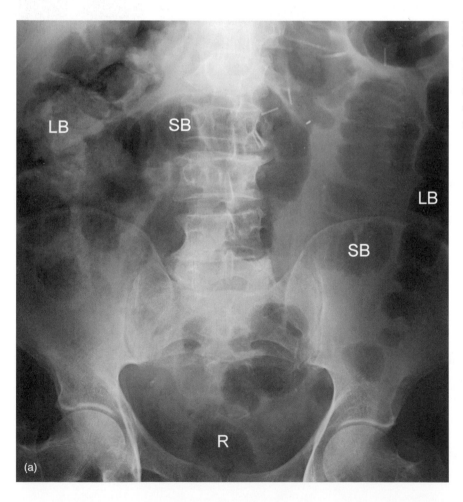

Fig. 6.10 *Generalized ileus. (a) Supine view shows dilated loops of both small (SB) and large bowel (LB). Gas is seen as far distally as the rectum (R) making a mechanical obstruction unlikely.*

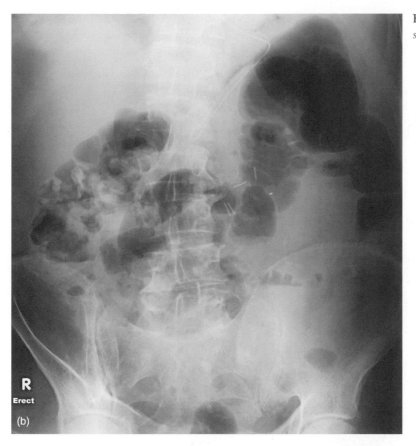

Fig. 6.10 (b) *Erect view showing only scattered fluid levels.*

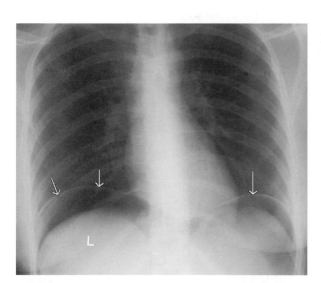

Fig. 6.11 *Free gas: chest X-ray. Free gas is seen beneath the diaphragm (arrows). Free gas separates the liver (L) from the right diaphragm.*

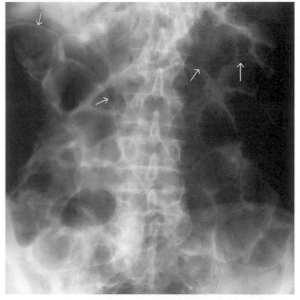

Fig. 6.12 *Free gas: abdomen X-ray. Free gas in the peritoneal cavity caused clear delineation of both sides of the bowel wall (arrows). Compare the appearances of these bowel loops with those visualized in other images in this chapter.*

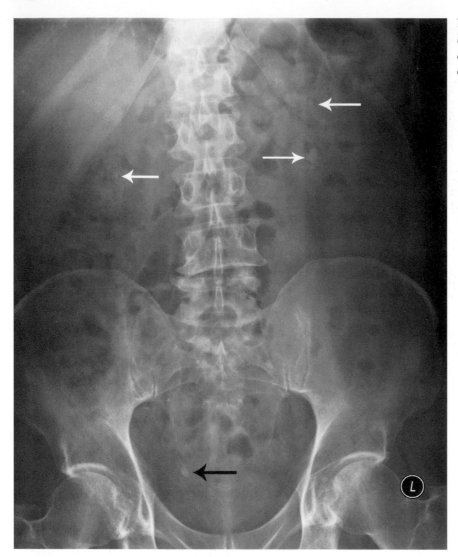

Fig. 6.13 *Renal calculi. Multiple bilateral renal calculi (white arrows) and right lower ureteric calculus (black arrow).*

also be performed after external shock wave lithotripsy or percutaneous calculus extraction to check for residual fragments in the urinary tract. About 90 per cent of renal calculi contain sufficient calcium to be radio-opaque, i.e. visible on AXR (Fig. 6.13). Cystine stones (3 per cent) are faintly opaque and may be visualized on AXR with difficulty. Urate stones (5 per cent) are lucent, i.e. not visible on AXR. The rare xanthine and matrix stones are also lucent. Note that opacities seen on AXR thought to be renal or ureteric calculi need to be differentiated from other causes of calcification, such as arterial calcification, calcified lymph nodes

and pelvic phleboliths. Phleboliths are small round calcifications in pelvic veins. They are extremely common, being visible on AXR in most adults.

ACUTE INFLAMMATORY CONDITIONS

Abdomen X-ray is unreliable for the diagnosis of most acute inflammatory conditions of the abdomen, being both non-specific and insensitive. It has been largely replaced in the diagnosis of most of these conditions by CT or US. However, AXR is often still performed as a first-line investigation in patients with acute abdomen. The astute observer may sometimes be able to suggest a

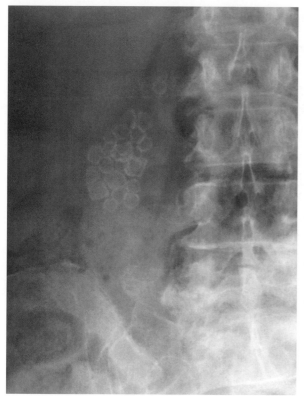

Fig. 6.14 *Gallstones. Multiple calcified gallstones seen in the right upper abdomen.*

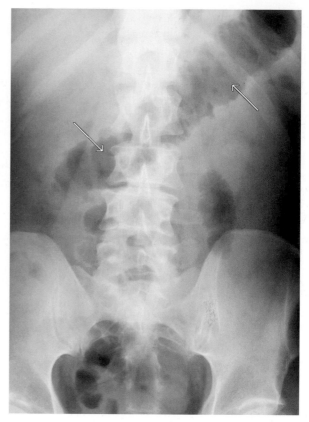

Fig. 6.15 *Toxic megacolon. Abdomen X-ray shows a dilated transverse colon (arrows) with thickening of the bowel wall.*

diagnosis and direct management based on recognition of some of the following signs on AXR.

Acute appendicitis

- Faecolith: calcified opacity usually in the right iliac fossa.
- Distal small bowel obstruction or localized paralytic ileus.
- Blurred right psoas margin and right properitoneal fat stripe.
- Lumbar scoliosis convex to the left.
- Decreased abdominal gas owing to vomiting and diarrhoea.
- Gas in the appendix.
- Appendix abscess: soft-tissue mass in the right iliac fossa which may separate gas-filled ascending colon from properitoneal fat stripe.

Acute cholecystitis

- Gallstones: only 10 per cent of gallstones contain sufficient calcium to be seen on AXR (Fig. 6.14).
- Soft-tissue mass in the right upper quadrant due to distended gallbladder.
- Paralytic ileus in the right upper quadrant.

Acute pancreatitis

- Paralytic ileus in the left upper quadrant.
- Generalized ileus.
- Loss of left psoas outline.
- Separation of greater curve of stomach from transverse colon.
- Pancreatic calcification with chronic pancreatitis.

- CXR signs that may be seen in association with acute pancreatitis include:
  (i) Left pleural effusion;
  (i) Atelectasis of left lower lobe;
  (i) Elevated left hemidiaphragm.

Abdominal abscess

- Mass, perhaps containing gas or even a fluid level on the erect view.
- Displaced bowel loops.
- Localized or generalized ileus.
- Loss of outline of adjacent structures, e.g. psoas muscle.
- CXR signs associated with subphrenic abscess:

  (i) Raised hemidiaphragm;
  (ii) Pleural fluid;

(iii) Lower lobe collapse;
(iv) Subdiaphragmatic fluid level.

Inflammatory bowel disease

- AXR signs of acute colitis:
  (i) Affected bowel shows wall thickening, blurred mucosal margins, absent haustral markings;
  (ii) Gasless colon strongly suggests severe disease.
- AXR signs of toxic megacolon:
  (i) Marked large bowel dilatation, most often of the transverse colon, often greater than 8 cm diameter (Fig. 6.15);
  (ii) May be complicated by perforation with free gas.

7

Gastrointestinal system

IMAGING INVESTIGATION OF THE GASTROINTESTINAL TRACT

ABDOMEN X-RAY

An abdomen X-ray (AXR) may be used for the assessment of acute abdomen, depending on the specific presentation. Particular indications for AXR include suspected bowel obstruction and perforation of the gastrointestinal tract (GIT). An AXR may also be used to monitor renal calculi and a number of less common indications will be encountered such as swallowed (or inserted) foreign body. For further notes on 'how to read an AXR' see Chapter 6. It is no longer recommended as a first-line investigation of abdominal masses, haematemesis, melaena, urinary tract infection or vague abdominal pain.

COMPUTED TOMOGRAPHY AND ULTRASOUND

Both computed tomography (CT) and ultrasound (US) are very commonly used in the assessment of abdominal pathology. Ultrasound has a long-established role in the diagnosis of biliary and hepatic pathology, particularly gallstones, biliary dilatation and hepatic masses. It is also used to screen for masses in other solid organs, free fluid and a wide range of gynaecological disorders that may present with acute abdominal pain. With the exception of acute cholecystitis it has less of a role in most acute abdominal disorders, although it should be used in young, thin patients for the diagnosis of acute appendicitis.

Computed tomography provides excellent delineation of the abdominal organs (Fig. 7.1) and is used in a wide range of clinical situations including abdominal

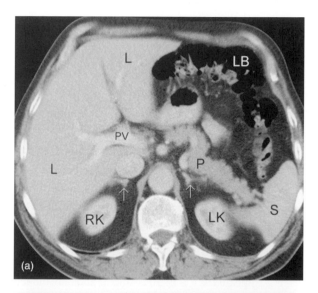

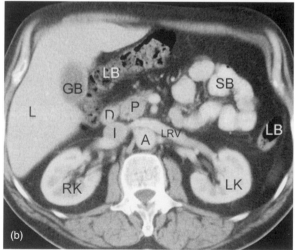

Fig. 7.1 *Normal abdomen: computed tomography (CT). Two separate transverse CT images of the upper abdomen showing the following structures: liver (L), portal vein (PV), right kidney (RK), left kidney (LK), spleen (S), pancreas (P), large bowel (LB), duodenum (D), inferior vena cava (I), aorta (A), left renal vein (LRV), small bowel (SB), adrenal glands (arrows).*

masses and acute abdominal pain. One of the primary imaging signs in acute abdomen is oedema in the fat adjacent to an inflamed organ. Because CT is able to demonstrate accurately peritoneal and retroperitoneal fat, it is extremely useful in the acute abdomen, as will be discussed below. It is less useful in this context in very thin or cachectic patients in whom fat planes may be absent or minimal.

CONTRAST STUDIES OF THE GASTROINTESTINAL TRACT

Barium swallow

Indications for barium swallow include dysphagia, swallowing disorders in the elderly following stroke or central nervous system (CNS) trauma, suspected gastro-oesophageal reflux, and post-oesophageal surgery.

The patient is asked to swallow contrast material and films are taken. Barium is usually used, although for checking of surgical anastomoses for leaks a water-soluble material, such as Gastrografin is preferable. Note that Gastrografin should not be used if pulmonary aspiration is suspected as it is highly osmolar and may induce pulmonary oedema if it enters the lungs.

Patients with swallowing disorders caused by CNS problems such as stroke or Parkinson's disease, or following laryngectomy may be assessed with modified barium swallow. This involves ingestion of liquids and solids of varying consistency under the supervision of a speech therapist and radiologist with video recording of swallowing.

Barium meal: examination of the stomach and duodenum

Given the ready availability of endoscopy, barium meal is less frequently performed than in the past. Where endoscopy is not available, barium meal may be useful for the investigation of dyspepsia, suspected upper GIT bleeding, weight loss or anaemia of unknown cause (Fig. 7.2). Water-soluble contrast material (Gastrografin) is used for assessment of anastomoses post-gastric surgery. The patient drinks a small amount of barium accompanied by gas-forming liquids. An antispasmodic agent

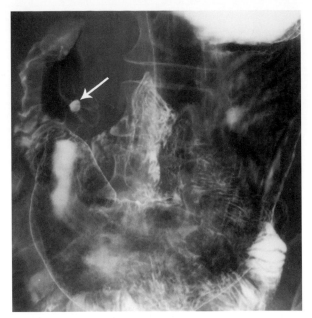

Fig. 7.2 *Duodenal ulcer: barium meal. The ulcer is seen as a small pocket of barium (arrow) in the first part of the duodenum.*

such as hyoscine (Buscopan) is commonly used to temporarily halt peristalsis and allow accurate imaging of the duodenum. The side-effects of hyoscine are rare and result from anticholinergic effects such as blurred vision and dry mouth. Hyoscine is contraindicated in patients with cardiac ischaemia or glaucoma and intravenous Glucagon may be used as an alternative antispasmodic agent in these cases.

Barium follow-through: examination of the small bowel

Barium follow-through or small bowel series is a simple procedure used to demonstrate small bowel pathology. The patient drinks a quantity of barium and films are taken until the contrast either reaches an obstruction or enters the large bowel. Gastrografin should be used if there is any suspicion of a perforation.

Small bowel enema (enteroclysis)

For enteroclysis a nasogastric tube is passed into the stomach and with the aid of a steering wire is then guided through the duodenum to the duodeno-jejunal flexure. A mixture of barium with either water or methyl cellulose is injected rapidly through the tube into the small bowel, giving a double-contrast effect. Advantages of this technique over simple barium follow-through include better assessment of the small bowel mucosal pattern and a quicker procedure. The major disadvantage is the use of a nasogastric tube, which is unpleasant to the patient. Indications for enteroclysis include Crohn's disease, malabsorption syndromes and miscellaneous small bowel conditions, such as tumour and Meckel diverticulum.

Barium enema: examination of the large bowel

Indications for barium enema include altered bowel habit, weight loss or anaemia of unknown cause, lower gastrointestinal tract (GIT) bleeding, and to screen for the presence of colorectal carcinoma or polyps in patients at risk. Most of these indications are better assessed with colonoscopy. Where colonoscopy is contraindicated barium enema may be useful, though it is being replaced by the newer technique of CT colography, also known as virtual colonoscopy (see below). Double-contrast barium enema technique with a combination of barium and air is required to diagnose most mucosal pathology as well as small mass lesions. Single-contrast enema studies with Gastrografin may be useful to outline and define a suspected large bowel obstruction, to define a suspected perforation or to check surgical anastomoses. The single-contrast technique may also be used in the very elderly or in children. Barium enema is contraindicated in the presence of acute colitis and toxic megacolon. Complications are very rare and consist of bowel perforation and transient bacteraemia; patients with artificial heart valves should receive antibiotic cover when having a barium enema.

SCINTIGRAPHY

Gastrointestinal bleeding study

- ^{99m}Tc-labelled red blood cells.
- Localize site of GIT bleeding.

Meckel diverticulum scan

- Free ^{99m}Tc (pertechnetate); taken up by gastric mucosa.
- Localize aberrant gastric mucosa in symptomatic Meckel diverticulum.

Gastrointestinal motility studies

- ^{99m}Tc-sulphur colloid in food preparation.
- Evaluate gastric and intestinal motility.
- Diagnose gastro-oesophageal reflux and pulmonary aspiration.

Hepatobiliary scan

- ^{99m}Tc-iminodiacetic acid (IDA); analogue of haem and taken up by the biliary system.
- Difficult cases of acute cholecystitis.
- Bile duct leak post-surgery including hepatic transplant or secondary to trauma.
- Neonatal jaundice to differentiate biliary atresia from neonatal hepatitis.

Tagged red cell scan

- ^{99m}Tc-labelled red blood cells.
- Confirm liver mass is a haemangioma

Liver–spleen scan

- ^{99m}Tc-sulphur colloid; taken up by reticuloendothelial cells in liver (Kupffer cells) and spleen.
- Investigation of liver function and hepatosplenomegaly.
- Confirm liver mass is focal nodular hyperplasia.
- Confirm presence of splenule or ectopic implantation of splenic tissue due to trauma (splenosis).

ANGIOGRAPHY

Indications for angiography in the abdomen include GIT bleeding, GIT ischaemia, posttraumatic bleeding, and preoperative demonstration of vascular supply of liver tumour ('surgical road map').

DYSPHAGIA

Dysphagia refers to the subjective feeling of swallowing difficulty caused by a variety of structural or functional disorders of the oral cavity, pharynx, oesophagus or stomach. Precise localization of the site of dysphagia by the patient may be difficult or inaccurate and as such, examination of all the above areas is often indicated.

BARIUM SWALLOW

In most instances barium swallow is the simplest and cheapest screening test for the investigation of dysphagia. For many conditions, barium swallow is sufficient for diagnosis; for others it will guide further investigations. Some of the more common conditions encountered on barium swallow are outlined below.

Pharyngeal pouch (Zenker's diverticulum)

Weakness of the posterior wall of the lower pharynx may lead to formation of a pharyngeal pouch. This is seen on barium swallow as a contrast-filled pouch that projects posteriorly and to the left above the cricopharyngeus muscle (Fig. 7.3). Pharyngeal pouches may become quite large with a fluid level seen on chest X-ray (CXR).

Achalasia

Achalasia is seen as dilated oesophagus that may also be elongated and tortuous with a smoothly tapered lower end. A CXR may show a mediastinal fluid level, absent gastric air bubble and evidence of aspiration pneumonia.

Sliding hiatus hernia

These range in size from a small, clinically insignificant hernia to the entire stomach lying in the thorax (i.e. thoracic stomach), which is at risk of volvulus. On CXR hiatus hernia may show as an apparent mass behind the heart containing an air–fluid level.

Carcinoma of the oesophagus

The appearances of oesophageal carcinoma depend on the pattern of tumour growth. Early lesions may show

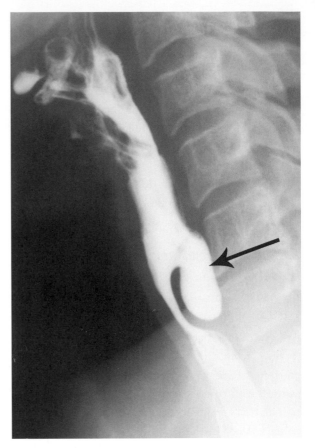

Fig. 7.3 *Pharyngeal pouch: barium swallow. A pharyngeal pouch (arrow) is seen on a lateral view projecting posteriorly from the lower pharynx.*

only an area of mucosal irregularity and ulceration. More advanced lesions present with irregular strictures with elevated margins. Further staging of carcinoma of the oesophagus consists of CT to assess local invasion and mediastinal lymphadenopathy, and to exclude liver and pulmonary metastases.

ENDOSCOPY AND BIOPSY

Endoscopy with biopsy is indicated as the primary investigation where there is a high clinical suspicion of oesophageal carcinoma. All strictures seen on barium swallow should undergo endoscopic assessment and biopsy, as should areas of ulceration and mucosal irregularity. Dysphagia in immunocompromised patients is usually caused by infectious oesophagitis. The commonest causative organism in human immunodeficiency virus (HIV)-positive patients is *Candida albicans* and dysphagia in these patients is often treated empirically with antifungal therapy. Other causes include herpes simplex and cytomegalovirus. If dysphagia fails to settle on antifungal therapy, endoscopy is indicated to obtain specimens for laboratory analysis.

ACUTE ABDOMEN

The common problem of acute abdominal pain encompasses a wide range of pathologies. A few key diagnostic points may be rapidly obtained from initial history and examination. These include the location of the pain, associated fever, a history of previous or recent surgery, prior history of similar pain, plus signs that may indicate intestinal obstruction such as abdominal distension, vomiting, and altered bowel habit. A full history and examination may be complemented with laboratory investigations such as white cell count and pancreatic enzymes.

Imaging may be used to complement, not replace clinical assessment. In the past, AXR has been the first line of imaging investigation for most patients with an acute abdomen. Signs to be searched for on the supine AXR of the patient with acute abdomen include abnormal bowel gas patterns such as small or large bowel obstruction, free gas indicating perforation of the GIT, gas in the biliary tree, abnormal calcifications such as renal calculi and pancreatic calcification, soft-tissue masses and foreign bodies. A CXR performed with the patient erect should accompany AXR for acute abdomen. The CXR may show free gas beneath the diaphragm, chest conditions which may present as acute abdomen, such as basal pneumonia, or chest complications of abdominal conditions, such as pleural effusion and basal atelectasis. Erect AXR should be reserved for cases of suspected intestinal obstruction or suspected perforation.

It is very important to emphasize that where the diagnosis is obvious on clinical grounds and/or AXR, more sophisticated imaging is not required. It is increasingly realized, however, that AXR may be negative or actually misleading in many of the common causes of acute abdomen. Other imaging modalities such as CT, US and contrast studies may be used where appropriate. Ultrasound is useful for assessment of the solid organs and for the diagnosis of gallstones. It is generally not useful for the diagnosis of bowel pathology and the central abdomen may be obscured by intestinal or free gas. Computed tomography provides excellent delineation of bowel wall thickening, soft-tissue masses and fluid collections, tiny amounts of free gas that may not be appreciated on AXR or CXR and sinus and fistula tracts.

Computed tomography has an increasing role in the assessment of acute abdominal pain. One of the most important reasons for this is the ability of CT to display inflammation or oedema in fat. Fat has a lower density than all other soft tissues and is therefore displayed on CT as a much darker shade of grey than all the other abdominal soft-tissue structures, including the solid organs, bowel wall and muscles. Inflammatory change in fat is very well shown on CT as streaky soft-tissue density or infiltration within the darker fat. This fatty infiltrative change is an extremely useful sign on CT. It often helps to localize pathology that may otherwise be overlooked and is the reason that even very subtle or early inflammatory change can be appreciated with CT. The importance of this sign is also one of the reasons that CT is less sensitive in the assessment of very thin or cachectic patients in whom abdominal fat planes may be absent.

SUSPECTED SMALL BOWEL OBSTRUCTION

The clinical presentation of small bowel obstruction may include abdominal pain and vomiting, progressing rapidly to fever and acute abdomen with abdominal distension and tenderness. The commonest causes are adhesions secondary to previous surgery, trauma or infection and hernias. Less common causes include small bowel neoplasm, gallstone ileus, intussusception and malrotation.

Abdomen X-ray is the primary investigation of choice in suspected small bowel obstruction. Situations where AXR may be less accurate include partial or early obstruction, and closed-loop obstruction. The majority of small bowel obstructions are diagnosed with clinical assessment and AXR. Computed tomography is the investigation of choice when clinical and AXR assessments are inconclusive. It is highly accurate for establishing the diagnosis of small bowel obstruction, defining the location and cause of obstruction, and diagnosing associated strangulation. The CT signs of small bowel obstruction include dilated small bowel loops measuring >2.5 cm diameter, with an identifiable transition from dilated to non-dilated or collapsed bowel loops (Fig. 7.4).

Oral contrast studies (small bowel follow-through) using barium or water-soluble contrast are often misleading, being unable to differentiate obstruction from paralytic ileus, and may in fact delay diagnosis. Enteroclysis (small bowel enema) is occasionally used for grading severity and location of partial obstruction.

SUSPECTED LARGE BOWEL OBSTRUCTION

Large bowel obstruction may have a subacute to chronic presentation with abdominal pain and distension and constipation. The commonest cause for such a presentation is colorectal carcinoma. More acute presentations may be seen with sigmoid or caecal volvulus and diverticulitis.

As for small bowel obstruction, the majority of large bowel obstructions are diagnosed with clinical assessment and AXR. Contrast enema may be helpful to localize the location of large bowel obstruction and to diagnose its cause (e.g. tumour or inflammatory mass). Contrast enema will also differentiate true large bowel obstruction from pseudo-obstruction. Pseudo-obstruction (non-obstructive large bowel dilatation) occurs most commonly in elderly patients and may be indistinguishable on AXR from mechanical obstruction.

Computed tomography is increasingly being used for the assessment of difficult or equivocal cases of large bowel obstruction (Fig. 7.5). In the majority of cases CT will diagnose the location and cause of obstruction. It has the added advantage of diagnosing other relevant findings such as liver metastases.

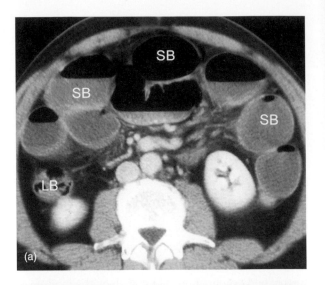

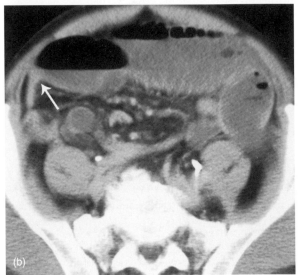

Fig. 7.4 *Small bowel obstruction: computed tomography. (a) Note dilated loops of small bowel (SB) containing fluid levels and non-dilated large bowel (LB). (b) Abrupt transition from dilated to nondilated small bowel (arrow) indicating mechanical small bowel obstruction.*

RIGHT UPPER QUADRANT PAIN

The primary diagnostic consideration in adult patients with right upper quadrant (RUQ) pain is acute cholecystitis. Ultrasound is the most sensitive investigation for the presence of gallstones and is therefore the investigation of choice for suspected acute cholecystitis. The diagnosis of acute cholecystitis is usually made

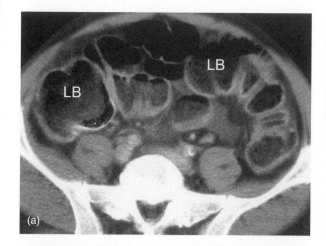

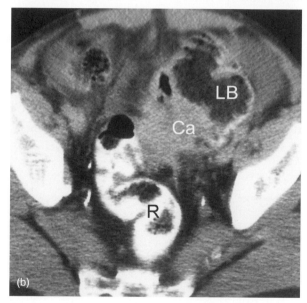

Fig. 7.5 *Large bowel obstruction caused by carcinoma: computed tomography. (a) Dilated loops of large bowel (LB). (b) Carcinoma (Ca) seen as a soft tissue mass in the sigmoid colon proximal to the rectum (R).*

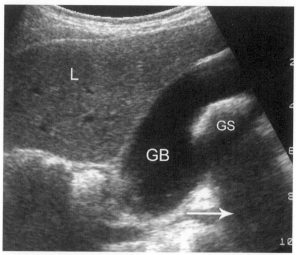

Fig. 7.6 *Gallstone: ultrasound. Note liver (L), gallbladder (GB) and gallstone (GS) casting an acoustic shadow (arrow).*

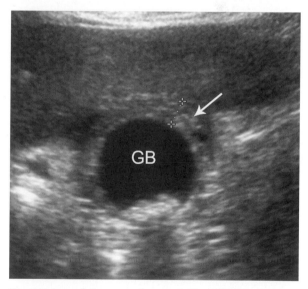

Fig. 7.7 *Acute cholecystitis: ultrasound. The gallbladder (GB) has a thickened wall (arrow) and contains multiple small gallstones.*

by confirming the presence of gallstones in a patient with RUQ pain and fever (Fig. 7.6). Other signs of acute cholecystitis that may be seen with US include thickening of the gallbladder wall, fluid surrounding the gallbladder and localized tenderness to direct probe pressure (Fig. 7.7).

Computed tomography is much less sensitive than US for the detection of gallstones. In a patient with acute cholecystitis CT may show signs of gallbladder inflammation such as thickening of the gallbladder wall with infiltrative streaking in adjacent fat.

Scintigraphy with ^{99m}Tc-IDA compounds (HIDA scan) has a limited role in difficult cases where clinical assessment and US are doubtful. Acute cholecystitis is indicated on a HIDA scan by non-visualization of the gallbladder with good visualization of the common bile duct and duodenum 1 hour after injection. Visualization of the gallbladder excludes acute cholecystitis.

RIGHT LOWER QUADRANT PAIN

The commonest cause of acute right lower quadrant (RLQ) pain is acute appendicitis. Differential diagnosis includes inflammatory bowel disease, mesenteric adenitis and gynaecological pathology in female patients. Most cases of acute appendicitis are confidently diagnosed on clinical grounds with typical history of pain and fever, and a raised white cell count. These cases do not require imaging. Imaging should be reserved for patients with atypical features on history or where gynaecological pathologies such as ectopic pregnancy or pelvic inflammatory disease are suspected.

Where imaging is required, US is the initial investigation of choice in children, thin patients and women of childbearing age. The accuracy of US is increased by the use of compression and colour Doppler imaging, and by concentrating the examination to the point of maximal tenderness as indicated by the patient (Fig. 7.8). Limitations of US are that the normal appendix

is often not visualized and retrocaecal appendicitis may be obscured. As such, the negative predictive value of a negative examination is not as high as for CT.

For most adult patients, excluding women of childbearing age, CT is the imaging investigation of choice in the assessment of RLQ pain (Fig. 7.9). Advantages of CT include its proven accuracy in the diagnosis of appendicitis and its ability to diagnose alternative causes of RLQ pain. The ability of CT to identify a normal appendix in the majority of patients plus its high level of sensitivity to even subtle inflammatory change mean that a negative CT has a very high negative predictive value.

LEFT LOWER QUADRANT PAIN

The primary diagnostic consideration for the patient with left lower quadrant (LLQ) pain is acute diverticulitis. The term 'acute diverticulitis' encompasses a range of inflammatory pathologies complicating diverticulosis with bowel wall and pericolonic inflammation and abscess formation, as well as formation of sinus or fistula tracts.

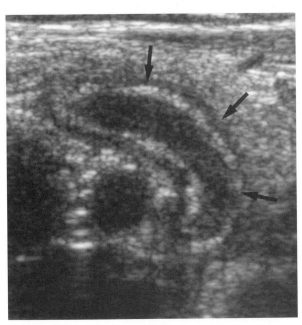

Fig. 7.8 *Acute appendix: ultrasound. Acutely inflamed appendix seen as a non-compressible blind-ending tubular structure (arrows) in the right iliac fossa.*

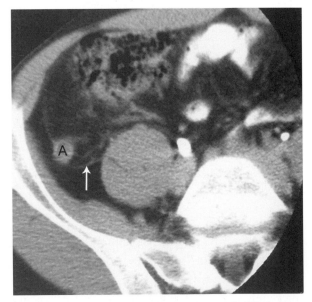

Fig. 7.9 *Acute appendicitis: computed tomography (CT). This shows a swollen appendix (A) with a soft tissue stranding pattern in adjacent fat (arrow). This stranding pattern is a highly useful sign on CT indicating oedema in fat adjacent to inflammation.*

Computed tomography is the investigation of choice for assessment of acute LLQ pain. Ultrasound should be used in women of child-bearing age in whom gynaecological pathology would be the main differential diagnosis. Computed tomography is highly accurate for the diagnosis of acute diverticulitis (Fig. 7.10). It is able to visualize intramural and pericolonic inflammation, and where diverticulitis is not present it may suggest alternative diagnoses such as small bowel obstruction, pelvic inflammatory disease, renal colic, etc. The CT signs of acute diverticulitis include localized bowel wall thickening and soft-tissue stranding or haziness in pericolonic fat. Gas in the bladder may indicate formation of a colovesical fistula.

ACUTE PANCREATITIS

Acute pancreatitis usually presents with severe acute epigastric pain. Risk factors for the development of acute pancreatitis include heavy alcohol intake and the presence of gallstones. The diagnosis may be confirmed by elevation of amylase and lipase levels. Computed tomography is the imaging investigation of choice for the diagnosis of acute pancreatitis. The CT signs in early pancreatitis may actually precede serum enzyme elevations. The CT signs of acute pancreatitis include diffuse or focal pancreatic swelling with indistinct margins and thickening of surrounding fascial planes (Fig. 7.11). Computed tomography scans performed during infusion of contrast material can differentiate necrotic non-enhancing tissue from viable enhancing tissue. This may have a major bearing on prognosis, as the presence of pancreatic necrosis is associated with a significantly increased mortality. Complications of pancreatitis such as phlegmon, abscess and pseudocyst are well shown on CT, which can be used to guide aspiration procedures and placement of drains.

ACUTE MESENTERIC ISCHAEMIA

Acute mesenteric ischaemia (AMI) is caused by abrupt disruption of blood flow to the bowel. It usually presents with sudden onset of severe abdominal pain and bloody diarrhoea. The goal of diagnosis and therapy is prevention or limitation of bowel infarction. Plain films are insensitive for AMI. The AXR signs, when present, usually indicate bowel infarction and include bowel wall thickening, dilated bowel loops, gas in the bowel wall and portal vein gas (Fig. 7.12). Prompt diagnosis requires a high index of suspicion and early referral for angiography in patients with clinical evidence of AMI. The

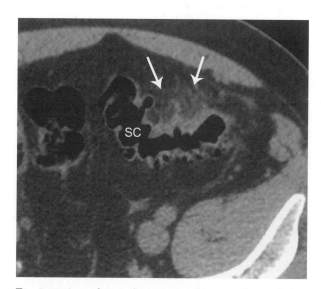

Fig. 7.10 *Acute diverticulitis: computed tomography. Multiple gas-filled diverticula arising from the sigmoid colon (SC). Note localized thickening of the bowel wall and adjacent fat stranding (arrows) indicating acute inflammation.*

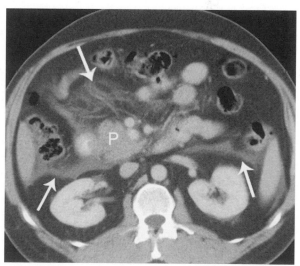

Fig. 7.11 *Acute pancreatitis: computed tomography. Pancreas (P) is swollen with adjacent fat stranding and thickening of fascial planes (arrows).*

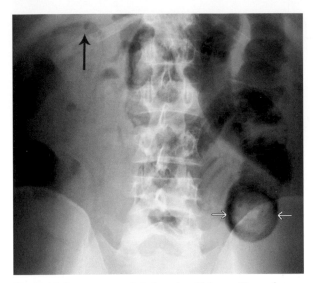

Fig. 7.12 *Acute mesenteric ischaemia. Abdomen X-ray shows gas in the bowel wall (white arrows) and portal vein (black arrow) indicating intestinal infarction.*

most common causes of AMI are superior mesenteric artery (SMA) embolus, SMA thrombosis and non-occlusive SMA vasospasm. In the case of SMA embolus the patient may have a history of cardiac disease, previous embolic event or simultaneous peripheral artery embolus. Thrombosis of the SMA is usually associated with an underlying stenotic atherosclerotic lesion in the SMA. Depending on the cause and clinical situation, particularly the presence or absence of peritoneal signs, treatment will be immediate surgery or interventional radiology. Interventional radiology consists of thrombolysis via a selective catheter, which may be followed by angioplasty of any underlying stenosis or papaverine infusion for SMA vasospasm.

FLANK PAIN AND RENAL COLIC

See Chapter 9.

INFLAMMATORY BOWEL DISEASE

The two diseases included in this section are Crohn's disease and ulcerative colitis. Crohn's disease is characterized by transmural granulomatous inflammation with deep ulceration, sinuses and fistula tracts. Crohn's disease may involve any part of the gastrointestinal tract from mouth to anus with small bowel involvement alone in 30 per cent, large bowel in 30 per cent and both small and large bowel in 40 per cent. Involvement is discontinuous with normal bowel between diseased segments ('skip lesions'). Ulcerative colitis is a disease of large bowel characterized by mucosal ulceration and inflammation. The rectum is involved in virtually all cases with disease extending proximally in the colon. Distribution of disease is continuous with no 'skip lesions'.

Patients with inflammatory bowel disease present with abdominal pain and diarrhoea. Extra-intestinal manifestations may occur including skin rashes, arthritis, ocular problems, and sclerosing cholangitis. The clinical course after initial presentation is usually intermittent episodes of diarrhoea or intestinal obstruction as well as infected sinus tracts and abscesses.

The main roles of imaging at initial presentation are to confirm the diagnosis and assess the distribution of disease. Initial diagnosis of inflammatory bowel disease involving the colon is usually by endoscopy, either sigmoidoscopy or colonoscopy, including biopsy. Where colonoscopy is unavailable or contraindicated barium enema may be performed. Signs of ulcerative colitis on barium enema include fine ulceration that gives the mucosa a granular pattern and loss of normal haustral markings. In later or more florid cases there may be pseudopolyp formation due to post-inflammatory granulation tissue and fibrosis. The rectum is involved with continuous retrograde involvement of the large bowel and no skip lesions.

Barium studies remain the primary imaging method for assessment of the small bowel, either small bowel follow-through or enteroclysis. Signs of Crohn's disease on barium studies include ulcers, strictures and 'cobblestoning' caused by fissures separating islands of intact mucosa with diseased segments separated by segments of normal bowel (Fig. 7.13).

Computed tomography is generally not used for the initial diagnosis. Abdomen X-ray is relatively insensitive and non-specific for the definitive diagnosis of inflammatory bowel disease. However, AXR is very

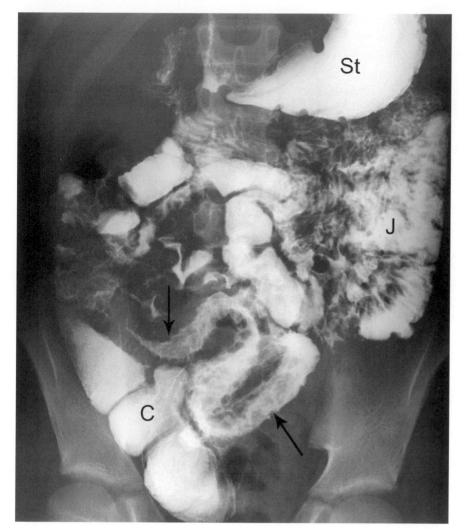

St

J

C

Fig. 7.13 *Crohn's disease: small bowel study. Barium study of the small bowel shows the following: stomach (St), jejunum (J), segment of distal small bowel with irregularity of the mucosal surface indicating multiple deep ulcers (arrows), caecum (C).*

useful in patients with severe symptoms for the diagnosis of toxic megacolon (Fig. 6.15), perforation or obstruction. Barium studies and colonoscopy are contraindicated by these findings.

In patients with known inflammatory bowel disease with recurrent symptoms or suspected complications CT is the investigation of choice. Computed tomography is used in inflammatory bowel disease to define the extent and site of bowel involvement, extracolonic inflammation and abscess formation, and sinus and fistula tracts. Magnetic resonance imaging may also be used for specific indications such as mapping of perirectal fistulas. Scintigraphy with ^{99m}Tc-HMPAO and ^{99m}Tc-labelled sucralfate may be useful in defining anatomical location

of disease, to a lesser extent in assessing disease severity, to diagnose relapse in patients with known inflammatory bowel disease and in acutely ill patients in whom barium studies are contraindicated.

GASTROINTESTINAL BLEEDING

Upper GIT bleeding is defined as any bleeding, from the oesophagus to the ligament of Treitz. Causes include peptic ulcer disease, erosive gastritis, varices, Mallory–Weiss tear and carcinoma. Common causes of acute lower GIT bleeding are angiodysplasia and diverticular disease. Although colonic diverticula are more prevalent in the sigmoid colon, up to 50 per cent of bleeding from diverticular disease occurs in the ascending colon. Less common causes of lower GIT bleeding include inflammatory bowel disease, colonic carcinoma, solitary rectal ulcer and post-polypectomy.

The goals of diagnosis and treatment of the patient with acute GIT bleeding are:

- Haemodynamic resuscitation.
- Localization and diagnosis of the source of bleeding.
- Control of blood loss by endoscopic haemostatic therapy, interventional radiology or surgery.

An upper GIT source for GIT bleeding is diagnosed by emergency upper GIT endoscopy in the majority of cases. Endoscopic haemostatic therapies include injection of sclerosants, injection of vasoconstrictors, thermal coagulation and mechanical methods.

Lower GIT bleeding is first investigated by sigmoidoscopy. If this is negative, scintigraphy and angiography are used to further assess the patient. Barium studies have no role in the patient with acute bleeding. Red blood cell (RBC) scintigraphy with ^{99m}Tc-labelled RBCs shows a GIT bleeding point as an area of increased activity (Fig. 7.14). Scintigraphy is more sensitive than angiography in that a lower rate of haemorrhage is required (0.1–0.2 mL/min) to produce a positive result. Scintigraphy is less anatomically specific than angiography. For this reason surgery based on RBC scintigraphy alone is not recommended. Rather, RBC scintigraphy should be seen as a screening test that will increase the accuracy of subsequent angiography. Red blood cell scintigraphy is therefore usually used in a complementary role to establish whether or not acute haemorrhage is occurring prior to angiography. A patient with clinical evidence of bleeding and negative scintigraphy should be investigated with elective colonoscopy.

Angiography is performed in acute GIT bleeding for two reasons:

1 To locate a bleeding point.
2 To achieve haemostasis by infusion of vasoconstrictors, or embolization.

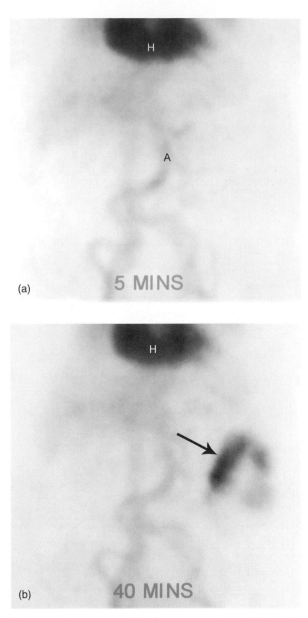

(a) 5 MINS

(b) 40 MINS

Fig. 7.14 *Gastrointestinal bleeding: scintigraphy. (a) The early phase of a labelled red blood cell study shows normal activity in the heart (H) and aorta (A). (b) A later scan shows accumulation of labelled red blood cells (arrow) in the left upper abdomen indicating bleeding into the large bowel. This was caused by angiodysplasia.*

Active haemorrhage is seen as extravasation of contrast material into the bowel if bleeding of 0.5–1.0 mL/min is occurring at the time of injection. Angiodysplasia is seen as a small nest of irregular vessels with early and persistent filling of a draining vein. Interventional radiology may be used when surgery is thought to be too risky, or for stabilization of bleeding prior to surgery. Options for the patient with GIT bleeding include selective infusion of vasoconstrictors such as vasopressin and embolization of small distal arterial branches following superselective catheterization.

CARCINOMA OF THE STOMACH

Endoscopy is usually performed in the assessment of symptoms suspicious for gastric carcinoma, including dyspepsia, upper abdominal pain, anaemia and weight loss. Barium meal is occasionally performed where endoscopy is not freely available. The appearance of a gastric tumour on barium meal depends on the pattern of growth. The following patterns may be seen:
- Gastric mass producing an irregular filling defect.
- Ulcer, usually with elevated margins.
- Mucosal infiltration with gastric fold thickening, mucosal irregularity and distorted gastric outline.
- 'Linitis plastica': small non-distensible stomach (Fig. 7.15).

Further imaging for staging of gastric carcinoma includes CT for liver metastases and lymphadenopathy, chest CT and CXR for pulmonary metastases, plus scintigraphy where bone metastases are suspected.

SMALL BOWEL NEOPLASMS

Small bowel neoplasms may present in a variety of ways and are often very difficult to diagnose. The patient may present with a quite specific clinical picture such as carcinoid syndrome or intussusception, or with less specific signs such as anaemia, weight loss or frank bleeding. The two principal imaging investigations are barium studies and CT. These studies are complementary in that barium studies show intraluminal and mucosal tumours while CT will image intramural tumours and extra-intestinal spread. Computed tomography will also show lymphadenopathy, liver metastases and tumour complications such as invasion of adjacent structures, fistula formation and intussusception.

The primary sign of a small bowel neoplasm on CT is asymmetric thickening of the bowel wall, usually >1.5 cm. This differs from bowel wall thickening in benign processes such as Crohn's disease or ischaemia; such thickening is usually concentric, symmetrical and may show a striped or 'target' appearance owing to mucosal oedema. Computed tomography is highly accurate for presence, site and size of tumour, as well as the presence of metastases. It is less accurate at predicting histology. The exception is lipoma where the fat content is well seen; carcinoid tumour may also have a fairly specific appearance. Benign tumours commonly present as the lead point in an intussusception.

COLORECTAL CARCINOMA

SCREENING FOR COLORECTAL CARCINOMA

Colorectal carcinoma (CRC) is the second leading cause of cancer death in Western society. It may present clinically with large bowel obstruction, GIT bleeding, or less specifically with weight loss or anaemia. A large

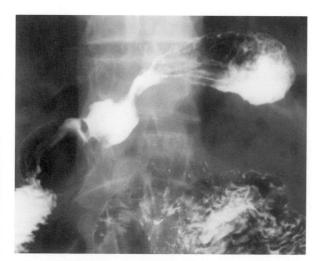

Fig. 7.15 *Linitis plastica: barium meal. The stomach is small and contracted because of diffuse infiltration of the gastric wall by tumour.*

percentage of CRC presenting clinically show locally invasive disease or distant metastases. The concept of the adenoma–carcinoma sequence illustrates the well-demonstrated fact that the vast majority of CRCs develop from small adenomatous polyps through a series of genetic mutations. The adenoma–carcinoma sequence is a slow process. It is estimated that an average of 5.5 years is required for large adenomas (greater than 10 mm diameter) to develop into CRC, with an average of 10–15 years for small adenomas (<5 mm). Colonic polyps are very common. Not all are adenomas and not all will develop cancer. Most polyps less than 5 mm are hyperplastic polyps or mucosal tags. These are not cancer precursors. Less than 1 per cent of adenomas up to 1 cm in diameter contain cancer, with cancer in small polyps (<5 mm) being extremely rare.

It is now generally agreed that screening for CRC is justified. Given the above concepts, it would seem logical that screening for CRC be targeted at detecting larger, more advanced adenomas with a high malignant potential, rather than trying to identify every single polyp regardless of size, the majority of which will never develop cancer. Various risk factors for the development of CRC have been identified allowing risk stratification into three categories:

- Average risk: age >50
- Moderate risk: past personal history of large adenoma or CRC or first-degree relative with large adenoma or CRC
- High risk: inflammatory bowel disease; hereditary non-polyposis CRC syndromes; familial polyposis syndromes.

Various screening strategies are available and include faecal occult blood testing, barium enema (double contrast), sigmoidoscopy and colonoscopy. All suffer from problems such as patient reluctance and lack of community awareness. Faecal occult blood testing gives a lot of false-positive results and will not detect adenomas or cancers that do not bleed. Sigmoidoscopy does not evaluate the entire colon. Barium enema has a relatively low sensitivity with detection rates of less than 50 per cent for polyps larger than 1 cm.

Colonoscopy provides the most complete and thorough examination and is the reference standard for evaluation of the colon. As well as detecting polyps and cancers with a high degree of accuracy, it also provides direct visualization of the mucosal surface and is able to diagnose the less common flat adenomas as well as inflammatory mucosal disease. Colonoscopy has the added benefit of being able to include biopsy and polypectomy. There are a number of limitations to colonoscopy. The most significant of these are the need for sedation and a failure rate of 5–10 per cent. Colonoscopy failure may result from tortuous loops of colon or colonic obstruction. Complications such as perforation and bleeding may also occur. These are rare, with a slightly increased incidence where polypectomy has been performed.

Computed tomography colonography, also known as virtual colonoscopy, is an evolving multidetector row CT technique with the potential to play a role in screening for CRC. For CT colonography, the colon is distended with room air or CO_2 administered through a rectal tube. One of the limitations of CT colonography is that retained faeces may simulate soft-tissue masses and polyps. For this reason, the patient's bowel is thoroughly cleansed before the procedure. This is usually easily done with commercially available preparation kits. The patient is then scanned lying supine and then prone, using a low radiation dose CT technique. The prone acquisition is to allow small faecal remnants to be differentiated from polyps. Faecal remnants are usually mobile and will shift with altered patient position, whereas polyps are adherent to the bowel wall. Furthermore, the use of the prone position allows more complete distension of parts of the colon that tend to be non-distended in the supine position. Images are reviewed on a computer workstation with software applications that allow instant multiplanar and 3D reconstructions as well as specialized algorithms for viewing the mucosal surface.

Computed tomography colonography has a sensitivity of over 90 per cent for the detection of polyps measuring 10 mm or more (Fig. 7.16). Limitations of CT colonography include the inability to reliably identify flat

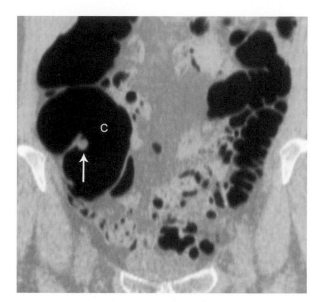

Fig. 7.16 *Adenomatous polyp of the colon: CT colography. The colon (C) is distended with air. This coronal view shows a round polyp (arrow) arising on a haustral fold in the right colon.*

adenomas or mucosal inflammation, plus low reported sensitivities for the detection of small polyps (<5 mm). Furthermore, biopsy and polypectomy cannot be performed. For these reasons, CT colonography cannot replace colonoscopy. Current indications for CT colonography include failed colonoscopy and evaluation of the colon proximal to an obstruction. It is also useful in patients for whom colonoscopy or sedation are contraindicated because of frailty or other factors. With improvements in technique and expertise it will probably play an increasing role in screening for CRC.

STAGING OF COLORECTAL CARCINOMA

Probably the most widely used classification of CRC is Kirklin's modification of Dukes' original system as below:

- Stage A: tumour confined to mucosa.
- Stage B1: tumour extension into, but not through, muscularis propria.
- Stage B2: tumour extension through muscularis propria but confined to bowel wall.
- Stage C1: stage B1 with lymph node metastases.

- Stage C2: stage B2 with lymph node metastases.
- Stage D: distant metastases.

As can be seen, the two most critical factors influencing survival data are depth of invasion of the bowel wall and the presence or absence of lymph node metastases. Unfortunately, two major limitations of imaging of CRC are assessment of depth of wall invasion and detection of microscopic metastases in non-enlarged lymph nodes. The exception to this is rectal CRC. Transrectal ultrasound (TRUS) is the investigation of choice for staging of rectal carcinoma. The layers of rectal wall are well seen and therefore TRUS is able to evaluate the depth of wall invasion. It may also be used for guided biopsy of perirectal lymph nodes. Limitations of TRUS include overstaging due to peritumoral inflammation mimicking invasion beyond the muscularis propria, as well as understaging due to microscopic tumour invasion too small to be seen with TRUS.

While accurate pretreatment staging of CRC is probably useful for planning of surgery, radiotherapy and chemotherapy, it remains controversial because of the limitations of imaging plus the fact that most patients with CRC will have surgery for either cure or palliation. Computed tomography of the abdomen is the imaging investigation of choice for detection of locally invasive disease, lymphadenopathy and distant metastases in patients with CRC. Colorectal carcinoma may be seen on CT as a mass or thickening of the bowel wall. Invasion beyond the bowel wall and invasion of adjacent structures are usually well demonstrated by CT. Computed tomography is unable to assess the depth of wall invasion or detect small metastases in non-enlarged lymph nodes. Therefore, CT is accurate for advanced disease, though less so for earlier non-invasive disease.

ABDOMINAL TRAUMA

Imaging plays an important role in the assessment of abdominal trauma. It should be emphasized that haemo-dynamically unstable patients should undergo immediate surgery. A specialized US technique known as FAST (focused abdominal sonography for trauma) is used in some centres for the rapid diagnosis of free intraperitoneal fluid. It is less sensitive than CT for the diagnosis of organ damage. Contrast-enhanced CT is the investigation of choice for suspected abdominal injuries in haemodynamically stable patients. Plain films are used to assess spinal and pelvic fractures. Angiography may occasionally be used in conjunction with embolization for localization and treatment of active bleeding, particularly in the pelvis.

Focused abdominal sonography for trauma

This consists of a rapid ultrasound assessment of the pelvis and abdomen looking for the presence of free fluid (Fig. 7.17). In many trauma and emergency centres focused abdominal sonography for trauma (FAST) is becoming the initial imaging investigation in the patient with abdominal trauma. It may be used to help decide which patients require immediate laparotomy or to indicate further investigation with CT. It may be

performed in a few minutes by experienced operators using small hand-held ultrasound units.

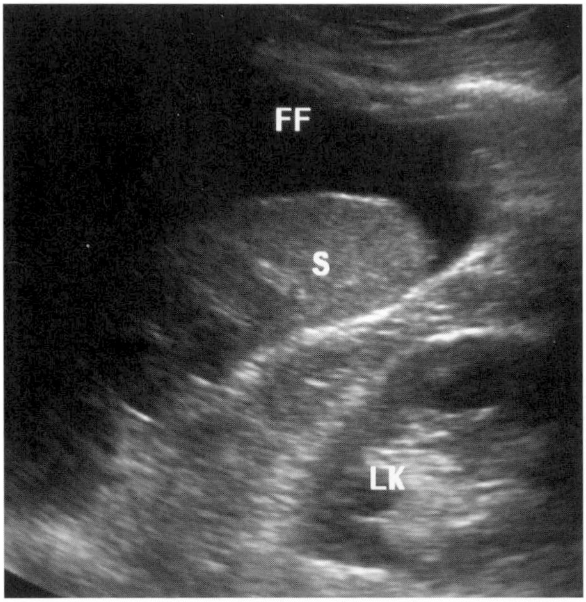

Computed tomography

Computed tomography provides excellent anatomical definition of intra-abdominal fluid collections and solid organ damage. For the assessment of abdominal trauma CT is usually performed with intravenous contrast material. This provides more accurate delineation of the liver, spleen, kidneys and pancreas. Free blood appears on CT as hypodense material in more dependent parts of the peritoneal cavity, i.e. pelvis, hepatorenal pouch and paracolic gutters. Splenic lacerations appear as hypodense lines separating more dense splenic fragments (Fig. 7.18). Hepatic trauma may be seen on CT as localized intrahepatic or subcapsular haematoma or lacerations seen as hypodense lines in the liver substance. Trauma to the kidney may result in renal haematoma or laceration. Lacerations involving the collecting system result in urine leaks and urinoma formation, seen on CT as active leakage of contrast material. A non-functioning kidney in a setting of acute trauma may be due to massive parenchymal damage, vascular pedicle injury or obstructed collecting system due to blood clot.

Fig. 7.17 *Free fluid: ultrasound (focused abdominal sonography for trauma, FAST). Free fluid (FF) is seen as anechoic material in the left upper abdomen adjacent to the spleen (S) and left kidney (LK).*

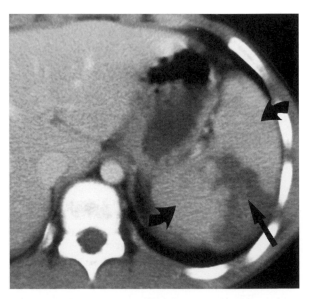

Fig. 7.18 *Splenic trauma: computed tomography. There is a large splenic laceration seen as a low attenuation cleft (straight arrow) between two splenic fragments (curved arrows).*

It is generally agreed that in most cases oral contrast material is not required for CT in abdominal trauma. Although free oral contrast material is a specific indicator of bowel perforation, it is not a sensitive sign. The presence of free fluid between bowel loops or at the base of the mesentery is a much more reliable CT sign in the diagnosis of bowel trauma. Bowel perforation may produce free intraperitoneal and retroperitoneal gas and CT may show haematoma in the bowel wall. None of these signs of bowel trauma require oral contrast.

Where bowel trauma is present, associated injuries such as solid organ damage or Chance fracture occur in over 50 per cent of cases. One of the advantages of multislice CT is that it may be used to assess the spine and bony pelvis by reviewing images in bony windows. In particular, instant sagittal reconstructions may be performed to provide a very rapid and accurate assessment of the spine.

Plain films: AXR

All patients with significant abdominal trauma should have a CXR. The CXR changes associated with abdominal trauma include pleural effusion, lower lobe collapse, ruptured diaphragm and rib fractures. With the wide availability of US and CT, AXR is often no longer performed in the setting of blunt abdominal trauma. It may be indicated in penetrating trauma to search for foreign material such as bullets or pieces of glass.

8

Liver

CHARACTERIZATION OF LIVER MASSES

Liver masses may present clinically in a number of ways. Large masses may cause upper abdominal pain, often described as 'dragging' in nature. Acute abdominal pain may be caused by sudden haemorrhage into a mass. A hepatocellular carcinoma occurring in a cirrhotic liver may cause a sudden deterioration in liver function or may present with increased ascites. Liver masses may also be detected during imaging screening of the liver for metastases in a patient with a known primary malignancy. A large proportion of liver masses are discovered as incidental findings during imaging investigation of unrelated symptoms. Characterization of liver masses, whether in the setting of a known malignancy or underlying cirrhosis is an important goal of diagnostic imaging.

The commonest benign liver masses are liver cysts and haemangiomas. Less common benign masses include focal nodular hyperplasia (FNH) and hepatic adenoma. Metastases and hepatocellular carcinoma (HCC) are the most common malignant liver masses. Most of the liver masses listed above have characteristic appearances on ultrasound (US), computed tomography (CT) and magnetic resonance imaging (MRI). Hepatic abscess may also present as a liver mass, though the diagnosis is usually suggested by the clinical setting of pyrexia and simple laboratory tests such as white cell count.

ULTRASOUND

Ultrasound is often the first investigation performed for a suspected liver mass, as it is non-invasive and relatively cheap. As with CT it gives good anatomical localization. It is highly sensitive for fluid-filled lesions such as cysts and abscesses, though less accurate than CT for characterization of solid lesions. Being non-invasive, US is particularly useful for masses requiring follow-up. A common example is suspected haemangioma where US is used to confirm lack of growth (Fig. 8.1). Intraoperative US with a high-frequency US probe directly applied to the surface of the liver may be used in the diagnosis and management of metastases.

Ultrasound is less accurate for detection of lesions high in the liver near the diaphragmatic surface. This is particularly the case where the liver lies high up under the rib cage. Another limitation of US is the fatty liver. Fatty infiltration produces an increasingly echogenic (bright) liver on US. Deeper parts of fatty

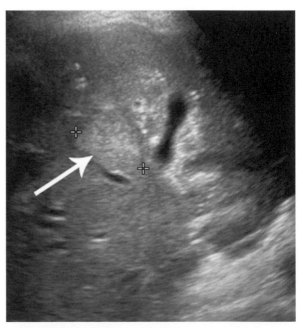

Fig. 8.1 *Haemangioma seen on ultrasound as a hyperechoic mass (arrow) in the liver.*

livers are difficult to examine with US, reducing the accuracy of lesion detection. Hepatic fat infiltration may occur in alcoholic liver disease. It is increasingly common today because of increased rates of obesity.

COMPUTED TOMOGRAPHY

Computed tomography is the imaging investigation of choice for assessment of most liver masses. Contrast-enhanced CT is the most sensitive technique for the detection of a mass. Computed tomography will reliably provide accurate anatomical localization and characterization of mass contents such as fluid, fat, or calcification. Complications of HCC such as invasion of the portal vein and arteriovenous shunting are well demonstrated with CT.

The ability to visualize a liver mass on CT relies on there being a difference in density between the mass and the surrounding liver. Lesions that are of low attenuation such as liver cysts are well seen on non-contrast enhanced CT. Lesions containing calcification such as mucin-producing metastases and hydatid cysts are also well seen. Unfortunately, a large percentage of liver malignancies are of equal or similar attenuation to liver tissue and are therefore difficult, if not impossible, to see with non-enhanced CT. Intravenous contrast material is used to improve lesion clarity. Modern helical and multislice CT scanners allow scanning of the entire liver during the various phases of contrast enhancement.

The liver receives a dual blood supply. The hepatic artery supplies 20 per cent of hepatic blood flow while the portal vein supplies the remaining 80 per cent. Three phases of contrast enhancement occur with intravenous injection of a bolus of contrast material. An early arterial phase begins at around 25 seconds following commencement of injection. After blood has circulated through the mesentery, intestine and spleen there is a later portal venous phase of enhancement beginning at around 70 seconds. Given that 80 per cent of the liver's blood supply is from the portal vein it follows that maximum enhancement of liver tissue will occur in the later portal venous phase. This is sometimes also referred to as the hepatic phase. After several minutes there is redistribution of contrast material to the extracellular space giving the third or equilibrium phase of contrast enhancement.

The hepatic artery supplies most liver tumours. Furthermore, most tumours are hypovascular, i.e. they receive less blood supply than surrounding liver. It follows then that maximum lesion clarity for most liver tumours, including metastases, will occur in the portal venous phase of contrast enhancement. (Please note that this is due to liver enhancement, not enhancement of the tumour.) These hypovascular tumours are seen as low-attenuation masses well-visualized against high-attenuation enhancing liver (Fig. 8.2). Portal phase CT

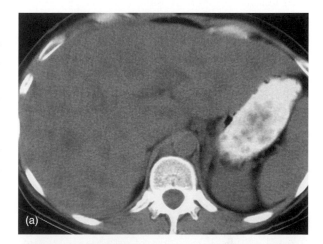

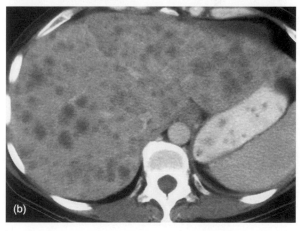

Fig. 8.2 *Hepatic metastases: computed tomography (CT). (a) Non-contrast CT of the liver shows subtle heterogeneity. (b) CT during the portal venous phase of contrast enhancement shows multiple low attenuation metastases throughout the liver; this is much more obvious than on the non-contrast scan.*

is the most sensitive imaging investigation for the detection of the majority of hepatic metastases.

Some liver tumours are hypervascular in that they receive more blood supply than surrounding liver. For these tumours maximum lesion clarity will occur in the arterial phase of contrast enhancement. (This is due to enhancement of the lesion, not the liver.) These lesions are seen as high-attenuation masses compared with the relatively low-attenuation liver tissue (Fig. 8.3). Examples of hypervascular lesions best seen in the arterial phase are small HCC, FNH and hypervascular metastases. The arterial phase is particularly useful for detection of a small enhancing HCC in a cirrhotic liver. Such lesions are often invisible in the portal venous phase. Hypervascular metastases are less common than hypovascular and may be seen with carcinoid tumour, renal cell carcinoma and melanoma.

As well as lesion detection, multiple-phase liver CT is often useful for liver mass characterization based on the contrast enhancement pattern. The most common example of this is for confirmation of hepatic haemangioma. Haemangioma is the most common benign hepatic mass and multiple haemangiomas are seen in up to 20 per cent of cases. Haemangioma is usually asymptomatic, though large lesions may bleed. The greatest significance in clinical practice is to differentiate haemangioma from a more sinister liver mass, especially in a patient with a known primary malignancy. For a suspected haemangioma detected initially on US it is suggested that CT be performed to define the enhancement pattern. Most haemangiomas show a typical peripheral nodular enhancement pattern in the arterial phase, and this is usually adequate for diagnosis (Fig. 8.4). Doubtful lesions may be followed up with a further CT or US in a few months' time to confirm lack of growth. Magnetic resonance imaging and/or scintigraphy may occasionally be used where immediate clarification is required.

MAGNETIC RESONANCE IMAGING

Magnetic resonance imaging is being used more commonly for liver lesion detection and characterization. Fast imaging sequences allow imaging of the liver during a single breath-hold. As with CT, scanning

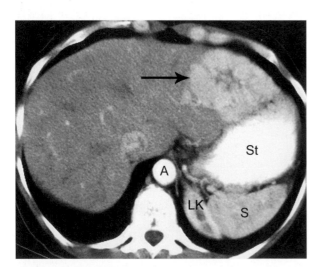

Fig. 8.3 *Focal nodular hyperplasia: computed tomography (CT). CT of the liver during the arterial phase of contrast enhancement shows the typical pattern of focal nodular hyperplasia with an intensely enhancing mass (arrow) containing a central non-enhancing scar. Note also aorta (A), left kidney (LK), spleen (S) and stomach (St).*

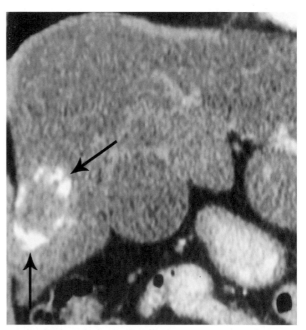

Fig. 8.4 *Haemangioma: computed tomography (CT). CT during the arterial phase of contrast enhancement shows the typical pattern of peripheral nodular enhancement indicating haemangioma (arrows).*

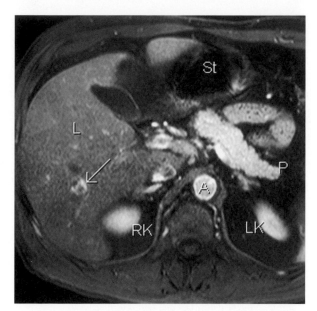

Fig. 8.5 *Haemangioma: magnetic resonance imaging (MRI). T1-weighted MRI during the arterial phase of contrast enhancement shows peripheral nodular enhancement indicating haemangioma (arrow). Note also stomach (St), pancreas (P), aorta (A), right kidney (RK) and left kidney (LK).*

may be performed during the arterial, portal venous, and equilibrium phases of contrast enhancement following intravenous injection of gadolinium. Magnetic resonance imaging is usually used to characterize lesions that do not have typical appearances on US or CT (Fig. 8.5). A common indication is to differentiate an atypical haemangioma from malignancy. The role of MRI for liver lesion characterization may expand further with the development of newer 'liver specific' contrast agents. These include:

- Iron oxide-based reticuloendothelial agents.
- Gadolinium-based hepatobiliary agents taken up by hepatocytes (Gd-EOB-DTPA and Gd-BOPTA/Dimeg).
- Mangafodipir trisodium (Mn-DPDP).

SCINTIGRAPHY

Two scintigraphic techniques are occasionally used for the characterization of liver masses. Tagged red cell scan with ^{99m}Tc-labelled red blood cells may be used to confirm that a liver mass is a haemangioma. Liver–spleen scan with ^{99m}Tc-sulphur colloid may be used to confirm the diagnosis of focal nodular hyperplasia. Most liver masses appear as filling defects except for focal nodular hyperplasia, which usually contains Kupffer cells and therefore shows tracer uptake.

IMAGING INVESTIGATION OF JAUNDICE

The causes of jaundice may be divided into two broad categories: mechanical biliary obstruction and intrahepatic biliary stasis, also known as hepatocellular or non-obstructive jaundice. Based on clinical findings, such as pain and stigmata of liver disease, plus biochemical tests of liver function the distinction between these categories can be made in most patients. Imaging has no significant role in non-obstructive jaundice, other than US guidance of liver biopsy. The use of US guidance both to localize the liver accurately and to avoid large vascular structures will increase the safety of liver biopsy.

Mechanical biliary obstruction may occur at any level from the liver to the duodenum. Causes include gallstones in the bile ducts, pancreatic carcinoma, cholangiocarcinoma, carcinoma of the ampulla of Vater or duodenum, iatrogenic biliary stricture, chronic pancreatitis, liver masses and sclerosing cholangitis. The roles of imaging are to determine the presence, level and cause of biliary obstruction.

Ultrasound is the first-choice imaging investigation for the jaundiced patient. If the bile ducts are not dilated, non-obstructive jaundice is considered and liver biopsy may be required. If the bile ducts are dilated on US without an obvious cause CT may be performed as this has a higher rate of diagnosis of the cause of biliary obstruction than US. Depending on the findings, US and CT may be followed by more definitive imaging of the biliary system with magnetic resonance cholangiopancreatography (MRCP), endoscopic retrograde cholangiopancreatography (ERCP) or percutaneous transhepatic cholangiography (PTC). In some centres, CT cholangiography and HIDA (hepatobiliary iminodiacetic acid) scans may also have a limited role.

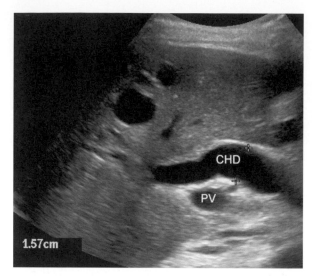

Fig. 8.6 *Biliary dilatation: ultrasound. Dilated common hepatic duct (CHD) seen as an anechoic tubular structure anterior to the portal vein (PV).*

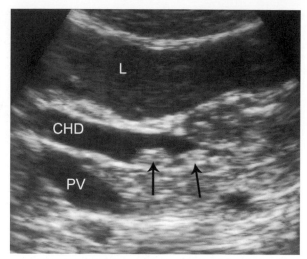

Fig. 8.7 *Choledocholithiasis: ultrasound. Biliary calculi are seen as hyperechoic foci (arrows) in the common hepatic duct (CHD). Note also liver (L) and portal vein (PV).*

ULTRASOUND

Ultrasound is the initial investigation of choice to identify dilated bile ducts and therefore confirm the presence of mechanical biliary obstruction (Fig. 8.6). Common bile duct diameter measurements are graded as follows:

- Normal <6 mm.
- Equivocal 6–8 mm.
- Dilated >8 mm.

The site and cause of obstruction are defined on US in only 25 per cent of cases as overlying duodenal gas often obscures the lower end of the common bile duct (Fig. 8.7). Associated dilatation of the main pancreatic duct suggests obstruction at the level of the pancreatic head or ampulla of Vater.

COMPUTED TOMOGRAPHY

Parameters of bile duct dilatation are as listed above for US (i.e. common bile duct >8 mm is dilated). As with US, main pancreatic duct dilatation localizes the obstruction to the lower common bile duct. The site and cause of bile duct obstruction may be suggested on CT in up to 90 per cent of cases (Fig. 8.8).

Computed tomography cholangiography involves a slow infusion of cholangiographic agent (Biliscopin) to opacify the bile ducts (Fig. 8.9). Helical CT scans and three-dimensional (3D) reconstructions are performed. Computed tomography cholangiography is a reasonably reliable method of imaging the biliary system where MRCP and the other more invasive methods listed below are contraindicated or not available. Limitations of CT cholangiography include poor bile duct opacification in jaundiced patients and risk of allergy to Biliscopin.

MAGNETIC RESONANCE CHOLANGIOPANCREATOGRAPHY

This has become a primary modality for the evaluation of biliary obstruction. It uses heavily T2-weighted images that show stationary fluids such as bile as high signal with moving fluids and solids as low signal. The bile ducts and gallbladder are therefore seen as bright structures on a dark background (Fig. 8.10). Magnetic resonance cholangiopancreatography is unaffected by bilirubin levels and may be combined with other sequences to provide more comprehensive imaging of the liver and pancreas. In many centres, MRCP has replaced diagnostic ERCP in the assessment of jaundiced

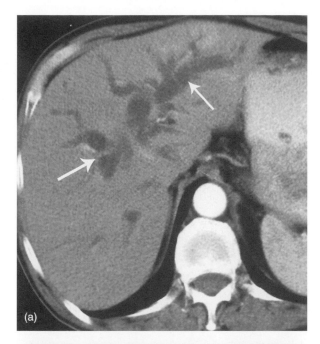

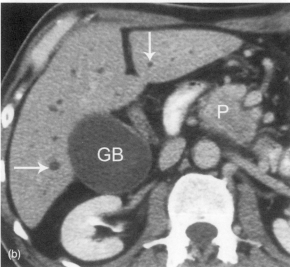

Fig. 8.8 *Biliary obstruction caused by carcinoma of the head of the pancreas: computed tomography (CT). (a) Dilated bile ducts seen on CT as a low attenuation branching pattern (arrows) in the liver. (b) Note enlargement of head of pancreas (P) by tumour, and distended gallbladder (GB).*

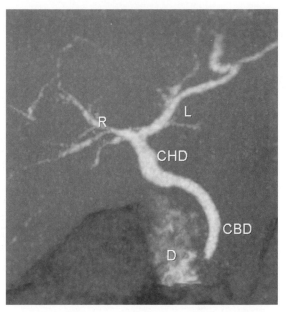

Fig. 8.9 *Normal bile ducts: computed tomography cholangiogram showing right and left hepatic ducts (R, L), common hepatic duct (CHD), common bile duct (CBD) and duodenum (D).*

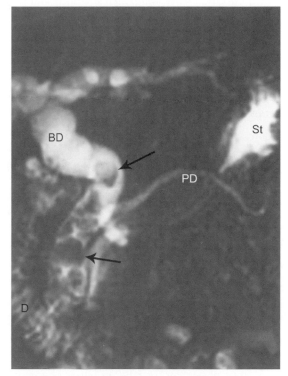

Fig. 8.10 *Choledocholithiasis: magnetic resonance cholangiopancreatography. Biliary calculi are seen as filling defects (arrows) within the dilated bile ducts (BD). Note also pancreatic duct (PD), stomach (St) and duodenum (D).*

patients with dilated bile ducts on US. Other indications for MRCP include prelaparoscopic cholecystectomy to diagnose bile duct calculi and bile duct variants, and to avoid intraoperative exploration of the common bile duct. Other advantages of MRCP are that it is non-invasive, does not involve ionizing radiation and does not require intravenous contrast material.

Disadvantages of MRCP include:

- Patients unsuitable for MRI, e.g. with cardiac pacemakers, claustrophobia.
- Limited spatial resolution, therefore difficulty visualizing stones <3 mm, tight biliary stenosis, small peripheral bile ducts and small side-branches of the pancreatic duct.
- No therapeutic applications, i.e. unable to perform sphincterotomy, insert stents, etc.

ENDOSCOPIC RETROGRADE CHOLANGIOPANCREATOGRAPHY

For ERCP, the ampulla of Vater is identified endoscopically and a small cannula passed into it under direct endoscopic visualization. Contrast material is then injected into the biliary and pancreatic ducts and films taken (Fig. 8.11). Where MRCP is not available, ERCP is used to assess biliary obstruction diagnosed on US or CT. It is still the investigation of choice for suspected distal biliary obstruction that may require sphincterotomy, basket retrieval of stones, biliary biopsy or biliary stent placement.

PERCUTANEOUS TRANSHEPATIC CHOLANGIOGRAPHY

This is indicated for assessment of high biliary obstruction at the level of the porta and where biliary obstruction cannot be outlined by ERCP because of previous biliary diversion surgery. For PTC a fine needle is passed into the liver and then slowly withdrawn as small amounts of contrast material are injected. Once a bile duct is entered, contrast is more rapidly injected to outline the biliary system. Percutaneous transhepatic cholangiography is often accompanied by biliary stent placement for relief of biliary obstruction. Patient preparation for PTC should include clotting studies and antibiotic cover to prevent septicaemia resulting from release of infected bile.

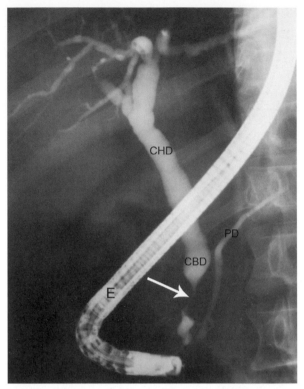

Fig. 8.11 *Cholangiocarcinoma: ERCP. Stricture (arrow) of the distal common bile duct (CBD) due to cholangiocarcinoma. Note also common hepatic duct (CHD), pancreatic duct (PD), and endoscope (E).*

SUMMARY OF INTERVENTIONAL PROCEDURES OF THE LIVER AND BILIARY TREE

LIVER BIOPSY

Liver biopsy may be performed under CT or US guidance. Core biopsy is often required, as fine-needle aspiration may not provide sufficient material for diagnosis. The two basic indications for guided liver biopsy are liver mass and diffuse liver disease. Not all liver masses should undergo biopsy. Bleeding may complicate biopsy of haemangioma. Seeding of tumour cells may occur along the needle track following biopsy of hepatocellular carcinoma. Most liver masses are characterized on imaging as above and managed surgically or non-surgically without biopsy. Biopsy of liver masses is restricted to a few specific indications. These would include a patient with liver metastases and an unknown primary tumour, or alternatively a patient with a known primary and a liver mass not able to be otherwise characterized. For liver biopsy in suspected diffuse liver disease imaging guidance is not strictly required but it may increase safety and diagnostic yield.

NON-SURGICAL MANAGEMENT OF BILE DUCT STONES

Non-surgical management of bile duct stones is normally done via ERCP, with widening of the lower end of the common bile duct (sphincterotomy) and removal of stones via a small wire basket. Occasionally, bile duct stones may be removed via a T-tube tract. This may be done by basket removal or flexible choledochoscope. For management of stones via T-tube, the T-tube should be *in situ* for at least 4 weeks postsurgery to ensure a 'mature' tract able to accept wires and catheters. Complications are rare but can include pancreatitis, cholangitis and bile leak.

NON-SURGICAL MANAGEMENT OF MALIGNANT BILIARY OBSTRUCTION

This section briefly describes a range of palliative procedures used to assist in the management of biliary obstruction caused by malignancies arising from the liver, bile ducts, pancreas and gallbladder. Indications are as follows:

- Symptomatic relief: relief of pruritus, pain, or cholangitis.
- Non-resectable tumour of bile ducts, head of pancreas or liver.
- Medical risk factors which make surgery impossible.

Methods vary with the type of tumour, its location and local expertise and preferences. Various methods include:
- Endoscopic: 'from below' for mid to low biliary obstruction.
- Percutaneous: 'from above' for high biliary obstruction or where the second part of duodenum

is inaccessible to endoscopy because of tumour or prior surgery (Fig. 8.12)
- Combined percutaneous–endoscopic methods.

Regardless of the approach to be used the basic technique is the same (Fig. 8.12). The bile ducts are opacified by ERCP or PTC, a wire is passed across the biliary obstruction and a stent or internal–external drain is inserted over the wire. Occasionally, in severe obstruction, a two-stage procedure is required. This involves placement of a drainage tube above the obstruction for a few days. After decompression of the biliary system, a wire is passed across the obstruction and a stent inserted. Internal biliary stents are made of plastic or self-expanding metal and are better accepted by patients as they avoid the potential problems of external biliary drains such as skin irritation, pain, bile leaks and risk of dislodgement.

PERCUTANEOUS CHOLECYSTOSTOMY (GALLBLADDER DRAINAGE)

Percutaneous cholecystostomy may be useful in the management of acute cholecystitis where the surgical risks are unacceptable. Percutaneous cholecystostomy is usually performed using US guidance. The gallbladder is punctured, a wire passed through the needle and a drainage catheter placed in the gallbladder over the wire. Non-resolution of pyrexia within 48 hours may indicate gangrene of the gallbladder, which requires surgery. A cholecystogram is performed once the acute illness has settled, with contrast material injected through the drainage catheter. Stones causing cystic duct obstruction may require surgery; otherwise the catheter is removed.

TRANSJUGULAR INTRAHEPATIC PORTOSYSTEMIC STENT SHUNTING

The transjugular intrahepatic portosystemic stent shunting (TIPSS) procedure is performed in the setting of portal hypertension for chronic, recurrent variceal haemorrhage not amenable to sclerotherapy. It is an

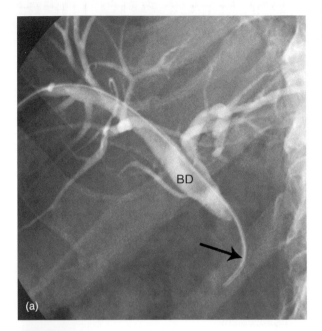

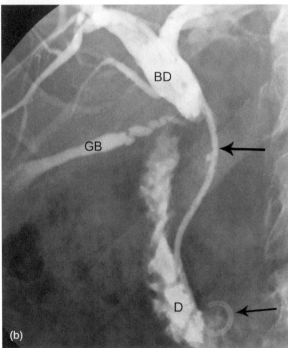

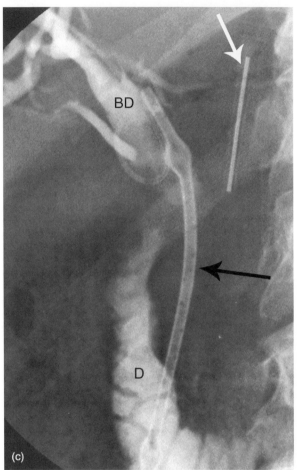

Fig. 8.12 (c) *A biliary stent (black arrow) is placed with its ends on either side of the biliary tumour. A radiographic marker (white arrow) assists with precise positioning of the stent.*

Fig. 8.12 *Biliary stent insertion. (a) percutaneous transhepatic cholangiography (PTC) shows obstruction of proximal bile ducts (BD) due to cholangiocarcinoma. A wire (arrow) is being passed through the obstruction.(b) A drainage catheter (arrows) has been passed over the wire into the duodenum (D). Note also the gallbladder (GB) now outlined by contrast material.*

interventional technique used to form a shunt from the portal system to the systemic venous circulation, thus lowering portal venous pressure. The patient is imaged with Doppler US before the procedure to exclude malignancy and confirm patency of the portal vein. The technique of TIPPS consists of jugular vein puncture, often under US control with a wire passed into the IVC and catheterization of a hepatic vein. A puncture device is passed through this catheter. Using US to select the most direct route, the portal vein is punctured and a wire passed. A tract from hepatic vein to portal vein is therefore formed. This tract is dilated and a stent inserted, usually a metallic prosthesis expanded by balloon.

Urinary tract and male reproductive system

9

IMAGING INVESTIGATION OF THE URINARY TRACT

COMPUTED TOMOGRAPHY, ULTRASOUND AND MAGNETIC RESONANCE IMAGING

As will be discussed below, computed tomography (CT) and ultrasound (US) are the main imaging investigations used for assessment of the urinary tract both in males and females. Magnetic resonance imaging (MRI) is increasingly used as a problem-solving modality in the characterization of renal and adrenal masses. It also has an increasingly accepted role in the staging of prostatic carcinoma.

SCINTIGRAPHY

Renogram

Renal scintigraphy with ^{99m}Tc-diethylenetriamine penta-acetic acid (DTPA) or ^{99m}Tc-mercaptoacetylglycine (MAG3) is performed to assess renal function and urodynamics, including calculation of the percentage of total renal function contributed by each kidney. Diuresis renography with injection of Furosemide is used to diagnose mechanical urinary tract obstruction. Angiotensin converting enzyme (ACE) inhibitor renography with injection of Captopril is used to diagnose renovascular hypertension. Renal transplant scintigraphy is used to assess renal perfusion and function, diagnose rejection or acute tubular necrosis, and detect urinary leak or outflow obstruction.

Renal cortical scintigraphy

Renal cortical scintigraphy with ^{99m}Tc-dimercaptosuccinic acid (DMSA) is used for the diagnosis of acute pyelonephritis in infants and young children, and to diagnose renal scars complicating urinary tract infection in children (see Chapter 16).

Radionuclide cystography

Radionuclide scintigraphy is used to detect, quantify and follow up vesicoureteric reflux (VUR) in children (see Chapter 16).

INTRAVENOUS PYELOGRAM

The method of performing intravenous pyelography (IVP) is as follows:
- Preliminary abdomen X-ray (AXR) to identify the kidneys and to visualize renal or ureteric calculi.
- Contrast material is then injected intravenously.
- Radiographs are taken to show the kidneys, the collecting systems, ureters and bladder.
- A post-micturition AXR confirms drainage of both ureters and emptying of the bladder.

For most indications, including renal colic, prostatism, urinary tract infection and renal cell carcinoma US, CT and scintigraphy have replaced IVP. Intravenous pyelography is still performed in some centres in the assessment of haematuria. Its principal advantage in this context is its ability to accurately outline the urinary tract, including the renal collecting systems and ureters. This enables the diagnosis of small transitional cell tumours that may otherwise be missed on CT or US. With the advent of multislice technology, CT is now able to delineate the renal collecting systems and ureters as well as IVP and, at the time of writing, CT is replacing IVP in the assessment of haematuria. In many centres IVP is only rarely performed for very specific indications such as sorting out complex congenital anomalies or following surgical repair or reconstruction of the ureters.

RETROGRADE PYELOGRAPHY

Retrograde pyelography (RPG) is usually performed in conjunction with formal cystoscopy. The ureteric orifice is identified and a catheter passed into the ureter. Contrast material is then injected via this catheter to outline the collecting system and ureter. A RPG may be performed to better delineate lesions of the upper renal tract identified by other imaging studies such as CT, or occasionally in a patient with haematuria where other imaging studies are normal or equivocal.

ASCENDING URETHROGRAPHY

Ascending urethrography is indicated prior to urethral catheterization in a male patient with an anterior pelvic fracture or dislocation, or with blood at the urethral meatus following trauma. It may also be performed to diagnose urethral strictures, which may be the result of previous trauma or inflammation. A small catheter is passed into the distal urethra and contrast material injected. Films are obtained in the oblique projection. The posterior urethra is often not opacified via the ascending method. Should this area need to be examined, a micturating cysto-urethrogram (MCU) will be required.

MICTURATING CYSTO-URETHROGRAPHY

Micturating cysto-urethrography is most commonly performed in children in the assessment of urinary tract infection (see Chapter 16). In adult males it is most commonly performed following radical prostatectomy to check the surgical anastomosis and the integrity of the bladder base. MCU may also be used to assess posterior urethral problems in male adults and stress incontinence in female adults.

The bladder is filled with contrast material via a urethral catheter. Images of the contrast-filled bladder are obtained. The catheter is then removed and films are taken during micturition.

INVESTIGATION OF A RENAL MASS

By far the commonest cause of a renal mass in an adult is a renal cyst. Renal cysts are usually small and asymptomatic, and usually discovered incidentally on CT or US examinations of the abdomen. Occasionally very large cysts may present with abdominal pain or a palpable abdominal mass. Most cysts are simple cysts with thin walls and clear fluid contents. A small percentage of benign cysts have more complex features and are classified as complex cysts. About 6 per cent contain turbid fluid resulting from haemorrhage or less commonly infection; 1 per cent of cysts contain calcification or thin soft-tissue septations. The presence of a soft-tissue mass in association with a cyst usually implies a cystic renal cell carcinoma.

Solid renal masses may be benign or malignant. The commonest benign renal mass is angiomyolipoma (AML). These are usually small and asymptomatic and as with cysts, are often discovered incidentally. Large AML may present as a palpable abdominal mass or may be complicated by haemorrhage giving acute abdomen and haematuria. Angiomyolipomas contain fat, giving them a characteristic appearance on US and CT. Eighty per cent of AMLs occur sporadically; 20 per cent occur in association with tuberous sclerosis and are often multiple.

The commonest malignant renal mass is renal cell carcinoma. Much less commonly, transitional cell carcinoma may produce a central mass centred in the collecting system and extending into the renal parenchyma. Other malignant cell types are much less common in the kidney. Renal cell carcinomas may be multiple at the time of presentation. The differential diagnosis for multiple non-fat-containing renal masses would include lymphoma and metastases.

The goals of imaging a suspected renal mass include:
- Confirmation of presence and site of mass.
- Classification into simple cyst, complicated cyst or solid mass.
- Assessment of contents, in particular the presence of fat.
- Differentiation of benign from malignant.
- Diagnosis of complications such as local invasion, venous invasion, lymphadenopathy and metastases.

Ultrasound

Ultrasound is the initial investigation of choice for assessment of a renal mass, followed by CT. Renal

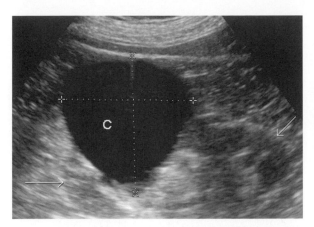

Fig. 9.1 *Simple renal cyst: longitudinal ultrasound (US) of left kidney (arrows). Note the US features of a simple cyst (C): anechoic contents, smooth wall and no soft tissue components.*

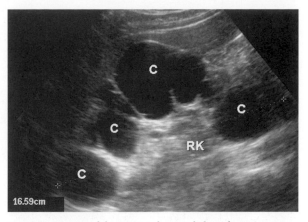

Fig. 9.2 *Autosomal dominant polycystic kidney disease: ultrasound. Multiple simple cysts (C) shown arising in the right kidney (RK).*

masses and cysts are also commonly found on US examinations being performed for other indications. Ultrasound will accurately characterize a mass as a simple cyst, complex cyst or a solid mass. A simple cyst will appear on US as a round anechoic (black) structure with a thin or invisible wall (Figs 9.1 and 9.2). If a simple cyst is found then no further imaging is required.

The term 'complex cyst' refers to a cyst with internal echoes which may be caused by haemorrhage or infection, soft-tissue septations, calcifications or an associated soft-tissue mass (Fig. 9.3). Causes of a complex cyst include a simple cyst complicated by haemorrhage or infection, benign cyst containing septations or calcifications, or a cystic tumour. A solid mass on US may show areas of increased echogenicity due to calcification or fat, or areas of decreased echogenicity due to necrosis. If a complex cyst or solid mass are found, further assessment will be needed and this is usually done with CT.

Where renal cell carcinoma is suspected, US is also used to look for specific findings such as invasion of renal vein and inferior vena cava (IVC), lymphadenopathy, and metastases in the liver and contralateral kidney.

Ultrasound may be used as a guide for:
- Biopsy of solid lesions or complicated cysts.
- Cyst aspiration for diagnostic and therapeutic purposes.

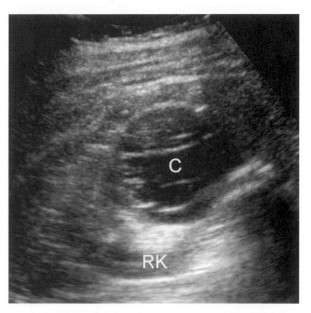

Fig. 9.3 *Complex renal cyst: ultrasound. Cyst (C) containing thin septations arising on the right kidney (RK).*

- Cyst ablation by injection of ethanol.
- Radiofrequency ablation of small tumours.

Computed tomography

Contrast-enhanced CT is used for further characterization of a solid lesion or complex cyst. Computed tomography is more accurate than US for characterization of internal contents of a mass, particularly to

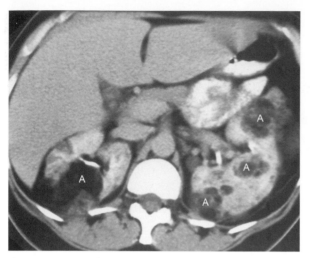

Fig. 9.4 *Angiomyolipoma: computed tomography (CT).*
Multiple angiomyolipomas (A) arising in both kidneys in a
woman with tuberous sclerosis. Note the typical low attenuation
fat content, well shown on CT.

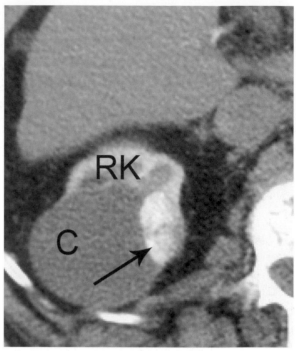

Fig. 9.6 *Renal cell carcinoma arising in a cyst: computed*
tomography. A cyst (C) arising on the right kidney (RK)
contains a soft tissue mass that enhances with intravenous
contrast (arrow). This is the typical appearance of a Bosniak
type 4 cyst and indicates malignancy.

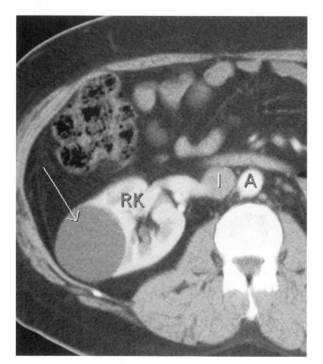

Fig. 9.5   *Simple renal cyst: computed tomography (CT).*
Note the CT features of a simple cyst (arrow) arising on the
right kidney (RK): homogenous low attenuation contents, thin
wall, and sharp demarcation from adjacent renal parenchyma.
Note also inferior vena cava (I) and aorta (A).

show areas of fat confirming the diagnosis of AML
(Fig. 9.4).

Based on their CT appearances, cystic renal lesions
may be classified according to the Bosniak system.
Simple cysts have thin walls and non-enhancing low-
density contents. Simple cysts are classified as Bosniak
type 1 and require no further follow-up (Fig. 9.5).
Cysts containing high-density fluid, thin septations or
fine calcifications are classified as Bosniak type 2.
These are regarded as benign although follow-up with
CT is recommended. Bosniak type 3 cysts contain
thicker septations or calcifications. About 50 per cent
of type 3 cysts are malignant and these are usually
treated surgically. Cysts containing an enhancing soft-
tissue mass are classified as Bosniak type 4 and regarded
as malignant (Fig. 9.6).

The more common appearance of renal cell carcinoma is a heterogeneous soft-tissue mass that enhances

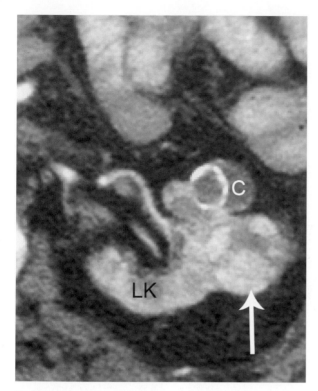

Fig. 9.7 *Renal cell carcinoma: computed tomography. Renal cell carcinoma seen as a small mass (arrow) arising on the left kidney (LK). Note also the presence of a partly calcified cyst (C).*

with intravenous contrast material (Fig. 9.7). Computed tomography is also used for staging of renal cell carcinoma. Factors relevant to staging detected on CT include invasion of local structures such as psoas muscle, vascular invasion of renal vein or IVC, lymphadenopathy, metastases in the liver and tumour in the other kidney.

Magnetic resonance imaging

Magnetic resonance imaging gives similar information to CT in the detection, classification and staging of renal cysts and tumours. Because MRI is able to define soft-tissue septations and masses, the Bosniak classification system may be used. The advantages of MRI in imaging renal masses include:

- Iodinated contrast material is not required, though gadolinium is injected.
- More accurate for assessing venous invasion.

- Multiplanar imaging gives more accuracy in assessing the renal poles, and for showing invasion of surrounding structures.

Angiography

Catheter angiography may be performed if tumour embolization is required before surgery. This may be done for haemorrhage complicating a large angiomyolipoma or with a highly vascular renal cell carcinoma.

Biopsy

Biopsy of renal masses is usually not indicated as tumour seeding may occur and histological interpretation is often difficult. Biopsy of a solitary renal mass may be indicated in the following uncommon situations:

- High suspicion for lymphoma.
- Known or previous primary carcinoma elsewhere, especially lungs, breast or stomach.
- Where a positive biopsy result would indicate a non-operative approach.

PAINLESS HAEMATURIA

Haematuria may be seen in association with urinary tract infection and ureteral stones. In these situations, other clinical symptoms and signs such as acute flank pain and fever are usually present. Glomerulonephritis is suspected where haematuria is accompanied by heavy proteinuria and red cell casts. Glomerulonephritis is confirmed with renal biopsy. Patients with glomerulonephritis should have a chest X-ray (CXR) to search for cardiac enlargement and pulmonary oedema, plus a renal US to screen for underlying renal morphological abnormalities. Renal biopsy is also best done under imaging guidance, usually US.

In the absence of compelling evidence of glomerulonephritis, painless haematuria should be considered to be caused by urinary tract tumour until proved otherwise. The imaging work-up of patients with painless haematuria is therefore directed at excluding or diagnosing renal cell carcinoma and transitional cell carcinoma (TCC). Occasionally, TCC may produce a central renal mass as described above. More commonly, however, TCC is a small tumour arising in the renal collecting systems, ureters and bladder. Furthermore, TCC is often a multifocal tumour. It follows from the above that the imaging assessment of painless haematuria requires visualization of the renal parenchyma to exclude a renal mass, plus visualization of the urothelium. This includes imaging of the collecting system, renal pelvis, ureters and bladder.

Until recently, the most commonly used initial tests were IVP plus cystoscopy. The main limitation of IVP in the setting of painless haematuria is that it will miss even moderate-sized renal cell carcinomas unless they cause significant deformity of the renal outline or collecting systems. Increasingly, multislice CT is replacing IVP as the initial imaging test for the patient with haematuria. A modified CT technique known as CT urography has been developed that provides excellent delineation of the renal collecting systems, ureters and bladder, as well as cross-sectional images of the kidneys and adjacent structures.

Although the precise method of performing CT urography may vary, the term refers to a contrast-enhanced CT scan with special reference to the urinary tract. The patient should be well hydrated. Computed tomography scans are performed with sufficient delay after contrast material injection to allow opacification of the collecting systems and ureters (Fig. 9.8). Multiplanar reconstructions in coronal and oblique planes allow precise definition of all areas. In some centres an abdominal radiograph is obtained immediately after the CT while the collecting systems and ureters are outlined by contrast material.

Regardless of the imaging tests used, cystoscopy is usually required in the assessment of painless haematuria to diagnose small bladder tumours and mucosal lesions.

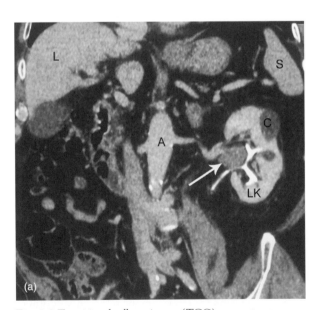

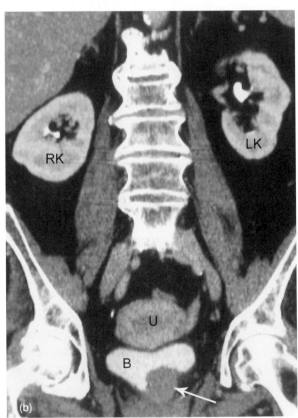

Fig. 9.8 *Transitional cell carcinoma (TCC): two separate cases of TCC diagnosed with computed tomography (CT) urography. (a) TCC of the left kidney (LK) seen as a central mass (arrow) on a coronal CT image. Note also liver (L), aorta (A), spleen (S), left renal cyst (C).*

Fig. 9.8 *(b) TCC of the bladder (B) seen as a soft tissue mass (arrow) on a coronal CT image. Note also both kidneys (RK, LK) and uterus (U).*

RENAL COLIC AND ACUTE FLANK PAIN

Acute flank pain describes pain of the posterolateral abdomen from the lower thorax to the pelvis. The most common cause of acute flank pain is ureteral obstruction caused by an impacted renal calculus. For this reason, the terms acute flank pain and renal colic are often used interchangeably. The term 'acute flank pain' more accurately reflects the fact that non-renal causes may produce similar symptoms to genuine renal colic. Non-renal causes of acute flank pain include appendicitis, torsion or haemorrhage of ovarian cyst, diverticulitis, inflammatory bowel disease and pancreatitis. Other renal causes of acute flank pain include acute pyelonephritis, TCC of the ureter causing obstruction and 'clot colic', i.e. ureteric colic caused by a blood clot complicating haematuria.

Computed tomography

In the patient with acute flank pain, initial assessment is directed towards confirming or excluding urinary tract obstruction secondary to a ureteric calculus. Helical CT without contrast enhancement is the imaging test of choice for acute flank pain. The helical acquisition means that the whole length of the urinary tract can be scanned without the possibility of missing small ureteric stones. Contrast material injection causes opacification of the renal collecting systems and ureters. This would obscure most renal or ureteric stones. For this reason, scans are done without contrast material (i.e. unenhanced).

In the past, IVP was performed for suspected renal colic. Unenhanced helical CT has a number of advantages over IVP in the assessment of acute flank pain:
- Speed:
  (i) CT usually takes about 5 min;
  (ii) IVP may take several hours where there is delayed renal function.
- Contrast material is not required.
- Virtually all stones are identified:

  (i) The only exceptions are stones resulting from precipitation of Indinavir crystals in human immunodeficiency virus (HIV) patients taking this medication;
  (ii) Cystine, urate, xanthine and matrix stones are all well seen on CT as high-attenuation foci.
- Stone position and size are accurately assessed:
  (i) The likelihood of a ureteric calculus passing spontaneously is largely related to size;
  (ii) A calculus of 5 mm or less will usually pass where a calculus of 10 mm or more is likely to become lodged.
- Non-renal causes of acute flank pain may be identified.

The CT signs of urinary tract obstruction consist of dilatation of the ureter above the calculus, dilatation of renal pelvis and collecting system and soft-tissue stranding in the perinephritic fat due to distended lymphatic channels (Fig. 9.9).

Plain films: KUB

A plain film of the abdomen done to diagnose and follow-up renal or ureteric calculi is termed KUB, for kidneys, ureter, and bladder. The KUB is no different from a supine AXR. Despite the use of CT, as described above, KUB still has a prominent role in the management of renal and ureteric calculi. Where possible, follow-up of ureteric or renal calculi should be with KUB, as this will give much less radiation than a repeat CT. About 90 per cent of renal calculi should be visible on KUB (see Fig. 6.13, page 100).

ADRENAL IMAGING

The adrenal gland is essentially made up of two separate organs, the adrenal cortex and the adrenal medulla. The adrenal cortex is an endocrine gland composed of fat-rich cells. It secretes cortisol, aldosterone and androgenic steroids. The adrenal medulla develops from the neural crest and secretes adrenaline

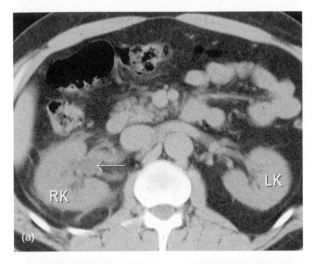

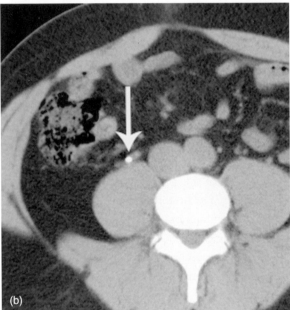

Fig. 9.9 *Ureteric calculus: computed tomography (CT). Non-enhanced CT performed in a patient with right renal colic. (a) Right kidney (RK), dilated right renal pelvis (arrow) and left kidney (LK). (b) Ureteric calculus (arrow).*

and noradrenaline. Imaging of the adrenal glands is performed for a number of applications as outlined below. Computed tomography is the investigation of choice for imaging of the adrenal glands. While adrenal masses may be seen on US, CT is more accurate for diagnosis and characterization. Magnetic resonance imaging and scintigraphy may occasionally be useful for specific indications. More specialized techniques, such as adrenal vein sampling and percutaneous biopsy, may rarely be required.

ENDOCRINE SYNDROMES

Imaging findings in Cushing syndrome are bilateral adrenal hyperplasia (70 per cent), unilateral adrenocortical adenoma (20 per cent) and adrenal carcinoma (10 per cent). Causes of primary hyperaldosteronism (Conn syndrome) are solitary unilateral adenoma (70 per cent), multiple adenomas (20 per cent), bilateral adrenal hyperplasia (10 per cent), and adrenal carcinoma (rare). When bilateral adrenal disease is seen on CT, or when CT is normal, bilateral selective adrenal vein sampling for aldosterone levels may be helpful in localizing a small abnormality and may therefore guide surgery. Primary adrenal insufficiency (Addison disease) is usually caused by idiopathic adrenal atrophy, probably autoimmune. Other causes include tuberculosis (TB), sarcoidosis, and bilateral adrenal haemorrhage caused by birth trauma, hypoxia and sepsis in neonates and anticoagulation therapy or sepsis in adults.

PHAECHROMOCYTOMA

Phaeochromocytoma is a tumour arising from chromaffin cells of the adrenal medulla. Ninety per cent occur in the adrenal gland with the other 10 per cent arising in ectopic extra-adrenal locations. Phaeochromocytoma usually presents with symptomatology related to excess catecholamine production. This includes paroxysmal or sustained hypertension, headaches, sweating, flushing, nausea and vomiting, and abdominal pain. Urine analysis reveals elevated levels of vanillylmandelic acid (VMA). Phaeochromocytoma may also be discovered in a hypertensive crisis brought on by surgery or some other stress. Ten per cent arise as part of a syndrome (e.g. multiple endocrine neoplasia, familial phaeochromocytomas, tuberous sclerosis, von Hippel–Lindau disease and neurofibromatosis); 10 per cent are malignant.

At the time of presentation phaeochromocytomas are usually large tumours measuring up to 12 cm with an average around 5 cm. Computed tomography of the abdomen, with particular attention to the adrenal glands is the initial imaging investigation of choice in the diagnosis of phaeochromocytoma.

In the past, there have been reports of hypertensive crisis precipitated by intravenous contrast material injection. It is now realized that this is extremely rare and that intravenous contrast material may be administered safely without routine premedication with α or β blockade.

When the adrenal glands are normal on CT and no obvious mass is seen elsewhere, whole-body scintigraphy with iodine-labelled metaiodobenzylguanidine (^{131}I-/^{123}I-MIBG) may be useful. Magnetic resonance imaging of the abdomen may also be diagnostic and may be used where MIBG is not available.

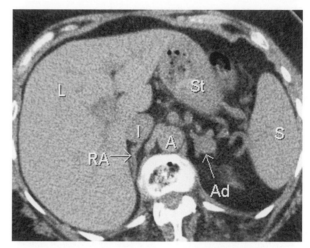

Fig. 9.10 *Adrenal adenoma: computed tomography (CT). A low attenuation mass (Ad) is seen arising on the left adrenal gland. Note also right adrenal gland (RA), liver (L), inferior vena cava (I), aorta (A), stomach (St) and spleen (S).*

THE INCIDENTALLY DISCOVERED ADRENAL MASS

Benign adrenal adenomas occur in 1–2 per cent of the population. Incidental adrenal masses are therefore a common finding on CT of the abdomen. It is important to differentiate benign from malignant, specifically adrenal adenoma from adrenal metastasis or carcinoma. An adrenal mass is a particularly significant finding where there is a history of malignancy. Tumours with a high incidence of metastasizing to the adrenal glands include melanoma, lung, breast, renal, GIT and lymphoma. It should be noted that about 50 per cent of adrenal masses seen in patients with primary carcinoma elsewhere are in fact benign adenomas, not metastases.

The CT features of a benign adrenal adenoma include small size (<3 cm), smooth contour and low density on unenhanced scans as a result of the high fat content of normal adrenal cells (Fig. 9.10). The CT features of adrenal carcinoma include relatively large size (>5 cm), higher density on unenhanced scans with low density centrally owing to necrosis, plus direct evidence of malignancy such as liver metastases, lymphadenopathy, venous invasion. Adrenal metastases tend to be larger in size (>3 cm) and of higher density on unenhanced scans.

Equivocal lesions may be further assessed with MRI. An MRI technique known as chemical shift imaging is particularly useful. Remember in Chapter 1 we discussed the precession of hydrogen atoms in a magnetic field. Hydrogen atoms in water precess at slightly different frequencies from those in fat. At certain intervals the hydrogen atoms in water and fat will be perfectly in phase and at other times, out of phase. A good analogy is to think of two children on swings in a playground, one swinging slightly faster than the other. At certain times both children will be at the top of their arcs at the same time. At other intervals the swings will be at opposite ends of their arcs. Where fat and water molecules are in close contact, such as in fat-rich adrenal cells, scans timed to detect the molecules in phase will show high signal, while scans timed to be out of phase will show reduced signal. With chemical shift MRI, normal adrenal tissue and adrenal adenomas show reduced signal on out of phase scans (Fig. 9.11). Adrenal metastases show relatively increased signal on the out-of-phase scans allowing differentiation from benign adrenal adenoma.

Occasionally, when imaging is unable to classify confidently an adrenal mass as either benign or

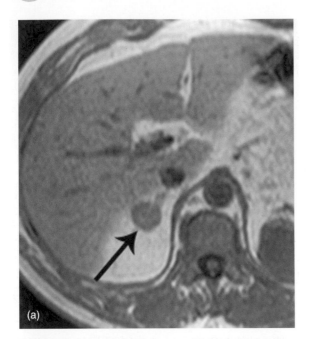

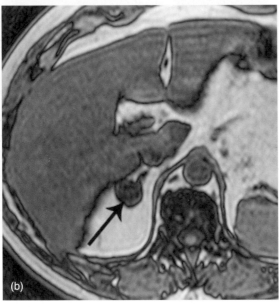

Fig. 9.11 *Adrenal adenoma: chemical shift magnetic resonance imaging. (a) In-phase gradient echo scan shows a small round mass on the right adrenal gland (arrow). (b) Out-of-phase gradient echo scan shows reduced signal intensity in the mass (arrow) typical of an adrenal adenoma.*

malignant, and where that adrenal mass is the only evidence of metastasis in a patient with a primary tumour, percutaneous biopsy under CT guidance may be required for definitive diagnosis.

TRAUMA TO BLADDER AND URETHRA

Suspected trauma to the lower urinary tract may be investigated by contrast examination of the bladder (cystoscopy) and contrast examination of the male urethra (urethrogram).

Bladder injury may be caused by blunt, penetrating or iatrogenic trauma. About 10 per cent of pelvic fractures have an associated bladder injury. Plain-film signs of bladder trauma include fracture/dislocation of the pelvis and soft-tissue mass in the pelvis resulting from leakage of urine. Air may be seen in the bladder following penetrating injury.

Urethral injury complicates about 15 per cent of anterior pelvic fractures in males. Before performing a cystogram for suspected bladder damage, the urethra must be examined. Urethral catheterization should not be attempted before urethrogram in any patient with an anterior pelvic fracture/dislocation, or with blood at the urethral meatus following trauma. Urethrogram is a simple procedure that can be performed quickly in the emergency room (Fig. 9.12). The proximal bulbous urethra is the most common site of urethral injury.

If the urethra is normal on urethrogram, a catheter can be passed into the bladder and a cystogram performed. Bladder deformity may be seen plus leakage of contrast. Leakage of contrast may be extraperitoneal in 80 per cent and intraperitoneal in 20 per cent. Extraperitoneal contrast leakage may extend into fat planes around the bladder and may track into the thigh or abdominal wall. Intraperitoneal ruptures occur with penetrating or iatrogenic trauma, with contrast leaking into the paracolic gutters and outlining loops of bowel.

IMAGING IN PROSTATISM

Prostatism refers to obstructive voiding symptoms due to prostatic enlargement. Nodular hyperplasia with enlargement of the central prostate is the commonest cause of symptomatic prostatic enlargement. The

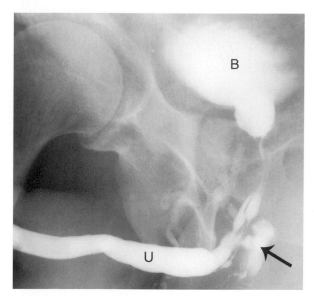

Fig. 9.12 *Urethral injury: urethrogram. Urethrogram outlines the bladder (B) and urethra (U) with leakage of contrast material (arrow) indicating a urethral tear.*

symptoms of prostatism include frequency, nocturia, poor stream, hesitancy and post-void fullness.

The primary imaging investigation in the assessment of prostatism is urinary tract US. Intravenous pyelogram is no longer recommended for routine use in prostatism. Urinary tract ultrasound includes assessment of prostate, bladder, and upper urinary tracts. Prostate diameters are measured and approximate volume calculated by a simple formula: height × width × length × 0.50 (Fig. 9.13).

The bladder is assessed for morphological changes indicating bladder obstruction, including bladder wall thickening and trabeculation, bladder wall diverticulum and bladder calculi (Fig. 9.14). Bladder volume is measured pre- and post-micturition. The kidneys are examined for hydronephrosis, asymptomatic congenital anomalies and tumours, and renal calculi.

ADENOCARCINOMA OF THE PROSTATE

Adenocarcinoma of the prostate is the second most common malignancy in males, its incidence increasing

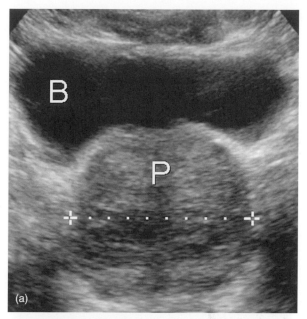

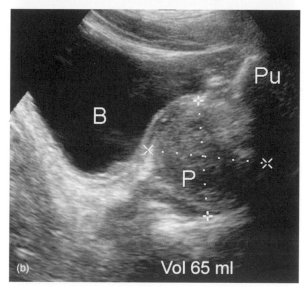

Fig. 9.13 *Prostate volume measurement: ultrasound. (a) Transverse plane. (b) Longitudinal plane. Note prostate (P), bladder (B), pubic bone (Pu).*

steadily with age. It may be diagnosed in a number of ways. Prostate carcinoma may also be diagnosed by histological examination of the tissue chips obtained by transurethral resection for presumed benign prostatic enlargement. Bone metastases may be the initial finding because of a specific presentation such as bone pain or spinal block. Multiple sclerotic metastases are

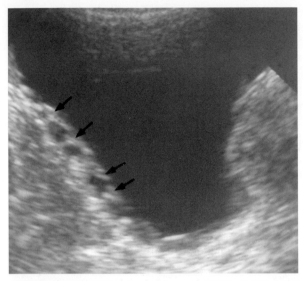

Fig. 9.14 *Bladder trabeculation: ultrasound (US). Bladder wall trabeculation caused by prostatomegaly seen on US as irregular thickening of the inner wall of the bladder (arrows).*

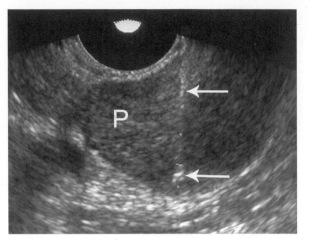

Fig. 9.16 *Prostate biopsy: transrectal ultrasound. Note the excellent visualization of the biopsy needle (arrows) within the prostate (P).*

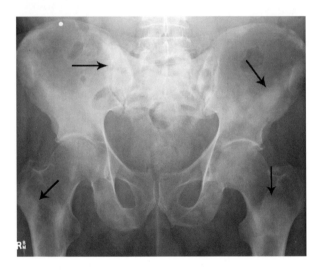

Fig. 9.15 *Bone metastases from prostate carcinoma seen as sclerotic deposits (arrows) in the skeleton.*

occasionally picked up as an incidental finding on an X-ray performed for unrelated reasons, e.g. pre-anaesthetic CXR or AXR for abdominal pain (Fig. 9.15).

Most prostate carcinomas are now diagnosed through screening. The current recommendation is that men over 50 have an annual digital rectal examination (DRE) and a prostate-specific antigen (PSA) blood assay. The PSA levels may be elevated in nodular

hyperplasia and chronic prostatitis, as well as prostatic carcinoma. An increasing PSA level in an individual patient is considered more significant than a single reading. If either DRE or PSA are abnormal, prostate biopsy is performed. This is done under transrectal ultrasound (TRUS) guidance (Fig. 9.16). Most operators perform six biopsies of the prostate (sextant biopsy). This consists of biopsy of the upper, mid and lower parts of the peripheral zone on each side. The peripheral zone is targeted, as this is where most tumours arise. Tumour is graded histologically using the Gleason scale from 2 (well differentiated) to 10 (anaplastic, highly aggressive).

The staging systems for adenocarcinoma of the prostate are the Jewett–Whitmore (A to D) and the TNM systems as follows:

- Stage A/T1: non-palpable tumour, confined to the prostate.
- Stage B/T2: palpable tumour, confined to the prostate.
- Stage C/T3: locally invasive disease with extension beyond the prostate capsule.
- Stage D/NM: distant metastases to lymph nodes and bone.

Screening with DRE and PSA has led to the diagnosis of more early-stage T1 and T2 tumours. Patients with stage T1 and T2 tumours may be offered curative therapy with either radical prostatectomy or radiotherapy. Patients with locally invasive disease, even with minor penetration of the prostate capsule are not offered surgery and are instead treated with palliative measures, including radiotherapy. Hormonal therapy is used for distant metastases. Given this current treatment regime, a key question when staging prostate carcinoma is whether or not there is invasion beyond the prostatic capsule. Computed tomography is not sensitive enough to answer this question. The two imaging tests that may be used to diagnose extracapsular extension are TRUS and MRI.

As described above TRUS is used for biopsy guidance. Prostate carcinoma may appear as a focal hypoechoic area in the peripheral zone. It is well recognized, however, that the majority of cancers are not visible on TRUS. Transrectal ultrasound is more accurate than CT in the diagnosis of extracapsular extension, though results may be somewhat variable. Magnetic resonance imaging is becoming the investigation of choice for local staging of prostate carcinoma. T2-weighted scans are able to display the architecture of the prostate with the central zone being of low signal partly surrounded by the high-signal peripheral zone. Carcinoma is seen as a low signal mass in the peripheral zone. Even small foci of extracapsular extension are well seen on MRI (Fig. 9.17). Some centres use endorectal coils to obtain high-resolution images. With modern scanners, adequate images can be obtained from surface body coils and the more invasive endorectal coils are used only for difficult or equivocal cases. The use of spectroscopy increases the accuracy of tumour detection with MRI, though has not replaced TRUS-guided biopsy.

Computed tomography is unable to reliably visualize stage T1 and T2 carcinomas, and is not sensitive enough to diagnose subtle extracapsular extension. However, more obvious locally invasive disease is well seen with CT, including invasion of seminal vesicles and invasion of the pelvic sidewall. Computed tomography is also highly accurate for the diagnosis of pelvic and abdominal lymphadenopathy. Scintigraphic bone scan is used to exclude bone metastases.

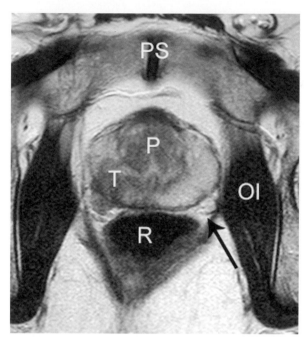

Fig. 9.17 *Locally invasive prostate carcinoma: magnetic resonance imaging (MRI). A transverse T2-weighted MRI image shows a prostatic carcinoma as a low signal tumour (T) in the posterior right peripheral zone of the prostate (P). Tumour tissue is extending through the prostate capsule and invading the right neurovascular bundle. By comparison, the normal left neurovascular bundle is well seen (arrow). Note also the pubic symphysis (PS) and obturator internus muscle (OI).*

The commonest approach to staging of prostate carcinoma is to first perform a bone scan plus CT of the abdomen and pelvis. If no bony or lymph node metastases are diagnosed, and if the CT shows no evidence of obvious locally invasive disease, MRI may be performed to exclude focal extracapsular extension.

INVESTIGATION OF A SCROTAL MASS

Ultrasound is the first investigation of choice for a scrotal mass. The primary role of US is to differentiate intratesticular from extratesticular masses; in most cases this is sufficient to distinguish malignant and benign lesions. Most (over 90 per cent) of intratesticular masses are malignant. Exceptions include testicular

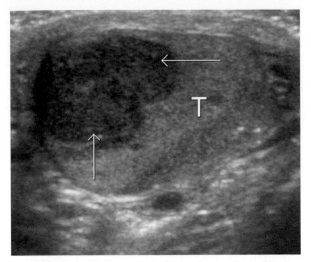

Fig. 9.18 *Seminoma: ultrasound (US). A seminoma is seen on US as a hypoechoic mass (arrows) arising in the testis (T).*

abscess, TB, sarcoidosis and benign tumour such as Sertoli–Leydig tumour.

Most intratesticular tumours are hypoechoic compared with surrounding testicle, although some may be hyperechoic, particularly in the presence of haemorrhage or calcification. Seminomas are usually hypoechoic and may be seen as a localized hypoechoic mass well outlined by surrounding hyperechoic testicular tissue (Fig. 9.18). Occasionally, with a large tumour, the entire testicle is replaced by abnormal hypoechoic tissue. Other tumour types such as choriocarcinoma, embryonal cell carcinoma, teratoma and mixed tumours usually show a heterogeneous echotexture. Lymphoma of the testis is hypoechoic and homogeneous, and may be focal or diffuse.

Further imaging for staging of testicular tumours consists of abdomen CT for retroperitoneal lymphadenopathy and chest CT for mediastinal lymphadenopathy and pulmonary metastases.

Most (90 per cent) of extratesticular lesions are benign. The most commonly encountered extratesticular masses are hydrocele, varicocele and epididymal cyst. Hydrocele is seen on US as anechoic fluid surrounding the testicle. Hydrocele may be congenital, idiopathic or secondary to inflammation, torsion, trauma or tumour. Epididymal cyst, also known as spermatocele,

is a common incidental finding on scrotal US. It appears on US as a well-defined anechoic simple cyst in the head of the epididymis (i.e. posterolaterally at the superior pole of the testis). Epididymal cyst may occasionally be large enough to present as a palpable mass.

A varicocele consists of dilated veins of the pampiniform plexus producing a tortuous nest of veins well seen on US. The vascular nature of the mass is confirmed with colour Doppler. Most varicoceles occur on the left and present with a clinically obvious mass or with infertility. Small asymptomatic varicoceles are common incidental findings on scrotal US. These are caused by venous incompetence in most cases. Varicoceles causing infertility or discomfort may be amenable to therapeutic embolization of the testicular vein. This is done via a femoral vein puncture with embolization of the testicular vein and collateral channels with steel coils.

ACUTE SCROTUM

Acute scrotum is defined as sudden unilateral scrotal swelling and is usually associated with significant pain. The main differential diagnosis in this situation is torsion versus acute epididymo-orchitis. The need for early exploration in suspected torsion gives imaging a role only in doubtful cases and where it is quickly available. Bacterial infection or mumps usually causes acute epididymo-orchitis. Scrotal haematoma, usually related to trauma, is the next most common cause of acute scrotum. Other causes include torsion of testicular appendages, strangulated hernia and haemorrhage into a testicular tumour.

Where imaging is required in the assessment of the patient with acute scrotum, US with colour Doppler is the investigation of choice. It is quick, non-invasive and highly accurate at differentiating torsion from inflammation. Acute epididymitis shows on US as an enlarged hypoechoic epididymis with increased blood flow on colour Doppler. Acute orchitis is seen as an enlarged hypoechoic testis with increased blood flow and surrounding fluid. With testicular torsion the testis may be normal in appearance or enlarged and hypoechoic. The key US signs are seen on colour Doppler with decreased spermatic cord Doppler signal and lack of blood flow in the testis.

In some centres scintigraphy is performed in the assessment of acute scrotum. Scintigraphy is a very quick method: ^{99m}Tc-pertechnetate is injected and immediate images are obtained during perfusion plus serial static images for 10 minutes. Epididymo-orchitis shows increased tracer uptake. Torsion shows a well-defined area of decreased uptake, sometimes with a surrounding 'halo' of increased uptake on the static images. Scintigraphy for the acute scrotum is now a rare examination given the high level of availability and accuracy of colour Doppler.

Once again, it should be emphasized that imaging should not hold up surgical exploration where torsion is suspected clinically.

INTERVENTIONAL RADIOLOGY OF THE URINARY TRACT

PERCUTANEOUS NEPHROSTOMY

Percutaneous nephrostomy refers to percutaneous insertion of a drainage catheter into the renal collecting system. Indications for percutaneous nephrostomy include:

- Relief of urinary tract obstruction, which may be caused by ureteric calculus, carcinoma of the bladder, ureteric TCC or carcinoma of the prostate.
- Pyonephrosis.
- Leakage of urine from upper urinary tract secondary to trauma or postsurgery.

Percutaneous nephrostomy may be performed with US and fluoroscopic guidance, or under CT control. Antibiotic cover is usually given. Local anaesthetic and sedation are usually adequate. General anaesthetic may be required in children or complicated cases.

Under imaging guidance the renal collecting system is punctured with a needle followed by passage of a guidewire and insertion of the nephrostomy catheter over the wire.

Complications may include haematuria, which is usually mild and transitory, and vascular trauma, which is very rare with imaging guidance.

URETERIC STENTS

Indications for ureteric stent insertion include:
- Malignant obstruction of urinary tract caused by carcinoma of the bladder, prostate or cervix.
- Pelviureteric junction obstruction.
- Other benign obstructions of the urinary tract, e.g. retroperitoneal fibrosis and ureteric stricture due to radiotherapy.
- Postureteric surgery.
- Extracorporeal shock wave lithotripsy (ESWL, see below) of large renal calculi, to promote passage of stone fragments and relieve ureteric obstruction by fragments.

Ureteric stent insertion may be either retrograde or antegrade. Retrograde insertion is done via cystoscopy. Antegrade insertion is performed where the lower ureter is occluded, making retrograde insertion impossible. With antegrade insertion the renal collecting system is punctured with a needle and a guide wire passed through the needle down the ureter and into the bladder. The stent is then passed over the guide wire and pushed into position. The upper pigtail of the stent should lie in the renal pelvis or upper pole calyx. The lower pigtail should lie in the bladder (Fig. 9.19).

SHOCK WAVE LITHOTRIPSY

Shock wave lithotripsy uses highly focused sound waves to fragment renal or ureteric stones. Where the shock waves are generated outside the body, the process is referred to as ESWL. Intracorporeal shock wave lithotripsy refers to shock waves generated inside the body through a ureteroscope. Shock wave lithotripsy is the technique of choice for most renal stones. Stones smaller than <1 cm are usually easily fragmented with ESWL.

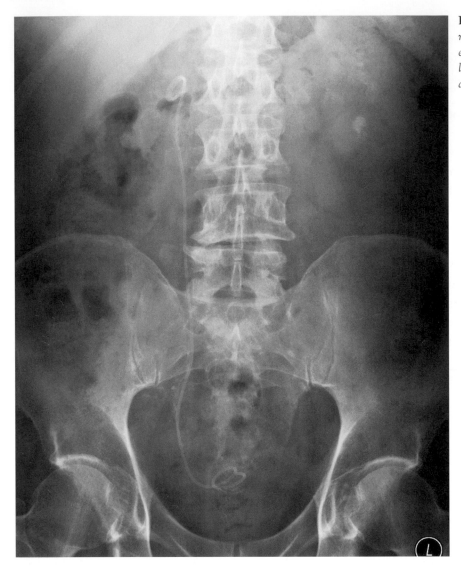

Fig. 9.19 *Ureteric stent. Note a right ureteric stent with its upper end in the right renal pelvis and its lower end in the bladder. Note also left renal calculi.*

PERCUTANEOUS NEPHROLITHOTOMY

Indications for percutaneous nephrolithotomy (PCNL) include failed ESWL, staghorn calculus and cystine or matrix calculus. It is usually performed under general anaesthetic. A retrograde ureteric catheter is inserted via cystoscopy to opacify the renal collecting system with contrast material and to prevent calculus fragments passing down the ureter. The renal collecting system is then punctured with a needle followed by passage of a guide wire. A tract into the collecting system is made with a series of dilators and the renal stone extracted by an endoscopist.

RENAL ARTERY EMBOLIZATION

Indications for renal artery embolization include:
- Control of urinary tract bleeding resulting from trauma, surgery or biopsy.
- Treatment of arteriovenous malformation (AVM) and arteriovenous fistula, which are most commonly seen as a complication of nephrostomy or biopsy.
- Palliation or preoperative reduction of vascular renal tumour, either renal cell carcinoma or large angiomyolipoma.

Female reproductive system

Ultrasound remains the mainstay of imaging in obstetrics and gynaecology. Either transabdominal or transvaginal ultrasound may be performed. Transabdominal ultrasound has a wider field of view and requires a full bladder to visualize the pelvic organs. Transvaginal ultrasound (TVUS) utilizes a transvaginal probe and higher frequency sound waves than the transabdominal approach. It provides better anatomical detail of the uterus and ovaries. A major limitation of TVUS is its smaller field of view and it is not appropriate for very young or elderly patients. Apart from these constraints, TVUS is more accurate than transabdominal ultrasound (US) in first trimester pregnancy and in most gynaecological conditions. It may be used to guide interventional procedures such as biopsy, cyst aspiration, abscess drainage and ovarian harvest. Magnetic resonance imaging (MRI) may occasionally be useful in second and third trimester pregnancy for sorting out complex fetal anomalies. Computed tomography (CT) and MRI are also used for staging gynaecological malignancies.

ULTRASOUND IN OBSTETRICS

FIRST TRIMESTER BLEEDING

First trimester bleeding occurs in around 25 per cent of pregnancies. In most cases it is a solitary event not accompanied by pain and is of no consequence. Bleeding accompanied by severe pain due to uterine contractions and a dilated cervix indicates a miscarriage and US is usually not indicated. Ultrasound may be helpful in threatened abortion, when bleeding and pain are mild and the cervix is closed. Differential diagnosis includes a normal pregnancy, missed abortion, blighted ovum, ectopic pregnancy and trophoblastic disease.

Ultrasound for first trimester bleeding should be performed with TVUS. The most important factors to establish are the presence and appearance of an intrauterine gestational sac. Knowledge of the human chorionic gonadotrophin (β-hCG) level may help to make sense of the findings. With TVUS, a gestational sac should become visible at a β-hCG level of 1000 mIU/ml (2nd International Standard). The yolk sac should become visible when the average diameter of the gestational sac is 8 mm; an embryo should be visible at 16 mm. Measurement of the length of the embryo gives the crown-rump length (CRL) (Fig. 10.1). This measurement correlates accurately with gestational age, especially if done at 6–10 weeks. Fetal heart beat should be visible on TVUS when the CRL is 5 mm.

If a gestational sac cannot be identified in the uterus despite a β-hCG level of 1000 mIU/ml or more, ectopic

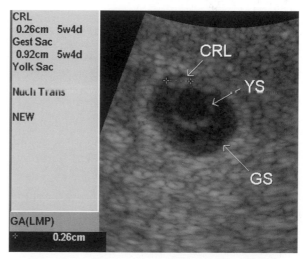

Fig. 10.1 *Early pregnancy: ultrasound. A gestational sac (GS) is seen as a round fluid filled structure in the uterus. It contains a yolk sac (YS) and a small fetal pole. Crown–rump length measurement (CRL) provides an accurate estimation of the stage of gestation.*

pregnancy should be considered. Clinical diagnosis of ectopic pregnancy is often difficult, with a history of a missed period present in only two-thirds of cases. The classic clinical triad of ectopic pregnancy consists of pain, vaginal bleeding and palpable adnexal mass. Like most classic triads, all three features occur in a minority of cases. Factors associated with an increased risk of ectopic pregnancy include increasing maternal age and parity, previous ectopic pregnancy, and previous fallopian tube surgery or infection. Transvaginal ultrasound may be able to directly visualize the ectopic gestation as a complex adnexal mass. On rare occasions fetal cardiac activity may be seen within the adnexal mass. Note, however, that an adnexal mass may not be visualized and therefore a normal pelvic US examination does not exclude ectopic pregnancy.

NUCHAL THICKNESS SCAN

Toward the end of the first trimester, a thin hypoechoic layer can be observed in the posterior neck of the fetus, deep to the skin. This is known as the nuchal translucency (Fig. 10.2). Thickening of this layer may be associated with fetal anomalies such as Down syndrome. An accurate risk assessment for the fetus having Down syndrome is calculated based on:

- Maternal age.
- Nuchal thickness.
- Presence or absence of the fetal nasal bone.
- Maternal levels of β-hCG and pregnancy-associated plasma protein-A (PAPP-A).

A chromosomal abnormality can only be confirmed by amniocentesis or chorionic villous sampling (CVS). These tests are invasive and each carries a risk of subsequent miscarriage of about 1 per cent. In general, amniocentesis or CVS are recommended if the risk as calculated from the above is 1 in 300 or more.

MULTIPLE PREGNANCY

Multiple pregnancy occurs in 2 per cent of pregnancies, with a rate of about 10 per cent for assisted conceptions. It is important to recognize multiple pregnancy as early as possible as there are a number of associated risks,

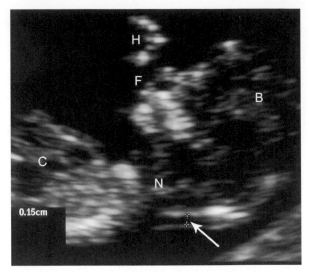

Fig. 10.2 *Nuchal fold thickness measurement: ultrasound. The nuchal fold is seen as a thin hypoechoic layer (arrow) at the back of the fetal neck (N). Note some other features of fetal anatomy: hand (H), face (F), chest (C) and brain (B).*

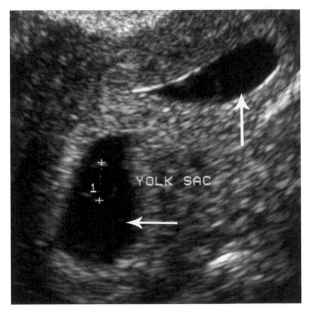

Fig. 10.3 *Twin gestation: ultrasound. This reveals two separate gestational sacs (arrows).*

as well as the social implications (Fig. 10.3). Risks to the fetuses include an increased incidence of congenital anomalies, intrauterine growth retardation and low birth weight, and premature labour. Risks to the mother include hyperemesis, cholestasis, antepartum haemorrhage, polyhydramnios, hypertension, and pre-eclampsia.

When twin pregnancy is recognized on US examination, it is important to try to classify as follows.

Dichorionic diamniotic

- May be dizygotic or monozygotic.
- Dizygotic may be different sex; monozygotic are same sex.
- Separating membrane seen between the fetuses.
- Separate placentas may be identified.
- Mortality rate 9 per cent.

Monochorionic diamniotic

- Monozygotic, therefore same sex.
- Separating membrane between the fetuses may be seen.
- Single placenta.
- Mortality rate 26 per cent.

Monochorionic monoamniotic

- Monozygotic, therefore same sex.
- No separating membrane.
- Single placenta.
- Mortality rate 50 per cent.

FETAL MORPHOLOGY SCAN

Whether a nuchal thickness scan was performed or not, a full fetal morphology scan is best performed at 19–21 weeks gestation. In Western society virtually all pregnant women will have an ultrasound scan. The obstetric scan should only be performed when the referring doctor and patient have a clear view of the benefits and limitations of the technique. The potential implications of an abnormal finding should be understood before the examination.

The fetal morphology scan provides an assessment of gestational age accurate to ±1 week, based on a number of measurements including:
- Biparietal diameter of the fetal skull (Fig. 10.4).
- Head circumference.
- Abdomen circumference.
- Femur length.

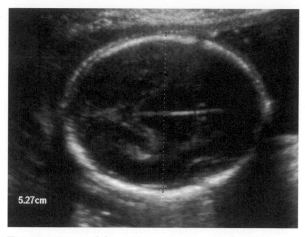

Fig. 10.4 *Biparietal diameter measurement: ultrasound.*

Placental position is documented, in particular the relationship of the lower placental edge to the internal os (i.e. diagnosis of placenta praevia). If placenta praevia is diagnosed on the fetal morphology scan a follow-up scan is performed. Owing to increased growth of the lower uterine segment in later pregnancy, the majority of placenta praevia will resolve spontaneously.

Amniotic fluid volume is assessed. Low amniotic fluid volume or oligohydramnios may be caused by intrauterine growth retardation secondary to placental insufficiency, chromosomal disorders, congenital infection and severe maternal systemic illness. Oligohydramnios may also indicate the presence of renal agenesis or obstruction of the fetal urinary tract. Common causes of high amniotic fluid volume or polyhydramnios include maternal diabetes, multiple pregnancy, neural tube defect, fetal hydrops and any disorder with impaired fetal swallowing, such as oesophageal atresia. In most cases, however, polyhydramnios is idiopathic, with no underlying cause found.

With modern US machines, a detailed assessment of fetal anatomy is possible. Most major fetal malformations are easily recognized. The fetal morphology scan also includes assessment of the fetal heart, with many congenital heart malformations able to be diagnosed at this time. Various 'soft signs' are known to be associated with an increased risk of chromosomal disorder.

SECOND AND THIRD TRIMESTER

Scans may also be required later in pregnancy for a variety of reasons.

Vaginal bleeding

Second or third trimester vaginal bleeding may be caused by premature delivery or placental problems, including placenta praevia, placental abruption and placenta accreta. Placental disorders are diagnosed with US, using a transabdominal approach. The only exception is placental abruption, which may be difficult to visualize because of the similar echogenicity of blood and placental tissue.

Follow-up of fetal abnormality

In some cases, a fetal abnormality diagnosed at the 20-week morphology scan may require follow-up. Reasons for this may include monitoring of hydronephrosis or of a soft-tissue mass such as sacrococcygeal teratoma.

Suspected growth retardation.

Clinical features suggestive of intrauterine growth retardation (IUGR) include small maternal size, slow weight gain, maternal hypertension or a history of complications in previous pregnancies such as pre-eclampsia. Intrauterine growth retardation may be confirmed by various US measurements of the fetus. As for the morphology scan, these include measurements of biparietal diameter, head circumference, abdomen circumference and femur length. The commonest cause of IUGR is placental insufficiency. In such cases the IUGR is asymmetric (i.e. the abdomen is disproportionately small compared with the head). The management of placental insufficiency is assisted with US assessment of fetal well-being. US parameters assessed include:

- Amniotic fluid volume.
- Doppler analysis of umbilical artery blood flow patterns.
- Fetal breathing movements.
- Fetal limb movements.
- Fetal heart rate.

Symmetrical IUGR (head and abdomen reduced in size to an equal degree) may be caused by chromosomal disorders including trisomy 13 or 18.

ULTRASOUND IN GYNAECOLOGY

Ultrasound is the primary imaging investigation of choice for assessment of gynaecological disorders. A variety of clinical presentations may occur, including pelvic mass, postmenopausal bleeding and irregular or painful periods in premenopausal women.

PELVIC MASSES

The first role of US in the assessment of a pelvic mass is to ascertain the organ of origin. The majority of solid masses arising from the uterus are fibroids. Fibroids are often multiple. They are usually seen on US as masses of variable echogenicity in the smooth muscle wall of the uterus (myometrium). Fibroids may project into the endometrial cavity. Alternatively, they may lie on the surface of the uterus or may even be attached by a stalk of tissue (pedunculated). Pedunculated fibroids may lie in the adnexa (in the pelvis lateral to the uterus) and may be difficult to distinguish from a solid ovarian tumour.

Most adnexal masses in women are ovarian in origin. Other possible causes of an adnexal mass would include bowel tumour, abscess or postoperative fluid collection. Ovarian masses may be classified on US as simple cysts, complex cysts (cyst complicated by soft-tissue septations or nodules) or solid. In addition to US, other data may be helpful in diagnosis, especially CA-125 (cancer antigen 125) levels.

Simple ovarian cysts

A cyst is classified as simple on US if it has anechoic fluid contents, a thin wall, and no soft-tissue components. Most simple cysts in premenopausal women are follicular cysts (Fig. 10.5). These may measure up to 5 cm and if asymptomatic require no further assessment. Similarly, a simple cyst less than 5 cm in a postmenopausal woman may be regarded as benign.

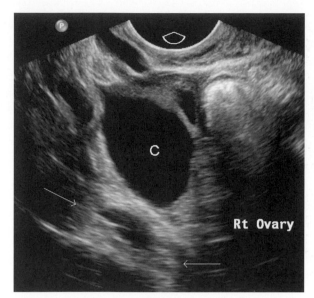

Fig. 10.5 *Simple ovarian cyst: ultrasound (US). Transvaginal US shows a simple cyst (C) arising on the right ovary and producing typical acoustic enhancement (arrows).*

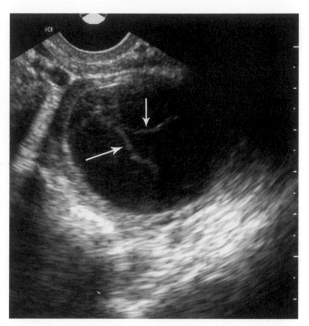

Fig. 10.6 *Complex ovarian cyst: ultrasound (US). This shows multiple soft tissue septations (arrows) in an ovarian cyst, thought to result from previous haemorrhage.*

Occasionally, simple cysts may be associated with mild pain or discomfort, in which case review in a few weeks time may be useful. Usually it is only those simple cysts that present with acute symptoms resulting from torsion or haemorrhage ('cyst accident') that require treatment.

Polycystic ovarian syndrome (PCOS) is a common cause of chronic anovulation and infertility. This refers to a spectrum of clinical disorders with the classic triad of oligomenorrhoea, obesity and hirsutism (Stein-Leventhal syndrome) being the best known. The 'Rotterdam criteria' for the diagnosis of PCOS have recently been established as follows:

- Anovulation.
- Hyperandrogenism.
- US findings of 12 or more follicles measuring 2–9 mm, and ovarian volumes of more than 10 cm^3.
- Exclusion of other possible aetiologies such as Cushing's disease or androgen secreting tumour.

Complex ovarian cysts

Complex ovarian cysts include all cysts that do not fulfil the US criteria for a simple cyst. This includes cysts with internal echoes or solid components such as soft-tissue septations, wall thickening, or associated soft-tissue mass.

In premenopausal women the differential diagnosis includes simple cysts complicated by haemorrhage giving echogenic fluid contents (Fig. 10.6). More complex lesions may be caused by ectopic pregnancy (see above), pelvic inflammatory disease, endometriosis and ovarian torsion. The most common ovarian tumour in this age-group is benign cystic teratoma or dermoid cyst. Dermoid cysts are bilateral in 10 per cent of cases. They contain fat, hair and sometimes teeth. Dermoid cysts are seen on US as complex cystic or solid lesions with markedly hyperechoic areas due to fat content (Fig. 10.7).

In postmenopausal women all complex cysts or simple cysts larger than 5 cm should be assessed by a specialist gynaecologist. Correlation with CA-125 levels may be helpful. Serous cystadenocarcinoma is the commonest type of ovarian malignancy. These are usually large (>15 cm) and seen on US as multiloculated

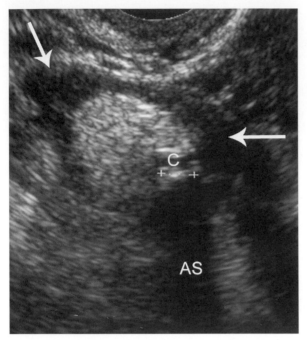

Fig. 10.7 *Dermoid cyst of the ovary: ultrasound. The right ovary (arrows) is enlarged because of the presence of a hyperechoic mass. The mass contains focal calcification (C) casting an acoustic shadow (AS).*

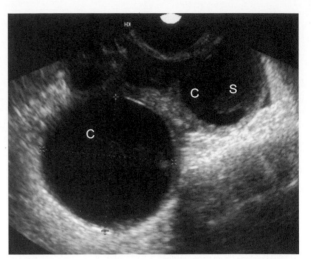

Fig. 10.8 *Cystadenocarcinoma of the ovary: ultrasound (US). Transvaginal US shows multiple cysts (C) arising on the ovary with associated solid components (S).*

cystic masses with thick, irregular septations and soft-tissue masses (Fig. 10.8). Ultrasound may also diagnose evidence of metastatic spread such as ascites and liver metastases. Other ovarian tumours seen on US as complex partly cystic ovarian masses include mucinous and serous cystadenoma, mucinous cystadenocarcinoma and endometrioid carcinoma.

Solid ovarian masses

Causes of a solid ovarian mass include fibroma, and Brenner tumour. A pedunculated fibroma may extend into the adnexa and mimic a solid ovarian mass.

ABNORMAL VAGINAL BLEEDING

As described above, abnormal vaginal bleeding may be caused by complications of pregnancy. In non-pregnant premenopausal women, abnormal vaginal bleeding is usually caused by hormonal imbalance and anovulatory cycles, treated with hormonal therapy. If

this does not control the bleeding, endometrial polyp is the primary diagnosis. Transvaginal ultrasound should be performed to measure endometrial thickness. The thickness of the normal endometrium varies with the phase of the menstrual cycle. Abnormal thickening may be caused by hyperplasia or an endometrial polyp. Saline infusion sonohysterography is a technique that enhances the accuracy of US assessment of the endometrium. A small catheter is placed in the uterus. Under direct visualization with TVUS, a small volume of sterile saline is injected to give a degree of distension of the uterine cavity. This produces excellent delineation of the two layers of endometrium and allows differentiation of endometrial masses from generalized endometrial thickening.

In postmenopausal women, atrophic endometrium is the commonest cause of abnormal vaginal bleeding. If bleeding persists despite a trial of hormonal therapy, endometrial carcinoma is the primary diagnosis. The diagnostic sign of endometrial carcinoma on US is endometrial thickening. An endometrial thickness of more than 5 mm in a postmenopausal woman is an indication for further assessment.

STAGING OF GYNAECOLOGICAL MALIGNANCIES

OVARIAN CARCINOMA

Ovarian carcinoma is the leading cause of death from gynaecological malignancy. This is because of the late stage at the usual time of diagnosis, with over 75 per cent of patients having metastatic disease beyond the ovaries. The staging system used is as follows

- Stage I: tumour confined to the ovary.
- Stage II: tumour involving one or both ovaries with pelvic extension.
- Stage III: intraperitoneal metastases and/or retroperitoneal or inguinal lymphadenopathy.
- Stage IV: distant metastases, e.g. liver metastases or malignant pleural effusion.

Most ovarian tumours are well seen with US (see above). Computed tomography of abdomen and pelvis is the investigation of choice for pretreatment staging of ovarian cancer. In particular, CT is used to search for signs of peritoneal spread such as ascites and peritoneal masses, liver metastases and lymphadenopathy. Chest X-ray (CXR) is also performed to detect pulmonary metastases and pleural effusion.

CARCINOMA OF THE CERVIX

Cervical cancer is the third most common gynaecological malignancy. The mortality from cervical cancer has decreased over the last 40 years as a result of the widespread use of the Papanicolaou (pap) smear.

The majority of cervical carcinomas are squamous cell carcinoma. The mode of spread is by local invasion plus involvement of lymph nodes. The staging system is as follows

- Stage 0: carcinoma *in situ*.
- Stage 1: confined to the uterus.
- Stage 2: local invasion beyond uterus not involving the lateral pelvic wall or lower third of vagina.
- Stage 3: more extensive invasion with involvement of pelvic wall or lower vagina or causing hydronephrosis.

- Stage 4: invasion of bladder or rectal mucosa or distant metastases, including pelvic and retroperitoneal lymph nodes.

Clinical assessment with examination under anaesthetic, colposcopy and ureteroscopy are used for initial diagnosis and assessment. Imaging is used to differentiate stage 1 tumours that can be treated with surgery from more advanced disease. Magnetic resonance imaging is the investigation of choice for measuring tumour size and assessing depth of uterine invasion and local tumour extension in the pelvis. The multiplanar capabilities of MRI are particularly useful for diagnosing tumour invasion of the pelvic sidewall and vaginal vault. Computed tomography of abdomen and chest is usually also performed to search for retroperitoneal lymphadenopathy, liver metastases and lung metastases.

ENDOMETRIAL CARCINOMA

Endometrial carcinoma is the most common gynaecological malignancy. Most tumours are adenocarcinomas, with a peak age of incidence of 55–65 years. The most common clinical presentation is postmenopausal bleeding. Fifteen per cent of women with postmenopausal bleeding will have endometrial carcinoma. The staging system for endometrial carcinoma is as follows

- Stage 0: carcinoma *in situ*.
- Stage I: tumour limited to the uterus.
- Stage IA: tumour limited to the endometrium.
- Stage IB: invasion of less than 50 per cent of the myometrium.
- Stage IC: invasion of more than 50 per cent of the myometrium.
- Stage II: invasion of the cervix with no extrauterine extension.
- Stage III: extension beyond the uterus, but not outside the pelvis.
- Stage IV: invasion of bladder or rectum, or distant metastases.

As can be seen from this staging system, the most important factor in early endometrial carcinoma is the degree of local invasion. Transvaginal ultrasound may be able to measure myometrial invasion, though in many cases not with sufficient accuracy. Magnetic resonance imaging is the investigation of choice for early stage disease. It is more accurate than US in the assessment of depth of myometrial invasion and invasion of the cervix.

BREAST IMAGING

Breast pathology may present clinically as a palpable breast mass, or less commonly with other symptoms such as nipple discharge. The two most common causes of a benign breast mass are simple cyst and fibroadenoma. Cysts occur most commonly in the decade before menopause and are uncommon in the very young and the elderly. Fibroadenoma accounts for 95 per cent of all breast masses in young women. Breast cancer is the most common malignancy in females and the second leading cause of cancer deaths in Western society. Various types of breast cancer are described. Invasive breast cancer accounts for 85 per cent with non-invasive breast cancer less common. Of the invasive cancers, the most common type is invasive ductal carcinoma, accounting for 65 per cent of all breast cancers. Invasive ductal carcinoma presents with a palpable mass or may be diagnosed on screening mammography as a non-palpable mass. The second most common breast cancer is invasive lobular carcinoma. Invasive lobular carcinoma is difficult to diagnose, being frequently missed on mammography and clinically. Of the noninvasive cancers, ductal carcinoma *in situ* (DCIS) is by far the most common type, with lobular carcinoma *in situ* accounting for most of the remainder. Ductal carcinoma *in situ* is usually diagnosed on screening mammography as focal clusters of irregular microcalcification. Imaging techniques used to evaluate breast pathology are outlined below.

Mammography

Mammography is a radiographic examination of the breast. Two types of mammography are performed,

diagnostic and screening. Diagnostic mammography is the first investigation of choice for a breast lump in women over 35 years of age. Diagnostic mammography may also be performed for other reasons such as nipple discharge, or to search for a primary breast tumour where metastases are found elsewhere. Screening mammography is performed to search for early cancers in asymptomatic women. The standard mammography examination consists of two views, craniocaudad (top to bottom) and mediolateral oblique. A range of further views may be used to delineate an abnormality seen on the two standard views. These include spot compression, magnification and angulated views. Mammography may be used to guide biopsy. It may also be used to position guidewires prior to surgical biopsy and removal of a non-palpable abnormality; this is known as localization. Most mammography systems use standard X-ray film developed in a processor or dark room. The newer technique of digital mammography uses digital radiographic systems, as described in Chapter 1.

Several signs of breast pathology are looked for on mammography. These include soft-tissue masses, calcifications and secondary signs such as distortion of breast architecture. Depending on their mammographic appearances, soft-tissue masses may be categorized as benign, probably benign, malignant, probably malignant or indeterminate. Similarly, calcification is a primary sign of early cancer, particularly DCIS. Most calcifications are small and therefore the term microcalcification is used. Many causes of benign microcalcification are also seen, including arterial calcification, calcification in cysts and calcification of benign masses such as fibroadenoma. The accuracy of mammography is variable according to the nature of the underlying breast tissue. Dense breast tissue may obscure a focal abnormality.

Ultrasound

High-resolution US now has multiple roles in breast imaging. It is the first investigation of choice for a palpable breast lump in a woman under 35 years of age, and in women that are pregnant or lactating. The traditional role for US has been differentiating cystic from solid lesions seen on mammography or found on palpation. As well as diagnosing cysts, breast US is useful for providing further definition of solid masses, specifically for differentiating benign and malignant lesions. It is also useful for assessment of mammographically dense breasts where small masses or cysts may be obscured by overlying breast tissue. Cyst aspiration, needle biopsy, guidewire localization and drainage placement are all easily and safely performed under US guidance. However, US is not able to characterize calcifications.

Magnetic resonance imaging

Magnetic resonance imaging using specific breast coils and contrast (gadolinium) injection is used in specialist centres for the detection and staging of breast cancer.

Scintigraphy

The most common application of scintigraphy in the context of breast disease is bone scintigraphy with ^{99m}Tc-methylene diphosphonate (MDP) for the detection of skeletal metastases (see Fig. 12.18).

The other major application is lymphoscintigraphy. Lymphoscintigraphy is based on identification of the sentinel lymph node. The sentinel lymph node is the first axillary lymph node that would receive tumour cells if there was metastatic spread via lymphatic channels. If the sentinel axillary lymph node can be identified and shown to be tumour free, then spread to any other axillary nodes is excluded with a high degree of accuracy. For lymphoscintigraphy, ^{99m}Tc-labelled colloid particles are injected around the breast tumour a few hours before surgery. The axillary region is imaged and the position of any positive sentinel nodes marked on the patient's skin. The surgeon may also localize the sentinel node in theatre with a hand-held gamma-detecting probe.

Breast biopsy

Breast biopsy is usually performed under imaging guidance, either mammography or US. For most masses, US is the quickest and most accurate method. With the 'freehand' technique, the US probe is held in one hand and the needle in the other. The needle is guided

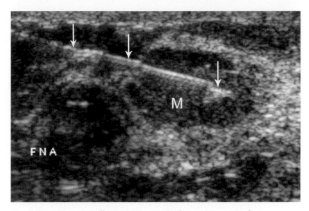

Fig. 10.9 *Fine needle aspiration of a breast mass under ultrasound guidance. The needle is seen as a hyperechoic line (arrows) passing into a hypoechoic mass (M). Cytology confirmed a fibroadenoma.*

into the mass under direct US visualization (Fig. 10.9). Cysts may be aspirated under US control. This is done to drain large cysts that are painful or to sample fluid from atypical cystic lesions. Ultrasound is unable to accurately visualize microcalcification. Therefore, for biopsy of microcalcification, mammographic guidance is used.

Several biopsy methods are used, including fine needle aspiration (FNA), core biopsy, vacuum-assisted core biopsy and open surgical biopsy requiring preoperative localization.

Fine needle aspiration is minimally invasive using 21–25 gauge needles. It is quick and relatively inexpensive, though requires an experienced cytopathologist for interpretation. Malignant lesions are usually more easily diagnosed with FNA; benign lesions may be more difficult to characterize, often leading to nonspecific reports such as 'no malignant cells seen'.

Core biopsy is performed with 14–18 gauge cutting needles that obtain a core of tissue for histological diagnosis. Best results are obtained using an automated core biopsy gun. Core biopsy may be performed under US or mammographic guidance. With core biopsy a definitive histological diagnosis is usually obtained, including benign lesions. A variation of core biopsy is vacuum assisted core biopsy (Mammotome). A Mammotome consists of an 11-gauge probe that is positioned under mammographic control. A vacuum pulls a small sample of breast tissue into the probe. This is cut off and transported back through the probe into a specimen chamber. This technique is particularly useful for microcalcification.

For open surgical biopsy non-palpable masses may be localized under US or mammographic control before surgery. Suspicious microcalcifications may be localized under mammographic control. A needle containing a hook-shaped wire is positioned in or near the breast lesion. Once correct positioning is attained, the needle is withdrawn leaving the wire in place. Either US or mammography of the excised specimen is performed to ensure that the mass or calcifications have been removed.

INVESTIGATION OF A BREAST LUMP

Palpable breast masses may be discovered by self-examination or clinical examination. It should be remembered that prominent glandular tissue may commonly mimic a breast mass in younger women. Benign solid masses and cysts tend to be mobile with well-defined smooth margins. Malignant masses tend to be firm to palpation with irregular margins and possible tethering to skin or deep structures. Mammography is the first investigation of choice for a breast lump in women over 35 years of age, with US used in younger women.

Mammographic features of a benign mass

Benign breast lesions, either cysts or fibroadenomas, tend to compress but not invade adjacent tissue. They are therefore round or oval in shape and well circumscribed, often with a surrounding dark halo caused by compressed fat. Calcification may occur in benign masses with various patterns seen:

- Large cyst: thin peripheral rim of wall calcification.
- Fibroadenoma: dense, coarse 'pop-corn' calcification (Fig. 10.10).
- Small cysts, adenosis, hyperplasia: multiple, tiny, pinpoint calcifications; milk of calcium in tiny cysts with multiple small fluid levels on the oblique view ('tea cupping').

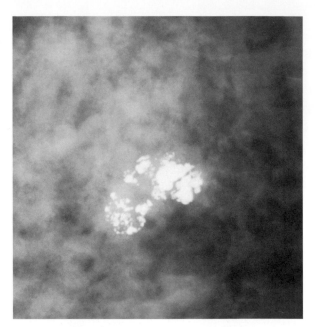

Fig. 10.10 *Fibroadenoma: mammogram. Small mass containing popcorn-like calcifications.*

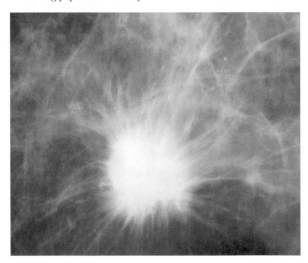

Fig. 10.11 *Breast carcinoma: mammogram. Typical mammographic appearance of a malignant mass with a dense centre and a spiculated margin.*

Mammographic features of a malignant mass

Carcinomas tend to invade adjacent tissue and often cause an irregular desmoplastic or fibrotic reaction. Carcinomas therefore tend to have irregular or indistinct margins, often described as spiculated or stellate (Fig. 10.11). There may be distortion of surrounding

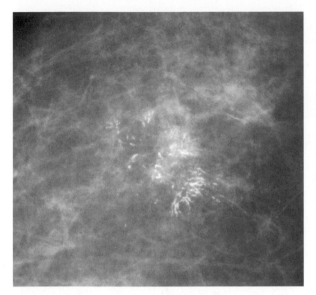

Fig. 10.12 *Ductal carcinoma in situ: mammogram. Note the typical features of malignant microcalcification: localized cluster of calcifications with an irregular branching pattern.*

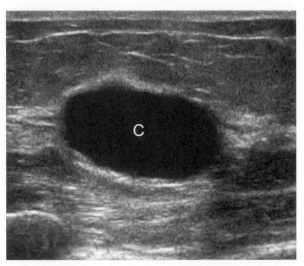

Fig. 10.13 *Simple cyst of the breast: ultrasound (US). Note the US features of a simple cyst (C): anechoic contents, smooth wall, no soft tissue components.*

breast tissue, known as architectural distortion. Secondary signs such as skin thickening and nipple retraction may be seen. Malignant microcalcification is commonly seen in association with a mass, or without a mass in the case of DCIS (Fig. 10.12). Malignant microcalcification has the following features:

- Irregular.
- Variable shape and size.
- Branching, ductal pattern known as 'casting'.
- Grouped in clusters.
- Variable density.

Ultrasound features of a simple cyst

Simple cysts are round with thin walls, anechoic contents and posterior acoustic enhancement (Fig. 10.13). Complicated cysts may have low-level internal echoes and slightly irregular walls because of infection, haemorrhage, or cellular and proteinaceous debris.

Ultrasound features of a fibroadenoma

Fibroadenoma is seen on US as a well-defined hypoechoic mass. The mass is usually ovoid in shape with its long axis parallel to the chest wall.

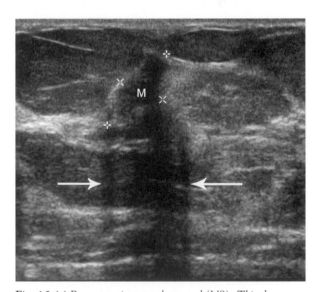

Fig. 10.14 *Breast carcinoma: ultrasound (US). This shows an irregular hypoechoic mass (M) with an acoustic shadow (arrows).*

Ultrasound features of a carcinoma

Breast carcinoma is seen on US as a focal mass with an irregular infiltrative margin and heterogeneous internal echoes. The mass is usually firm and noncompressible with a prominent posterior acoustic shadow (Fig. 10.14).

INVESTIGATION OF NIPPLE DISCHARGE

Radiological investigation is particularly useful if nipple discharge is unilateral, from a single duct, or bloodstained. First, mammography and US should be performed to exclude any obvious mass or suspicious microcalcification. If these are negative, galactography may be required.

Galactography is a procedure whereby the mammary duct orifice is gently cannulated and a small amount of contrast material injected. With gentle palpation, a small amount of discharge fluid can usually be 'milked' as a guide to which duct to inject. Also, the discharging duct is usually slightly dilated. Intraduct papilloma shows on galactography as a smooth or irregular filling defect; these may be multiple. Invasive carcinoma shows as an irregular duct narrowing with distal dilatation.

BRIEF NOTES ON BREAST SCREENING

Screening mammography refers to mammographic examination of asymptomatic women to diagnose early-stage breast cancers. Various trials have shown that screening mammography is of benefit in reducing mortality from breast cancer in women aged 50–69 years. Women in this age-group are actively recruited in countries that offer screening services. Practices vary for women aged 40–49 years. In Australia, women in this age group may choose to be screened but are not actively recruited. Screening is recommended every 2 years. For women with risk factors such as strong family history, annual mammography may be required. A dedicated team is essential to the screening process and includes radiographer, radiologist, surgeon, pathologist and counselling nurse. Mammography is the only validated screening test for breast cancer. Strict quality control over equipment, film processing and training of personnel is essential to provide optimum images and maximize diagnostic efficiency.

An abnormality on initial screening leads to recall of the patient and a second stage of investigation comprising any or all of the following

- US.
- Further mammographic views including magnification.
- Clinical assessment.
- FNA or core biopsy.

If, after this second stage a lesion is found to be malignant the patient is referred for appropriate management. About 10 per cent of recalled women will be found to have a breast cancer. The overall rate of cancer diagnosis in screening programmes is about 0.5 per cent.

11

Skeletal trauma

RADIOGRAPHIC ANATOMY OF BONE

Before exploring the general principles of bony trauma, it is important to understand some of the anatomical terms used in the skeletal system (Figs 11.1 and 11.2).

Mature bones consist of a dense cortex of compact bone and a central medulla of cancellous bone. The cortex is seen radiographically as the white periphery of a bone. The central medulla is less dense. The cancellous bone that makes up the medulla consists of a sponge-like network of thin bony plates known as trabeculae. The trabeculae support the bone marrow and are seen radiographically as a latticework of fine white lines in the medullary cavity. The bone cortex tends to be thicker in the shafts of long bones. Where these bones flare at their ends the cortex is thinner and the trabeculae in the medulla are more obvious.

Bones also have various surface features. Elevations and projections provide attachments for tendons and ligaments. A large projection is known as a process (e.g. coracoid process of the scapula); a rounded projection may be a tuberosity (lesser and greater tuberosities of the humerus) or a trochanter (greater and lesser trochanters of the femur). Articular surfaces lie at synovial articulations with other bones. Articular surfaces

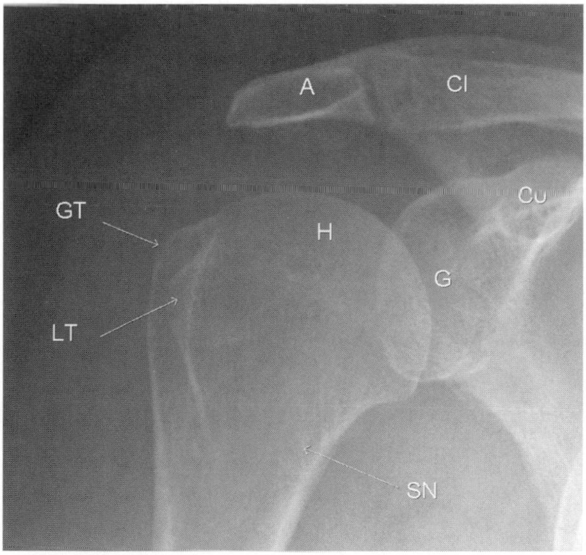

Fig. 11.1 *Normal shoulder. Note greater tuberosity (GT), lesser tuberosity (LT), surgical neck (SN), humeral head (H), glenoid (G), acromion (A), clavicle (Cl) and coracoid process (Co).*

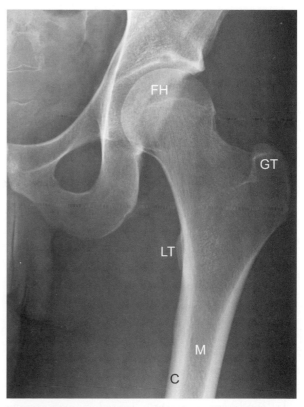

Fig. 11.2 *Normal upper femur. Note femoral head (FH), greater trochanter (GT), lesser trochanter (LT), cortex (C) and medulla (M).*

consist of smooth bone covered with hyaline cartilage. Rounded articular surfaces are termed condyles (femoral condyles); flat articular surfaces are termed facets. An epicondyle is a projection close to a condyle providing attachment sites for the collateral ligaments of the joint (humeral and femoral epicondyles). Some bones have expanded proximal ends known as the head (humerus, radius and femur).

Bones also have depressions and holes. A hole in a bone is termed a foramen (foramen ovale in the skull base). A long foramen is known as a canal (infraorbital canal). A long depression is known as a sulcus (humeral bicipital sulcus between lesser and greater tuberosities). A wider depression is termed a fossa (acetabular fossa).

Most cartilages in the body are hyaline or fibrocartilage. Smooth hyaline cartilage is more common and is found covering the articular surfaces in synovial joints. A rim of fibrocartilage known as the labrum also surrounds the articular surfaces of the acetabulum and glenoid. Fibrocartilage is also found in the articular discs or menisci of the knee and temporomandibular joint, and in the triangular fibrocartilage complex of the wrist.

GROWING BONES IN CHILDREN

Bones develop and grow through primary and secondary ossification centres (Fig. 11.3). Virtually all primary centres are present at birth. The part of bone ossified from the primary centre is termed the *diaphysis*. In long bones the diaphysis forms most of the shaft. Secondary ossification centres occur later in growing bones, with most appearing after birth. The secondary centre at the end of a growing long bone is termed the *epiphysis*. The epiphysis is separated from the shaft of the bone by the epiphyseal growth cartilage or physis. An *apophysis* is another type of secondary ossification centre that forms a protrusion from the growing bone. Examples of apophyses include the greater trochanter of the femur and the tibial tuberosity. The *metaphysis* is that part of the bone between the diaphysis and the physis. The diaphysis and metaphysis are covered by periosteum, and the articular surface of the epiphysis is covered by articular cartilage.

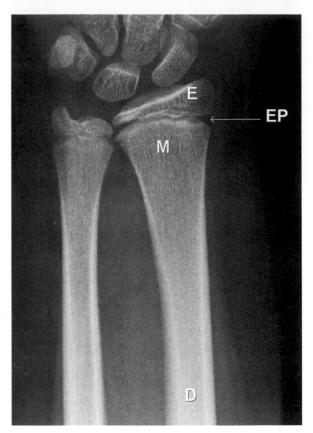

Fig. 11.3 *Normal wrist in a child. Note epiphysis (E), epiphyseal plate (EP), metaphysis (M) and diaphysis (D).*

FRACTURES AND DISLOCATIONS: GENERAL PRINCIPLES

RADIOGRAPHY OF FRACTURES

High-quality radiographs are required for the assessment of bony trauma. Fine bony detail should be visible, including crisp cortical surfaces and visible bony trabeculae. Soft-tissue planes should also be visible such that fat planes between muscles as well as small soft-tissue calcifications and foreign bodies are visible. Where a joint is being examined, the articular surfaces should be visible with radiographs angled to show minimal overlap of adjacent bones. Some bony overlap is unavoidable in complex areas and multiple views with different angulations may be required. A minimum requirement for trauma radiography is that two views be taken of the area of interest. These views should be perpendicular to each other. Most trauma radiographs therefore consist of a lateral view and a front-on view, usually anteroposterior (AP). Where long bones of the arms or legs are being examined, the radiographs should include views of the joints at each end. For example, where a midshaft fracture of the tibia is suspected, the radiographs must include views of the knee and ankle. Similarly for fractures of midshaft radius and ulna the elbow and wrist must be included.

For suspected ankle trauma three standard views are performed, AP, lateral and oblique. In other areas, extra views may be requested depending on the clinical context. These may include:

- Acromioclavicular joint: weight-bearing views.
- Elbow: oblique view for radial head.
- Wrist: angled views of the scaphoid bone.
- Hip: oblique views of the acetabulum.
- Knee: intercondylar notch view; skyline view of the patella.
- Ankle: angled views of the subtalar joint; axial view of the calcaneus.

Occasionally, stress views of the ankle or thumb may be performed to diagnose ligament damage, though usually not in the acute situation.

CLASSIFICATION OF FRACTURES

Fractures may be classified in a number of ways and are usually described by using a combination of the following terminology.

Fracture type

Common fracture types include:
- Complete.
- Incomplete.
- Avulsion.
- Stress.
- Insufficiency.
- Pathological.

Complete fractures traverse the full thickness of a bone. Depending on the orientation of the fracture

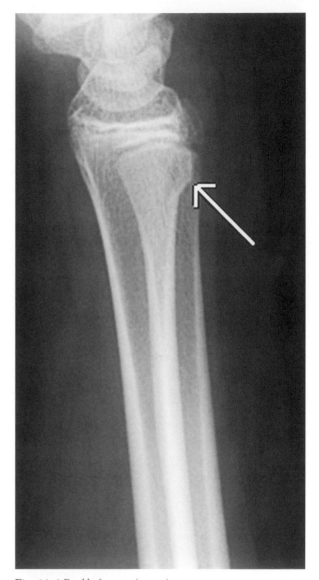

Fig. 11.4 *Buckle fracture (arrow).*

line, complete fractures are described as transverse, oblique, or spiral.

Incomplete fractures are classified as buckle or torus, greenstick and plastic or bowing. Incomplete fractures occur most commonly in children, as they have softer, more malleable bones. Buckle (torus) fracture refers to a bend in the bony cortex without an actual cortical break (Fig. 11.4). With greenstick fracture only one cortex is broken with bending of the other cortex (Fig. 11.5). Plastic or bowing fracture refers to bending of a long bone without an actual fracture line (Fig. 11.6).

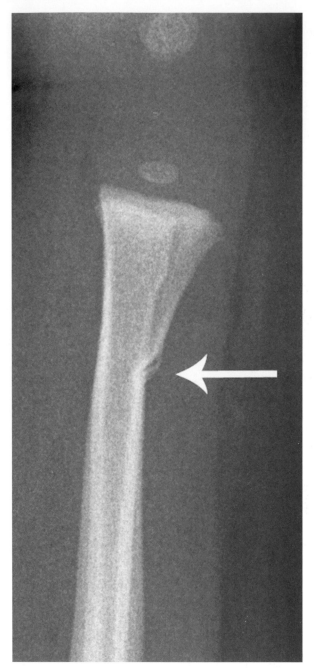

Fig. 11.5 *Greenstick fracture (arrow).*

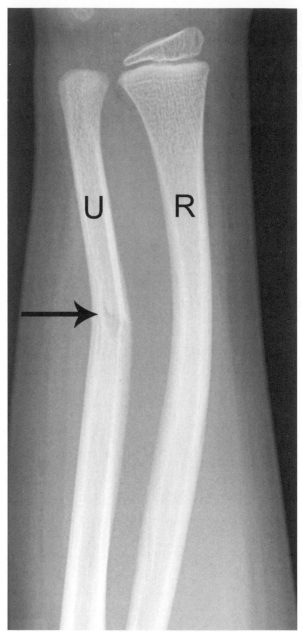

Fig. 11.6 *Bowing fracture. Undisplaced fracture (arrow) of the ulna (U), plus bowing of the radius (R).*

Avulsion fractures occur because of distraction forces at muscle, tendon and ligament insertions. They are particularly common around the pelvis in athletes, for example at the ischial tuberosity (hamstring origin) and anterior inferior iliac spine (rectus femoris origin).

Avulsion fractures also occur in children at major ligament insertions such as the insertion of the cruciate ligaments into the upper tibia (Fig. 11.7). In children, the softer bone is more easily broken than the tougher ligament, whereas in adults the ligaments will tend to tear leaving the bony insertions intact.

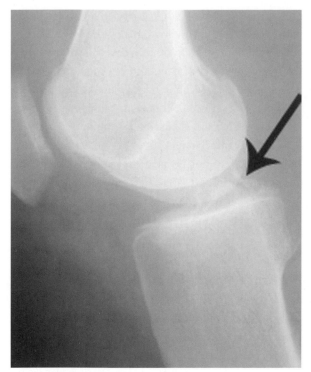

Fig. 11.7 *Avulsion fracture. Lateral view of the knee showing a small bone fragment above the posterior tibia (arrow). This is an avulsion of the tibial insertion of the posterior cruciate ligament.*

Stress fractures are caused by repetitive trauma to otherwise normal bone. Stress fractures are common in athletes and other active people. Certain types of stress fracture occur in certain activities (e.g. upper tibial stress fractures in runners and metatarsal stress fractures in marchers). Radiographs are often normal at the time of initial presentation. After 7–10 days, a localized sclerotic line with periosteal thickening is usually visible (Fig. 11.8). Scintigraphy with ^{99m}Tc-methylene diphosphonate (MDP) is usually positive at the time of initial presentation. Computed tomography is useful for stress fractures in complex areas difficult to see with radiographs.

Insufficiency fracture is a type of stress fracture in which weakened bone fractures with minor stress. A common example is insufficiency fracture of the sacrum in patients with severe systemic illnesses.

Pathological fracture is a fracture through a weak point in a bone caused by the presence of a bone

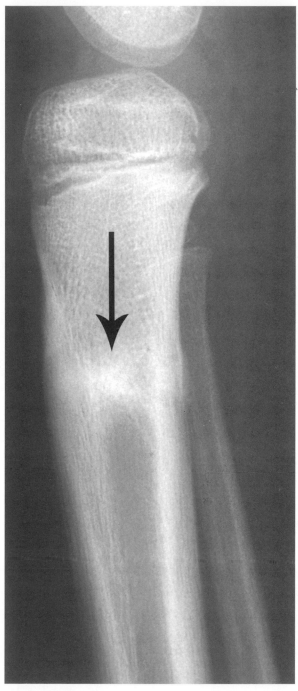

Fig. 11.8 *Stress fracture. A stress fracture of the upper tibia is seen as a band of sclerosis posteriorly (arrow).*

abnormality. Pathological fractures may occur through benign bone lesions such as bone cysts or Langerhans cell histiocytosis (Fig. 11.9). They may also be seen in association with primary bone neoplasms and skeletal

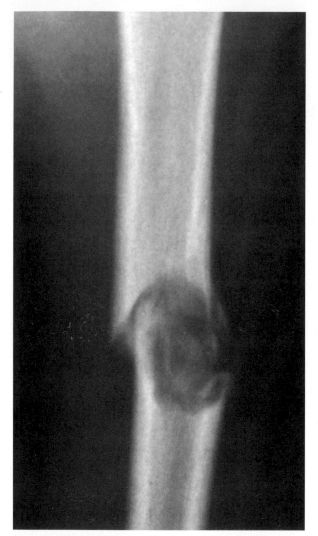

Fig. 11.9 *Pathological fracture: Langerhans cell histiocytosis. The history is of acute arm pain following minimal trauma in an 8-year-old child. Radiograph shows an undisplaced fracture through a slightly expanded lytic lesion in the humerus.*

metastases. In some cases, the underlying bone lesion may be obscured on radiographs by the fracture. The clue to a pathological fracture is that the bone injury is out of proportion to the amount of trauma.

Bone bruise is a type of bone injury caused by compression. The term bone bruise actually refers to bone marrow oedema in association with microscopic fractures of bony trabeculae, without a visible fracture line. Bone bruises cannot be seen on radiographs or computed tomography (CT). They are seen on magnetic resonance imaging (MRI) and may show areas of mildly increased activity on scintigraphy.

Bone involved and position

A description of a fracture should include naming the bone involved. The part of the bone should also be included (e.g. midshaft or distal shaft). Fracture lines involving articular surfaces are important to recognize as more precise reduction and fixation may be required. Fractures in and around the epiphysis in children, also known as growth plate fractures, may be difficult to see and are classified by the Salter–Harris system (Fig. 11.10) as follows:

- Salter–Harris 1: epiphyseal plate (cartilage) fracture.
- Salter–Harris 2: fracture of metaphysis with or without displacement of the epiphysis.
- Salter–Harris 3: fracture of epiphysis only.
- Salter–Harris 4: fracture of metaphysis and epiphysis.
- Salter–Harris 5: impaction and compression of the epiphyseal plate.

Types 1 and 5 are the most difficult to appreciate as the bones themselves are intact. Type 2 is the most

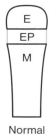
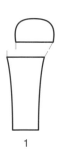
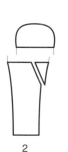
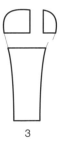
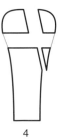
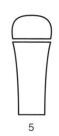

Normal   1   2   3   4   5

Fig. 11.10 *Schematic diagram illustrating the Salter–Harris classification of growth plate fractures. Note the normal anatomy: epiphysis (E), cartilage epiphyseal plate (EP) and metaphysis (M).*

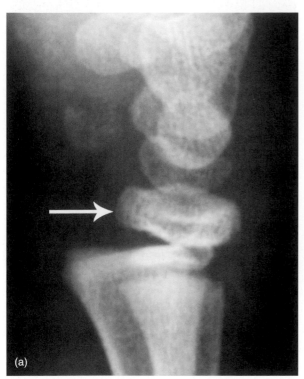

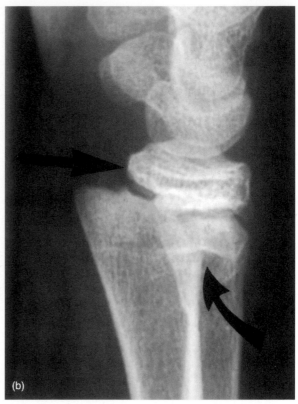

Fig. 11.11 *Salter–Harris fractures. (a) Salter–Harris 1 fracture of the distal radius with posterior displacement of the epiphysis (arrow). (b) Salter–Harris 2 fracture of the distal radius with fracture of the metaphysis (curved arrow) and posterior displacement of the epiphysis (straight arrow).*

common form (Fig. 11.11). It is important to diagnose growth plate fractures since untreated disruption of the epiphyseal plate may lead to problems with growth of the bone.

Comminution

A simple fracture has two fracture fragments only. A comminuted fracture is a fracture associated with more than two fragments. The degree of comminution is important to assess as this partly dictates the type of treatment required. A good example is fracture of the calcaneus. Fractures with three or four major fragments are usually amenable to surgical reduction and fixation. A severely comminuted fracture of the calcaneus with multiple irregular fragments may be impossible to fix, the only option being fusion of the subtalar joint.

Closed or open (compound)

A compound or open fracture is usually obvious clinically. Where a bone end does not project through an open wound, air in the soft tissues around the fracture or in an adjacent joint may be a useful radiographic sign of a compound injury (Fig. 11.12).

Degree of deformity

The degree of displacement refers to the separation of the bone fragments. Undisplaced fractures are often referred to as 'hairline' fractures. Oblique fractures of the long bones can be especially difficult to recognize, particularly in paediatric patients. A classic example of this is the undisplaced spiral fracture of the tibia in the 1-3 years age-group (the so-called 'toddler's fracture'). Undisplaced fractures through the waist of the scaphoid can also be difficult in the acute phase.

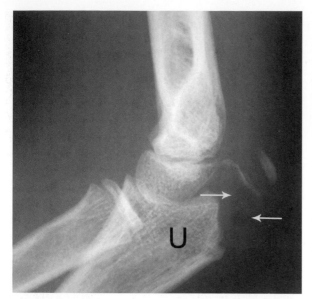

Fig. 11.12 *Compound fracture. Fracture of the proximal ulna (U) with avulsions of the triceps tendon insertion. Gas in the soft tissues (arrows) indicates a compound injury.*

Other types of deformity may also occur at fracture sites, including angulation and rotation. Angulation may occur with or without displacement.

FRACTURE HEALING

Fracture healing is also referred to as union and occurs in three overlapping stages. First is the inflammatory phase characterized by haematoma and swelling at the fracture site. Next is the reparative phase with proliferation of new blood vessels and increased blood flow around the fracture site. Collagen is laid down with early cartilage and new bone formation. This reparative tissue is known as callus. Finally comes the remodelling phase, with continued new bone formation bridging the fracture.

A major part of fracture management is knowing when to cease immobilization and when to allow unrestricted activity. The definition of union may be quite difficult in individual cases and is usually made with a combination of clinical and radiographic assessments. Different stages of union are recognized. Early union (incomplete repair) is indicated radiographically by densely calcified callus around the fracture, with the fracture line still visible (Fig. 11.13). Clinical assessment

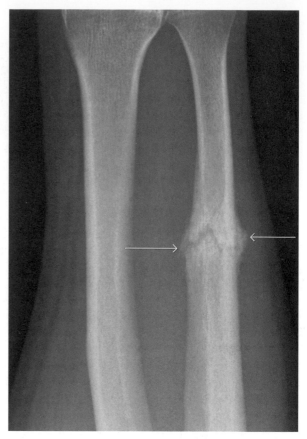

Fig. 11.13 *Early union. Subperiosteal new bone formation adjacent to the fracture (arrows).*

will usually reveal an immobile fracture site, though with some tenderness with palpation and stress. Fracture immobilization can generally be ceased at this stage, although return to full activity is not recommended. Late union (complete repair or consolidation) is indicated radiographically by ossification of callus producing mature bone across the fracture (Fig. 11.14). The fracture line may be invisible or faintly defined through the bridging bone. Clinically, the fracture is immobile with no tenderness. No further restriction or protection is necessary.

Owing to variable biological factors, it is impossible to precisely predict fracture healing times in individual cases. Spiral fractures unite faster than transverse fractures. In adults, spiral fractures of the upper limb unite in 6–8 weeks. Spiral fractures of the tibia unite in 12–16 weeks and of the femur in 16–20 weeks.

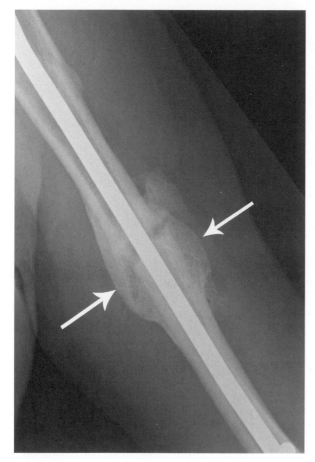

Fig. 11.14 *Late union. Dense new bone bridging the fracture margins (arrows).*

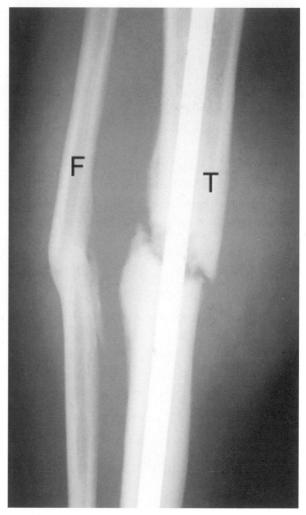

Fig. 11.15 *Non-union. Fracture of the tibia (T) 6 months previously. The fracture margins are rounded and sclerotic indicating non-union. The adjacent fracture of the fibula (F) has united.*

Transverse fractures take about 25 per cent longer to unite. Union is much quicker in children, and generally slower in the elderly

PROBLEMS WITH FRACTURE HEALING

Delayed union

Delayed union is defined as union that fails to occur within the expected time, as outlined above. Delayed union may be caused by incomplete immobilization, infection at the fracture site, pathological fractures or vitamin C deficiency, or may occur in elderly patients.

Non-union

The term 'non-union' implies that the bone will never unite without some form of intervention. Non-union is diagnosed radiographically with sclerosis (increased density) of the bone ends at the fracture site. The fracture margins often have rounded edges and the fracture line is still clearly visible (Fig. 11.15). A variation of non-union may be seen where there is mature bone formation around the edge of the fracture with failure of healing of the central fracture line. This may be difficult to recognize radiographically and CT may be required for diagnosis. This form of non-union may be suspected where there is ongoing pain despite apparently solid radiographic union.

Traumatic epiphyseal arrest

Traumatic epiphyseal arrest refers to premature closure of a bony growth plate due to failure of recognition or inadequate management of a growth plate fracture. An example of this is fracture of the lateral epicondyle of the humerus leading to premature closure of the growth plate and alteration of the carrying angle of the elbow.

Malunion

In malunion complete bone healing has occurred, and if in a poor position it leads to bone or joint deformity, and often to early osteoarthritis (Fig. 11.16).

OTHER COMPLICATIONS OF FRACTURES

Associated soft-tissue injuries

There are many examples of soft-tissue injuries associated with fractures. These are often of more clinical significance than the bony injuries. For example, pneumothorax may complicate rib fractures. Significant haemorrhage may occur in association with fractures of the pelvis and femur.

Complications of recumbency

Complications such as pneumonia and deep venous thrombosis (DVT) are common complications of recumbency, especially in the elderly.

Arterial injury

Arterial laceration and occlusion causing acute limb ischaemia may be seen in association with displaced fractures of the femur or tibia, and in the upper limb with displaced fractures of the distal humerus and elbow dislocation.

Nerve injury

Nerve injury following fracture or dislocation is a relatively rare event. The best-known examples are listed below:
- Shoulder dislocation: axillary nerve.
- Fracture midshaft humerus: radial nerve.
- Displaced supracondylar fracture humerus: median nerve.

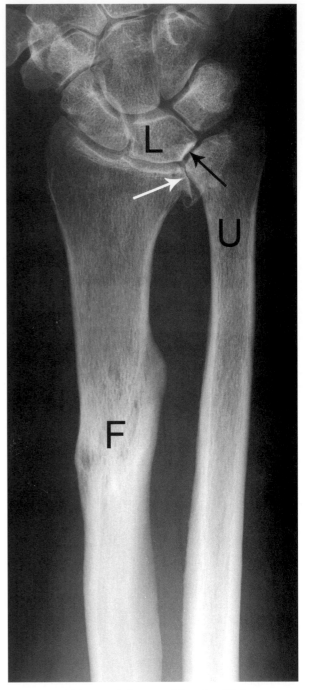

Fig. 11.16 Malunion. A fracture of the radius (F) has united with shortening of the radius. As a result the ulna (U) is relatively longer than the radius (positive ulnar variance) and is contacting the lunate (L, black arrow). This is known as ulnar abutment and is a cause of wrist pain. There is also secondary osteoarthritis of the distal radio-ulnar joint (white arrow).

- Elbow dislocation: ulnar nerve.
- Hip dislocation: sciatic nerve.
- Knee dislocation: tibial nerve.
- Fractured neck of fibula: common peroneal nerve.

Avascular necrosis

Traumatic avascular necrosis (AVN) occurs most commonly in three sites: proximal pole of scaphoid, femoral head and body of talus. In these sites, AVN is caused by interruption of blood supply, as may occur in fractures of the waist of the scaphoid, femoral neck and neck of talus. New bone is laid down on necrosed bone trabeculae causing the non-vascularized portion of bone to become sclerotic on radiographs over 2–3 months. Because of weight bearing, the femoral head and talus may show deformity and irregularity as well as sclerosis.

Reflex sympathetic dystrophy (Sudeck's atrophy):

Reflex sympathetic dystrophy may follow trivial bone injury. It occurs in bones distal to the site of injury and is associated with severe pain and swelling. Radiographic changes include a marked decrease in bone density distal to the fracture site, with thinning of the bone cortex. Scintigraphy shows increased tracer uptake in the limb distal to the trauma site.

Myositis ossificans

Myositis ossificans refers to posttraumatic non-neoplastic formation of bone within skeletal muscle, usually within 5–6 weeks of trauma. Myositis ossificans may occur at any site, though the muscles of the anterior thigh are most commonly affected. It is seen radiographically as bone formation in the soft tissues. This bone has a striated appearance conforming to the structure of the underlying muscle.

FRACTURES AND DISLOCATIONS: SPECIFIC AREAS

In the following section radiographic signs of the more common fractures and dislocations will be discussed.

Those lesions that may cause problems with diagnosis will be emphasized. Most fractures and dislocations are diagnosed with radiographs. Other imaging modalities will be described where applicable.

SHOULDER

Fractured clavicle

Fractures of the clavicle usually involve the middle third. The outer fragment usually lies at a lower level than the inner fragment with the acromioclavicular joint intact.

Acromioclavicular joint dislocation

With acromioclavicular joint dislocation there is widening of the joint space with elevation of the outer end of the clavicle. The underlying pathology is tearing of the coracoclavicular ligaments seen radiographically as increased distance between the under-surface of the clavicle and the coracoid process. Radiographic signs may be subtle and weight-bearing views may be useful in doubtful cases (Fig. 11.17).

Anterior dislocation of the shoulder

With anterior dislocation the humeral head lies anterior to the glenoid fossa. This is easily seen on a lateral radiograph. On the AP view the humeral head overlaps the lower glenoid and the lateral border of the scapula (Fig. 11.18). Associated fractures occur commonly and include:

- Wedge-shaped defect in the posterolateral humeral head (Hill–Sachs deformity).
- Fracture of the inferior rim of the glenoid (Bankart lesion).
- Fracture of the greater tuberosity (Fig. 11.18).
- Fracture of the surgical neck of the humerus.

Recurrent anterior dislocation may be seen in association with fracture of the glenoid, fracture of the anterior cartilage labrum and laxity of the joint capsule and glenohumeral ligaments. These injuries are diagnosed with MRI (see Chapter 12).

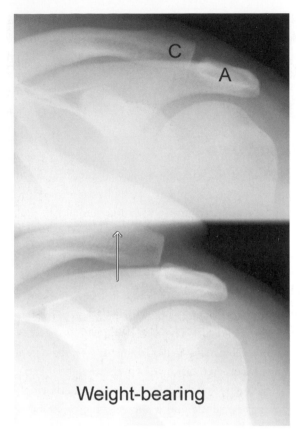

Weight-bearing

Fig. 11.17 *Acromioclavicular joint dislocation. Note: acromion (A) and clavicle (C). At rest the acromioclavicular joint shows normal alignment. A radiograph performed with weight-bearing shows upward dislocation of the clavicle (arrow).*

Posterior dislocation of the shoulder

Posterior shoulder dislocation is a rare injury, representing only 2 per cent of shoulder dislocations. It is easily missed on radiographic examination. Signs on the AP film are often subtle and include loss of parallelism of the articular surface of the humeral head and glenoid fossa. There is medial rotation of the humerus so that the humeral head looks symmetrically rounded like an ice-cream cone or an electric light bulb (Fig. 11.19). On the lateral film the humeral head is seen posterior to the glenoid fossa.

HUMERUS

Proximal fractures commonly involve the surgical neck of the humerus. These fractures are often significantly

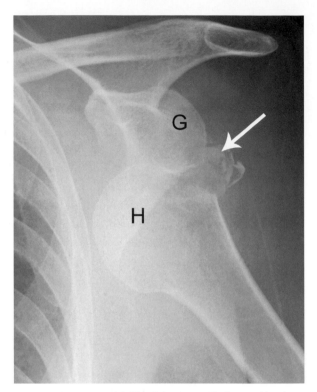

Fig. 11.18 *Anterior shoulder dislocation. The humeral head (H) lies anterior and medial to the glenoid (G). Associated fracture of greater tuberosity (arrow).*

displaced or impacted. Less commonly, fractures of the greater tuberosity or lesser tuberosity may be seen. With severe injuries, combinations of the above may occur. Humeral shaft fractures may be transverse, oblique, simple or comminuted.

ELBOW

Elbow joint effusion

Fat pads lie on the anterior and posterior surfaces of the distal humerus at the attachments of the synovium of the elbow joint. On a lateral view of the elbow these fat pads are usually not visualized, though occasionally the anterior fat pad may be seen applied to the anterior surface of the humerus. With an elbow joint effusion the fat pads are lifted off the humeral surfaces and are seen on lateral radiographs of the elbow as dark-grey triangular structures (Fig. 11.20). There is a high rate of association of elbow joint effusion with fracture. Recognition of such effusions is therefore very important in the

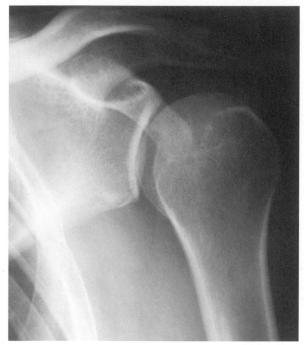

Fig. 11.19 *Posterior shoulder dislocation. In posterior dislocation the humeral head is internally rotated with the articular surface of the humerus facing posteriorly. As a result, the humeral head has a symmetric round configuration likened to a light bulb or ice cream cone. Compare this with the normal appearance in Figure 11.1, page 157.*

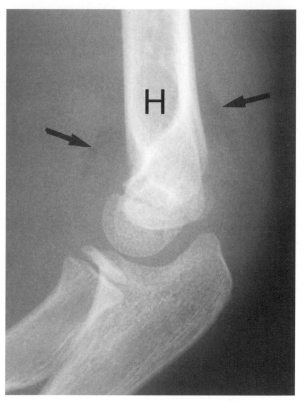

Fig. 11.20 *Elbow joint effusion. Elbow joint effusion causes elevation of the anterior and posterior fat pads producing triangular lucencies (arrows) anterior and posterior to the distal humerus (H).*

diagnosis of subtle elbow fractures. Where an elbow joint effusion is present in a setting of trauma and no fracture can be seen on standard elbow films, consider an undisplaced fracture of the radial head or a supracondylar fracture of the distal humerus. In this situation, either perform further oblique views or treat and repeat radiographs in 7–10 days.

Supracondylar fracture

Supracondylar fracture of the distal humerus may be undisplaced or displaced anteriorly or posteriorly. Posterior displacement is the most common and when severe may be associated with injury to brachial artery and median nerve (Fig. 11.21).

Fracture and separation of the lateral condylar epiphysis

Fracture of the lateral humeral epicondyle in children may be missed on radiographs or may look deceptively

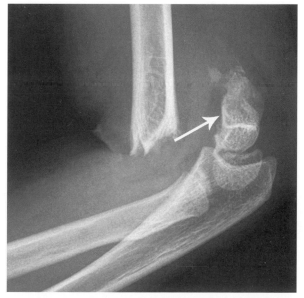

Fig. 11.21 *Supracondylar fracture, distal humerus. The distal fragment is displaced posteriorly (arrow).*

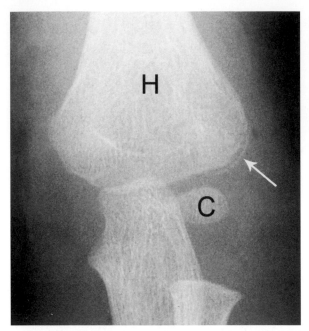

Fig. 11.22 *Lateral humeral condyle fracture. Note the normal appearance of the humerus (H) and growth centre for the capitulum (C) in an 18-month-old child. A fracture of the lateral humeral condyle is seen as a thin sliver of bone adjacent to the distal humerus (arrow).*

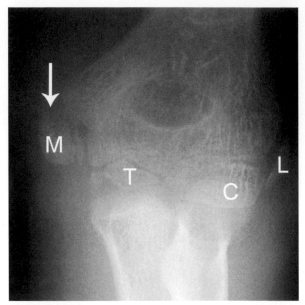

Fig. 11.23 *Medial humeral epicondyle fracture. Note the normal growth centres in a 12-year-old child: capitulum (C), trochlea (T), lateral epicondyle (L). The growth centre for the medial epicondyle (M) is displaced with a small adjacent fracture fragment (arrow). Although subtle, this represents a significant elbow injury.*

small, as the growth centre may be predominantly cartilage (Fig. 11.22). Adequate treatment is vital as this fracture may damage the growth plate and the articular surface, leading to deformity.

Fracture of the head of the radius

Three patterns of radial head fracture are commonly seen: vertical split, small lateral fragment or multiple fragments. Radial head fracture may be difficult to see and elbow joint effusion may be the only radiographic sign initially.

Fracture of the olecranon

Two patterns of olecranon fracture are commonly seen, either comminuted fracture or a single transverse fracture line with separation of fragments due to unopposed action of the triceps muscle.

Other elbow fractures

'T'- or 'Y'-shaped fracture of the distal humerus with separation of the humeral condyles. Fracture

separation of the capitulum usually results in the capitulum being sheared off vertically. Fracture and separation of the medial epicondylar apophysis may occur in children and may be difficult to recognize (Fig. 11.23).

RADIUS AND ULNA

Midshaft fractures usually involve both radius and ulna. They may be transverse, oblique, angulated or displaced. Isolated fracture of the midshaft of either radius or ulna should be diagnosed with caution. More commonly there is associated disruption of wrist or elbow joint. Two patterns are seen:

- Monteggia fracture: anteriorly angulated fracture of upper third of the shaft of the ulna is often associated with anterior dislocation of the radial head (Fig. 11.24).
- Galeazzi fracture: fracture of the lower third of the shaft of the radius may be associated with subluxation or dislocation of the distal radio-ulnar joint.

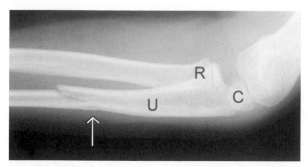

Fig. 11.24 *Monteggia fracture–dislocation. Fracture of the ulna (arrow). The head of the radius (R) is displaced from the capitulum (C) indicating dislocation.*

The distal radius is the most common site of radial fracture. The classical Colles' fracture consists of a transverse fracture of the distal radius with the distal fragment angulated and/or displaced posteriorly, usually associated with avulsion of the tip of the ulnar styloid process. The less common Smith's fracture refers to anterior angulation of the distal radial fragment. The distal radius is a common fracture site in children with buckle, greenstick or Salter–Harris type 2 fractures particularly common. Comminuted fracture of the distal radius is a common injury in adults. Fracture lines may extend into the articular surfaces. Computed tomography may be used for planning of surgical reduction of these complex fractures (Fig. 11.25).

WRIST AND HAND

Scaphoid fracture

Two common patterns of scaphoid fracture are seen:
- Transverse fracture of the waist of the scaphoid.
- Fracture and separation of the scaphoid tubercle.

Undisplaced fracture of the waist of the scaphoid may be difficult to see on radiographs at initial presentation, even on dedicated oblique views (Fig. 11.26).

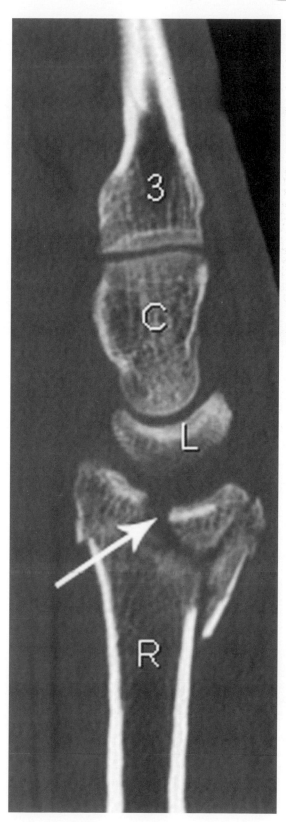

Fig. 11.25 *Distal radius fracture: computed tomography (CT). Multidetector CT sagittal image shows the anatomy of a complex comminuted fracture of the distal radius (arrow). Note also lunate (L), capitate (C) and third metacarpal (3).*

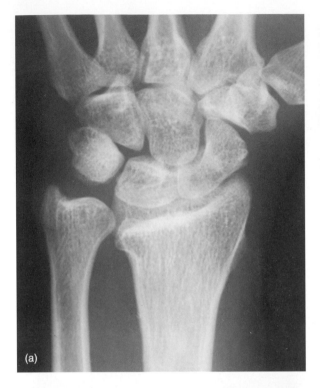

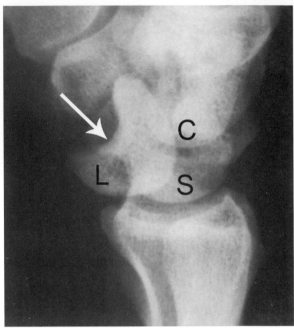

Fig. 11.27 *Lunate dislocation. Lateral radiograph of the wrist showing the capitate (C) and scaphoid (S) in normal position with the lunate (L) displaced anteriorly. Note the distal articular surface of the lunate (arrow). This would normally articulate with the capitate.*

Further investigations may be required to confirm the diagnosis. This usually consists of a repeat radiograph after 7–10 days of immobilization. If immediate diagnosis is required, scintigraphic bone scan will be positive within 24 hours.

Lunate dislocation

Lunate dislocation refers to anterior dislocation of the lunate. This may be difficult to appreciate on the frontal film, though is easily seen on the lateral view with the lunate rotated and displaced anteriorly (Fig. 11.27).

Perilunate dislocation

In perilunate dislocation, the lunate articulates normally with the radius, with the remainder of the carpal bones displaced posteriorly. On the frontal radiograph there is abnormal overlap of bone shadows, with dissociation of articular surfaces of the lunate and capitate. The lateral film shows minimal, if any, rotation of the lunate with

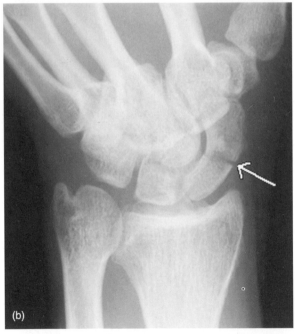

Fig. 11.26 *Scaphoid fracture. (a) Frontal radiograph of the wrist shows no fracture. (b) Oblique view of the scaphoid shows an undisplaced fracture (arrow). This example demonstrates the need to obtain dedicated scaphoid views where scaphoid fracture is suspected.*

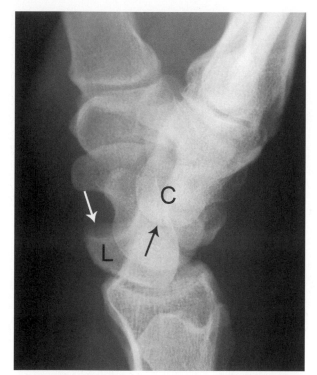

Fig. 11.28 *Perilunate dislocation. Lateral radiograph of the wrist showing the lunate (L) in normal position with the capitate (C) and other carpal bones displaced posteriorly. Note the separation of the distal articular surface of the lunate (white arrow) from the proximal articular surface of the capitate (black arrow).*

posterior displacement of the remainder of the carpal bones (Fig. 11.28). Perilunate dislocation may be associated with scaphoid fracture (trans-scaphoid perilunate dislocation), or fracture of the radial styloid.

Other carpal fractures

Avulsion fracture of the posterior surface of the triquetral is seen only on the lateral view as a small fragment of bone adjacent to the posterior surface of the triquetral.

Fracture of the hook of hamate is a common injury in golfers and tennis players.

Ligament and cartilage injuries

The wrist is an anatomically complex area with several important ligament and cartilages supporting the carpal bones. The most commonly injured structures are scapholunate ligament, triquetrolunate ligament, and triangular fibrocartilage complex. Suspected ligament and cartilage injuries may be investigated with stress radiographs to demonstrate carpal instability and MRI.

Hand fractures

Fractures of the metacarpals and phalanges are common. Fracture through the neck of the fifth metacarpal is the classic 'punching injury'. Fractures of the base of the first metacarpal are usually unstable. Two patterns of fracture are seen: either a transverse fracture of the proximal shaft, with lateral bowing, or an oblique fracture extending to the articular surface at the base of the first metacarpal. Avulsion fracture of the distal extensor tendon insertion at the base of the distal phalanx may result in a flexion deformity of the distal interphalangeal joint (Mallet finger) (Fig. 11.29).

PELVIS

Pelvic ring fracture

In general, fractures of the pelvic ring occur in two separate places, though there are exceptions. Three common patterns of injury are seen:
- Separation of the pubic symphysis with widening of a sacroiliac joint, or fracture of the posteromedial aspect of the iliac bone.
- Fractures of the superior and inferior pubic rami, which may be unilateral or bilateral.
- Unilateral fracture of the pubic rami anteriorly, and the iliac bone posteriorly.

Pelvic ring fractures have a high rate of association with urinary tract injury (see Chapter 9) and with arterial injury causing severe blood loss. Angiography and embolization may be required in such cases.

Hip dislocation

Anterior dislocation is a rare injury easily recognized radiographically and not usually associated with fracture. Posterior dislocation is the most common form of hip dislocation. The femoral head dislocates posteriorly and superiorly. Posterior dislocation is usually associated with small or large fractures of the posterior acetabulum, and occasionally fractures of the femoral head.

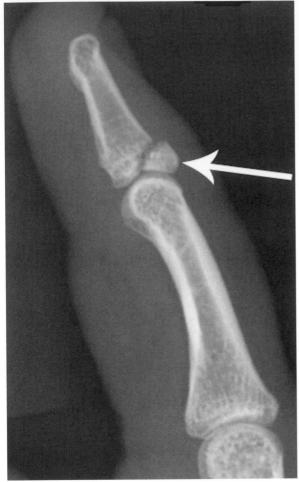

Fig. 11.29 *Mallet finger. Lateral radiograph shows an avulsion fracture (arrow) at the dorsal base of the distal phalanx at the distal attachment of the extensor tendon. As a result, the distal interphalangeal joint cannot be extended.*

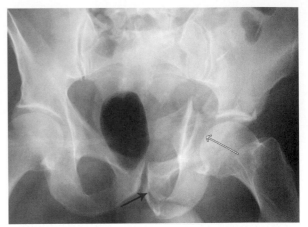

Fig. 11.30 *Acetabulum fracture. A comminuted fracture of the acetabulum with central impaction of the femoral head (white arrow). Note also a fracture of the pubic bone (black arrow).*

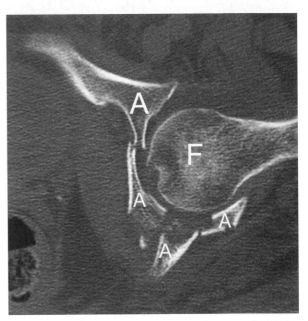

Fig. 11.31 *Acetabulum fracture: computed tomography (CT). The precise anatomy of an acetabular fracture is demonstrated with CT. Note multiple acetabular fragments (A) and the femoral head (F).*

Fractures of the acetabulum

Three common acetabular fracture patterns are seen:

- Fracture through the anterior acetabulum associated with fracture of the inferior pubic ramus.
- Fracture through the posterior acetabulum extending into the sciatic notch associated with fracture of the inferior pubic ramus.
- Horizontal fracture through the acetabulum.

Acetabular fractures are difficult to define radiographically because of the complexity of the anatomy and overlapping bony structures (Fig. 11.30). Computed tomography with multiplanar and three-dimensional (3D) reconstructions is useful for definition of fractures and for planning of operative reduction. Combinations of the above fracture patterns may be seen as well as extensive comminution and central dislocation of the femoral head (Fig. 11.31).

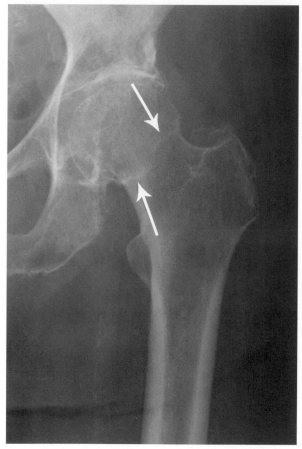

Fig. 11.32 *Neck of femur fracture. An undisplaced fracture of the neck of femur is seen as a sclerotic line (arrows).*

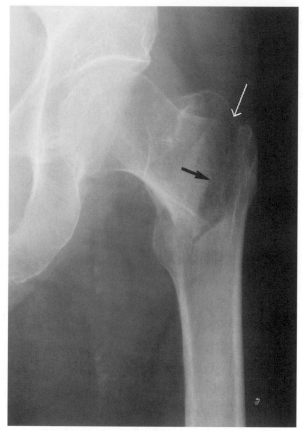

Fig. 11.33 *Intertrochanteric fracture. A fracture line is seen extending from the greater trochanter (white arrow) inferiorly through the intertrochanteric region (black arrow).*

FEMUR

Fractures of the upper femur (also known as hip fractures) are particularly common in the elderly and have a strong association with osteoporosis. Femoral neck fracture usually consists of a fracture across the femoral neck with varying degrees of angulation and displacement. The occasional undisplaced or mildly impacted fracture may be difficult to recognize radiographically. Look for a faint sclerotic band passing across the femoral neck (Fig. 11.32). Fracture of the femoral neck is complicated by avascular necrosis in 10 per cent of cases, with a higher rate for severely displaced fractures. Intertrochanteric fracture varies in appearance from an undisplaced oblique fracture to comminuted fractures with marked displacement of the lesser and greater trochanters (Fig. 11.33). Subtrochanteric fracture refers to fracture below the lesser trochanter.

Fractures of the femoral shaft are easily recognized radiographically. Common patterns include transverse, oblique, spiral and comminuted fractures with varying degrees of displacement and angulation. Femoral shaft fractures are often associated with severe blood loss and occasionally with fat embolism.

KNEE

Lower femur

The most common distal femoral fracture is the supracondylar fracture. This usually consists of a transverse fracture above the femoral condyles with posterior angulation of the distal fragment best appreciated on the lateral radiograph. Fracture and separation of a femoral condyle may also occur. 'T'- or 'Y'-shaped distal femoral fracture may also be seen, with a vertical

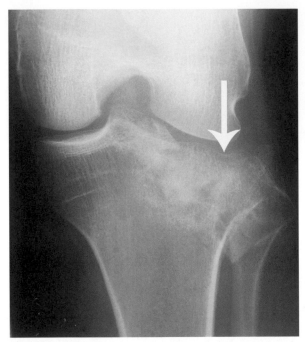

Fig. 11.34 *Tibial plateau fracture. Note an inferiorly impacted fracture of the lateral tibial plateau (arrow).*

fracture line extending upwards from the articular surface causing separation of the femoral condyles.

Patella

Three common patterns of patellar fractures are seen:
- Undisplaced fracture.
- Displaced transverse fracture.
- Complex comminuted fracture.

All patterns may be associated with haemarthrosis. Fracture of the patella should not be confused with bipartite patella. This is a common anatomical variant with a fragment of bone separated from the superolateral aspect of the patella. Unlike an acute fracture, the bone fragments in bipartite patella are corticated (i.e. they have a well-defined white margin).

Tibial plateau

Common patterns of upper tibial injury include:
- Crush fracture of the lateral tibial plateau (Fig. 11.34).

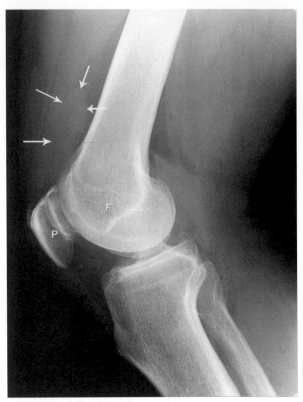

Fig. 11.35 *Knee joint effusion. Lateral radiograph shows fluid distending the suprapatellar recess of the knee joint (arrows) extending superiorly between the patella (P) and the femur (F).*

- Fracture and separation of one or both tibial condyles.
- Complex comminuted fracture of the upper tibia.

Minimally crushed or displaced fractures of the upper tibia may be difficult to recognize radiographically. Often the only clue is the presence of a joint effusion or lipohaemarthrosis (Figs 11.35 and 11.36). Oblique views may be required to diagnose subtle fractures; CT with multiplanar reconstructions is often performed to define the injury and assist in the planning of surgical management.

TIBIA AND FIBULA

Fracture of the tibial shaft is usually associated with fracture of the fibula. Fractures may be transverse, oblique, spiral, and comminuted with varying degrees of displacement and angulation. Fractures of the tibia

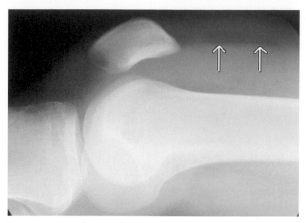

Fig. 11.36 *Lipohaemarthrosis. Lateral radiograph obtained with the patient supine shows distension of the suprapatellar recess of the knee joint. A fluid level (arrows) results from the presence of fat floating on more dense blood. This finding is virtually always associated with a fracture.*

are often open (compound) with an increased incidence of osteomyelitis, compartment syndrome, and vascular injury. In particular, injury to the popliteal artery and its major branches requires emergency angiography and treatment.

Isolated fracture of the tibia is a relatively common injury in children aged 1–3 years (toddler's fracture). These fractures are often undisplaced and therefore very difficult to see. They are usually best seen as a thin oblique lucent line on the lateral radiograph (Fig. 11.37). Scintigraphic bone scan may be useful in difficult cases.

Isolated fracture of the shaft of the fibula may occur secondary to direct trauma. More commonly, an apparently isolated fracture of the upper fibula is associated with disruption of the syndesmosis between the distal tibia and fibula. This combination is known as a Maissoneuve fracture.

ANKLE AND FOOT

Common ankle fractures

Injuries may include fractures of the distal fibula (lateral malleolus), fractures of distal tibia medially (medial malleolus) and posteriorly, talar shift and displacement, fracture of the talus, separation of the distal tibiofibular joint and ligament rupture with joint instability.

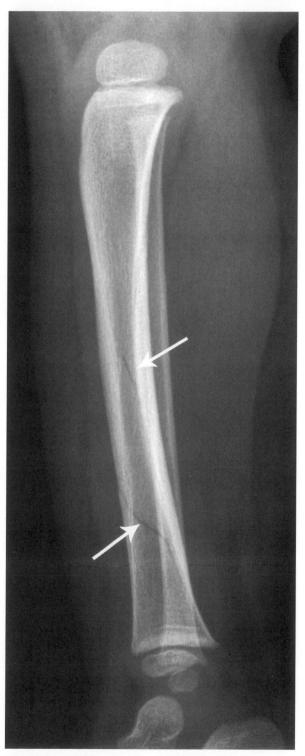

Fig. 11.37 *Toddler's fracture. Undisplaced spiral fracture of the tibia (arrows).*

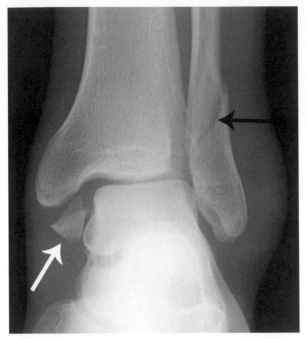

Fig. 11.38 *Ankle fracture due to external rotation. Note: spiral fracture of distal fibula (black arrow), avulsion of medial malleolus (white arrow), lateral shift of talus, widening of the space between distal tibia and fibula indicating syndesmosis injury.*

Salter–Harris fractures of the distal tibia and fibula are common in children. The pattern of fracture seen on X-ray depends on mechanism of injury:

- Adduction: vertical fracture of the medial malleolus, avulsion of the tip of the lateral malleolus and medial tilt of the talus.
- Abduction: fracture of the lateral malleolus, avulsion of the tip of the medial malleolus and separation of the distal tibiofibular joint.
- External rotation: spiral or oblique fracture of the lateral malleolus and lateral shift of the talus (Fig. 11.38).
- Vertical compression: fracture of the distal tibia posteriorly or anteriorly and separation of the distal tibiofibular joint.

Fractures of the talus

Small avulsion fractures of the talus are commonly seen in association with ankle fractures and ligament

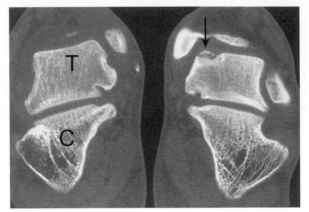

Fig. 11.39 *Osteochondral fracture of the talus: coronal CT of both ankles. Note the normal appearance of right talus (T) and calcaneus (C). A defect in the cortical surface of the left talar dome is associated with a loose bone fragment (arrow).*

damage. Osteochondral fracture of the upper articular surface of the talus (talar dome) is a common cause of persistent pain following an inversion ankle injury. Osteochondral fractures of the medial talar dome tend to be characterized by rounded defects in the cortical surface, often with loose bone fragments that generally require surgical fixation. Osteochondral fractures of the lateral talar dome are usually small bone flakes. These fractures may be difficult to see on radiographs and often require CT or MRI for diagnosis (Fig. 11.39).

Fracture of the neck of the talus may be widely displaced, associated with disruption of the subtalar joint and complicated by avascular necrosis.

Fractures of the calcaneus

Fractures of the calcaneus may show considerable displacement and comminution, and may involve the subtalar joint. Boehler's angle is the angle formed by a line tangential to the superior extra-articular portion of the calcaneus and a line tangential to the superior intra-articular portion. Boehler's angle normally measures 25–40°. Reduction of this angle is a useful sign of a displaced intra-articular fracture of the calcaneus as these fractures may be difficult to see on radiographs (Fig. 11.40). Computed tomography is useful to define fractures and to assist in planning of surgical reduction.

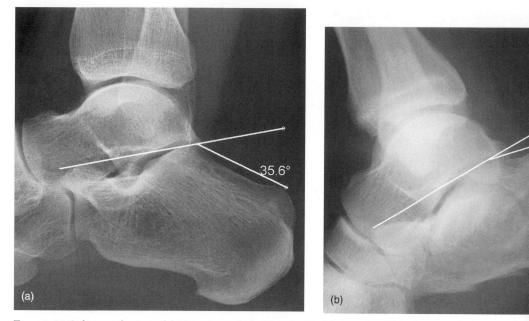

Fig. 11.40 *Calcaneus fracture. (a) Note the method of drawing Boehler's angle. (b) In this example there is reduction of Boehler's angle associated with multiple fractures of the calcaneus.*

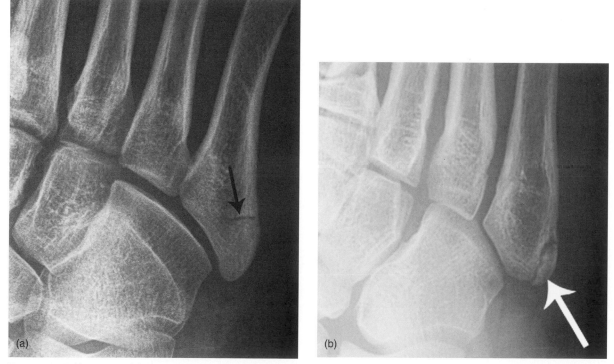

Fig. 11.41 *Fifth metatarsal fracture. (a) Transverse fracture of the base of the fifth metatarsal (arrow). (b) Normal growth centre at the base of the fifth metatarsal (arrow). This is aligned parallel to the long axis of the bone and should not be confused with a fracture.*

Calcaneal fractures, particularly when bilateral, have a high association with spine and pelvis fractures.

Other fractures of the foot

The Lisfranc ligament is a major stabiliser of the mid-foot. It joins the distal lateral surface of the medial cuneiform to the base of the second metatarsal. The Lisfranc fracture/dislocation refers to disruption of this ligament, with midfoot instability. Radiographic signs may be difficult to appreciate and include widening of the space between the bases of the first and second metatarsals and associated fractures of metatarsals, cuneiforms and other tarsal bones. Computed tomography may be required to confirm the diagnosis.

Metatarsal fractures are usually transverse. The growth centre at the base of the fifth metatarsal lies parallel to the shaft and should not be mistaken for a fracture; fractures in this region usually lie in the transverse plane (Fig. 11.41).

Stress fractures of the foot are common particularly involving the metatarsal shafts, and less commonly the navicular and talus.

12

Musculoskeletal system

IMAGING INVESTIGATION OF THE MUSCULOSKELETAL SYSTEM

RADIOGRAPHS

Conventional radiographs remain the most commonly performed imaging investigations for the musculoskeletal system. They are indicated in all fractures and dislocations and are sufficient for diagnosis in the majority of cases. Most general bone conditions such as Paget's disease are diagnosed on radiographs. The vast majority of bone tumours and other focal bone lesions are characterized by clinical history and plain radiographs. More sophisticated tests such as magnetic resonance imaging (MRI) and computed tomography (CT) are performed to look for specific complications of these lesions but usually add little to the diagnostic specificity of radiographs.

A major limitation of radiography is insensitivity to early bony changes in conditions such as osteomyelitis and stress fractures.

COMPUTED TOMOGRAPHY

Multidetector row CT is increasingly used for further delineation of complex fractures. Common indications include depressed fracture of the tibial plateau, comminuted fracture of the calcaneus, and various other fractures involving articular surfaces. Computed tomography may also be used to diagnose non-union of fractures. It may assist in staging bone tumours by looking for specific features such as soft-tissue extension and cortical destruction.

SCINTIGRAPHY

Bone scintigraphy is performed with diphosphonate-based radiopharmaceuticals such as ^{99m}Tc-methylene diphosphonate (MDP). Bone scintigraphy is highly sensitive and therefore able to demonstrate pathologies such as subtle undisplaced fractures, stress fractures and osteomyelitis prior to radiographic changes becoming apparent. Scintigraphy is also able to image the entire skeleton and is therefore the investigation of choice for screening for skeletal metastases and other multifocal tumours. The commonest exception to this is multiple myeloma, which may be difficult to appreciate on scintigraphy. Skeletal survey (radiographs of the entire skeleton) or whole-body MRI are indicated to assess the extent of multiple myeloma.

The major limitation of bone scintigraphy is its non-specificity. Areas of increased uptake may be seen commonly in benign conditions, such as osteoarthritis. Correlative radiographs are often required for definitive diagnosis.

ULTRASOUND

Musculoskeletal ultrasound (MSUS) is used to assess the soft tissues of the musculoskeletal system i.e. tendons, ligaments and muscles. It is able to diagnose muscle and tendon tears. Musculoskeletal ultrasound is also used to assess soft-tissue masses and is able to provide a definitive diagnosis for much common pathology such as ganglion and superficial lipoma. It is highly sensitive for the detection of soft-tissue foreign bodies, including those not visible on radiographs such as thorns, splinters and tiny pieces of glass. Bony pathology cannot be visualized with MSUS. It is also unsuitable for most internal joint derangements.

MAGNETIC RESONANCE IMAGING

Magnetic resonance imaging is able to visualize all of the different tissues of the musculoskeletal system, including cortical and medullary bone, hyaline and fibrocartilage, tendon, ligament and muscle. As such, it has a wide diversity of applications, especially internal derangements of joints. It may also be helpful in the staging assessment of bone and soft-tissue tumours.

INTERNAL JOINT DERANGEMENT: METHODS OF INVESTIGATION

Joint pain may result from a number of causes, including trauma, internal derangement and arthropathy. Skeletal trauma was discussed in Chapter 11 and an approach to arthropathies is discussed below.

WRIST

Persistent wrist pain following trauma or post-traumatic carpal instability may be caused by ligament or cartilage tears. The two most commonly injured internal wrist structures are the scapholunate ligament and the triangular fibrocartilage complex (TFCC). The scapholunate ligament stabilizes the joint between the medial surface of the scaphoid and the lunate. The TFCC is a triangular wedge of fibrocartilage joining the medial surface of the distal radius to the base of the ulnar styloid process. Radiographs of the wrist, including stress views, may be useful to confirm carpal instability, in particular widening of the space between the scaphoid and lunate with disruption of the scapholunate ligament (Fig. 12.1). Magnetic resonance imaging is the investigation of choice to confirm tears of internal wrist structures (Fig. 12.2).

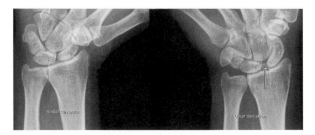

Fig. 12.1 *Scapholunate ligament tear: stress views of the wrist. With ulnar deviation there is widening (arrow) of the gap between scaphoid (S) and lunate (L), indicating a tear of the scapholunate ligament.*

SHOULDER

Rotator cuff disease

Calcific tendinitis caused by hydroxyapatite crystal deposition is particularly common in the supraspinatus tendon. Calcific tendinitis occurs in young to middle-aged adults and usually presents with acute shoulder pain accentuated by abduction. Tears of the rotator cuff most commonly involve the supraspinatus tendon. Rotator cuff tear is usually the result of 'wear and tear'. It most commonly presents in elderly patients with persistent shoulder pain worsened by abduction. The pain is often quite bad at night with interruption of sleep being a common complaint.

For suspected rotator cuff disease, radiographs of the shoulder are used to diagnose calcific tendinitis (Fig. 12.3) and to exclude underlying bony pathology as a cause of shoulder pain. Ultrasound (US) is the investigation of choice for suspected rotator cuff tear. Ultrasound of the rotator cuff is highly accurate when performed by radiologists experienced in the technique (Fig. 12.4). Magnetic resonance imaging provides excellent views of the muscles and tendons of the rotator cuff and is a problem-solving tool for difficult or equivocal cases.

Glenohumeral joint instability (recurrent dislocation)

Dislocation of the glenohumeral (shoulder) joint is a common occurrence and in most cases recovery is swift and uncomplicated. In a small percentage of cases, tearing of stabilizing structures may cause glenohumeral instability with recurrent dislocation. Magnetic resonance imaging is the investigation of choice for assessment of glenohumeral instability. The accuracy of MRI may be enhanced by the intra-articular injection of a dilute solution of contrast material (gadolinium) (Fig. 12.5, page 184).

HIP

Hip pain is a common problem and may occur at any age. Hip problems in children are discussed in Chapter 16.

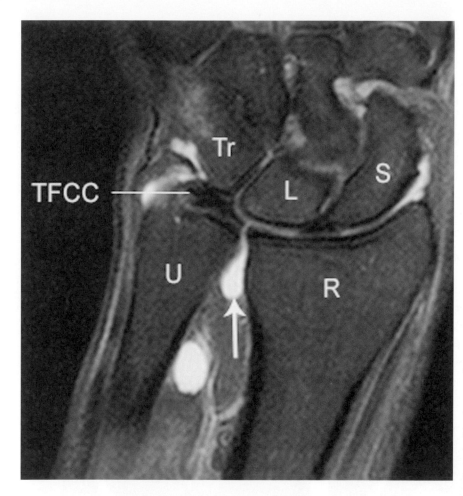

Fig. 12.2 *Triangular cartilage complex tear: magnetic resonance imaging of the wrist, coronal plane. Fluid is seen passing into the distal radio-ulnar joint (arrow) through a perforation of the radial insertion of the triangular fibrocartilage complex (TFCC). Note also triquetral (Tr), lunate (L), scaphoid (S), ulna (U) and radius (R).*

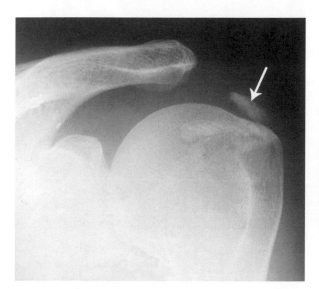

Fig. 12.3 *Calcific tendinitis. A focal calcification is seen above the humeral head (arrow) in the supraspinatus tendon.*

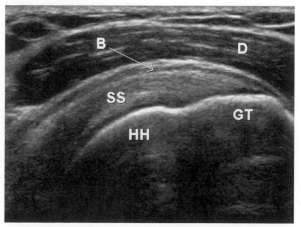

Fig. 12.4 *Normal rotator cuff: ultrasound. A scan of the shoulder in an oblique coronal plane shows the following: deltoid muscle (D), subdeltoid bursa (B), supraspinatus tendon (SS), humeral head (HH) and greater tuberosity (GT).*

In young active adults a tear of the fibrocartilage-nous labrum may present with hip pain plus an audible 'clicking'. In elderly patients, osteoarthritis is a common cause of hip pain. Less commonly hip pain may be caused by bone disorders such as avascular necrosis (AVN), and a history of risk factors such as steroid use may be relevant. Radiographs are usually sufficient for the diagnosis of osteoarthritis of the hip. Magnetic resonance imaging is the investigation of choice for suspected labral tear. As with the shoulder, the accuracy of MRI in this context may be increased by intra-articular injection of dilute gadolinium. It is also the investigation of choice for AVN.

KNEE

Radiographs are performed for the assessment of most causes of knee pain. Magnetic resonance imaging is the investigation of choice in the assessment of most internal knee derangements, including meniscus injury (Fig. 12.6), cruciate ligament tear, collateral ligament

tear, osteochondritis dissecans, etc. Ultrasound is useful in the assessment of periarticular pathology such as popliteal cysts and patellar tendinopathy.

ANKLE

There are numerous indications for imaging of the ankle. Persistent pain post-trauma may be caused by delayed healing of ligament tears or osteochondral fracture of the articular surface of the talus. Magnetic resonance imaging is the investigation of choice in the assessment of persistent post-traumatic ankle pain. Tendinopathy and tendon tears are common around the ankle joint. The most commonly involved tendons are

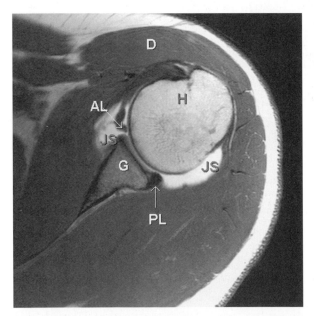

Fig. 12.5 *Anterior labral tear: magnetic resonance arthrogram of the shoulder, transverse plane. Note the following: deltoid muscle (D), humerus (H), glenoid (G), posterior labrum (PL), joint space distended with dilute gadolinium (JS) and anterior labrum (AL). Joint fluid is seen between the base of the anterior labrum and the glenoid indicating an anterior labral tear.*

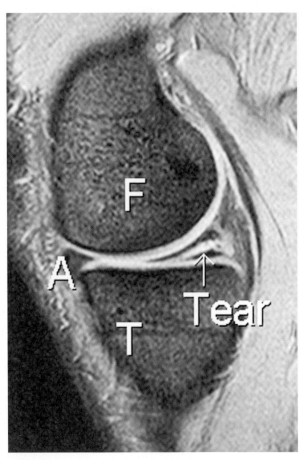

Fig. 12.6 *Meniscus tear: magnetic resonance imaging of the knee, sagittal plane. Note the femur (F), tibia (T), and the normal low signal triangular outline of the anterior horn of the medial meniscus (A). A tear of the posterior horn is seen as a high-signal line through the meniscus.*

the Achilles tendon, tibialis posterior and peroneus longus and brevis. These tendons are well assessed with US and MRI.

APPROACH TO ARTHROPATHIES

Many classifications of joint diseases are available based on differing criteria such as aetiology and radiographic appearances. I find it most useful to decide first whether there is involvement of a single joint (monoarthropathy), or multiple joints (polyarthropathy). This is fine as long as one remembers that a polyarthropathy may present early with a single painful joint. Polyarthropathies may be divided into three large categories:

- Inflammatory.
- Degenerative.
- Metabolic.

A detailed discussion of the clinical features and biochemical testing for arthropathies is beyond the scope of this book. Outlined below is a summary of radiographic manifestations of the more commonly encountered arthropathies.

MONOARTHROPATHY

A common cause for a single painful joint is trauma. There will usually be an obvious history and radiographs may show an associated fracture and joint effusion.

In cases of septic arthritis the affected joint may be radiographically normal at the time of initial presentation. Later, a joint effusion and swelling of surrounding soft tissues may occur, followed by bone erosions and destruction. Scintigraphy with ^{99m}Tc-MDP is usually positive at time of presentation.

Other causes of a monoarthropathy are polyarthropathy presenting in a single joint and include osteoarthritis, gout and rheumatoid arthritis.

INFLAMMATORY POLYARTHROPATHY

Inflammatory arthropathies present with painful joints and associated soft-tissue swelling.

Rheumatoid arthritis

Rheumatoid arthritis (RA) affects predominantly the small joints, especially metacarpophalangeal, metatarsophalangeal, carpal, and proximal interphalangeal joints, usually with a symmetrical distribution. Soft-tissue swelling overlying joints is an early sign. Bone erosions occur in the feet and hands. Bone erosions are best demonstrated in the metatarsal and metacarpal heads, articular surfaces of phalanges and carpal bones (Fig. 12.7). Other radiographic signs of RA include reduced bone density adjacent to joints (periarticular osteoporosis) and abnormalities of joint alignment with subluxation of metacarpophalangeal (MCP) joints giving ulnar deviation and subluxation of

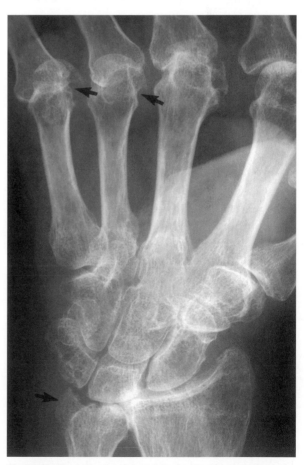

Fig. 12.7 *Rheumatoid arthritis of the hand and wrist. Bone erosions are seen involving the metacarpals and the ulnar styloid process (arrows).*

metatarsophalangeal (MTP) joints producing lateral deviation of toes. Axial involvement is rare apart from the cervical spine where erosion of the odontoid peg is the most significant feature.

Other connective tissue (seropositive) arthropathies

Other ('non-RA') seropositive arthropathies include systemic lupus erythematosus (SLE), systemic sclerosis, CREST (calcinosis, Raynaud's, eosophageal dysfunction, sclerodactyly and telangectasia), mixed connective tissue disease, polymyositis and dermatomyositis. These arthropathies tend to present with symmetrical arthropathy involving the peripheral small joints, especially the metacarpophalangeal and proximal interphalangeal joints. Radiographic signs may be subtle and include soft-tissue swelling and periarticular osteoporosis. Erosions are less common than with RA. Soft-tissue calcification is common, especially around joints. Resorption of distal phalanges and joint contractures are prominent features of systemic sclerosis.

Seronegative spondyloarthropathy

The seronegative spondyloarthropathies (SpAs) are asymmetrical polyarthropathies, usually involving only a few joints. The SpAs have a predilection for the spine and sacroiliac joints. Five subtypes of SpA are described with shared clinical features including association with HLA-B27:

- Ankylosing spondylitis.
- Reactive arthritis.
- Arthritis spondylitis with inflammatory bowel disease.
- Arthritis spondylitis with psoriasis.
- Undifferentiated spondyloarthropathy (uSpA).

Clinical features of SpA may include inflammatory back pain, positive family history, acute anterior uveitis and inflammation at tendon and ligament insertions (enthesitis). Enthesitis most commonly involves the distal Achilles tendon insertion and the insertion of the plantar fascia on the under-surface of the calcaneus. Features of inflammatory back pain include

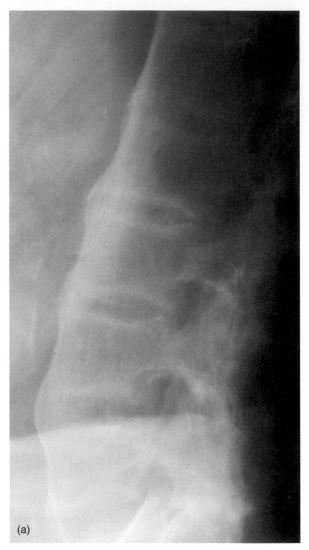

(a)

Fig. 12.8 *Ankylosing spondylitis. (a) Lateral view of the lumbar spine showing fusion (ankylosis) of the vertebral bodies.*

insidious onset, morning stiffness and improvement with exercise.

Ankylosing spondylitis is the most common SpA. Radiographic changes in the spine include vertically orientated bony spurs arising from the vertebral bodies (syndesmophytes) and later fusion or ankylosis of the spine giving the 'bamboo spine' appearance (Fig. 12.8(a)). Sacroiliac joint changes include erosions producing an irregular joint margin, with sclerosis and joint fusion later in the disease process (Fig. 12.8(b)).

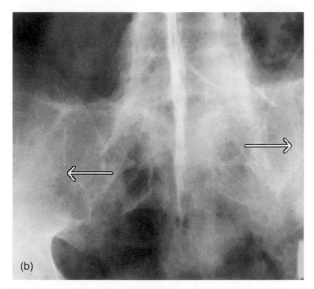

Fig. 12.8 *(b) Frontal view of the pelvis showing fused sacroiliac joints (arrows).*

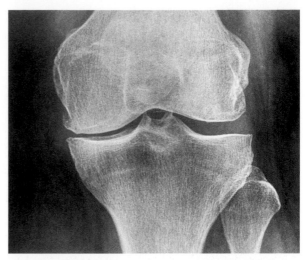

Fig. 12.9 *Osteoarthritis of the knee. Note narrowing of the medial joint compartment caused by thinning of articular cartilage.*

Psoriatic arthropathy is an asymmetrical arthropathy, predominantly affecting the small joints of the hands and feet. Radiographic changes seen in the peripheral joints include periarticular erosions and periosteal new bone formation.

DEGENERATIVE ARTHROPATHY: OSTEOARTHRITIS

Primary osteoarthritis (OA) refers to degenerative arthropathy with no apparent underlying or predisposing cause. Secondary OA refers to degenerative change complicating underlying arthropathy such as RA, trauma, or Paget's disease. Primary OA is an asymmetric process involving the large weight-bearing joints, hips and knees, lumbar and cervical spine (see Chapter 13), distal interphalangeal, first carpometacarpal and lateral carpal joints.

The dominant pathological process in OA is loss of articular cartilage. This results in joint space narrowing and abnormal stresses on joint margins with osteophyte formation (Fig. 12.9). Other radiographic changes include sclerosis of joint surfaces, periarticular cyst formation and loose bodies in joints due to detached osteophytes and ossified cartilage debris.

METABOLIC ARTHROPATHIES

Gout

Gouty arthropathy involves the first metatarsophalangeal joint in 70 per cent of cases. Other joints of lower limbs may be affected, including ankles, knees and intertarsal joints. Gout is usually asymmetric in distribution and often monoarticular. Acute gout refers to soft-tissue swelling, with no visible bony changes. Chronic gouty arthritis occurs with recurrent acute gout. Radiographic features include:

- Bone erosions: usually set back from the joint surface (para-articular).
- Calcification of articular cartilages, especially the menisci of the knee.
- Tophus: soft-tissue mass in the synovium of joints, the subcutaneous tissues of the lower leg, Achilles tendon, olecranon bursa at the elbow, helix of the ear.
- Calcification of tophi is an uncommon feature.

Calcium pyrophosphate deposition disease

Also known as pseudogout, calcium pyrophosphate deposition disease (CPPD) may occur in young adults as an autosomal dominant condition, or sporadically in older patients. It presents with intermittent acute

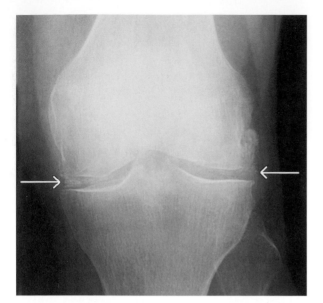

Fig. 12.10 *Chondrocalcinosis of the knee. Calcification of the lateral and medial menisci of the knee (arrows) caused by calcium pyrophosphate deposition.*

joint pain and swelling. It may affect any joint, most commonly knee, hip, shoulder, elbow, wrist and ankle. Radiographic signs of CPPD include calcification of intra-articular cartilages, especially the menisci of the knee and the triangular fibrocartilage complex of the wrist (Fig. 12.10). Secondary degenerative change may occur with subchondral cysts and joint space narrowing.

Calcium hydroxyapatite crystal deposition disease

Calcium hydroxyapatite crystal deposition presents with monoarticular or polyarticular joint pain, with reduced joint motion in patients aged 40–70 years. The most common site of involvement is the shoulder, with calcific tendinitis of the supraspinatus tendon (Fig. 12.3, page 183). Virtually any other tendon in the body may be affected, though much less commonly than supraspinatus. The classical radiographic sign of calcium hydroxyapatite deposition is calcification in the supraspinatus tendon. In acute cases, the calcification may be semi-liquid and difficult to see radiographically.

SOME COMMON BONE CONDITIONS

PAGET DISEASE

Paget disease is an extremely common bone disorder, occurring in elderly patients, characterized by increased bone resorption followed by new bone formation. The new bone thus formed has thick trabeculae and is softer and more vascular than normal bone. Common sites include the pelvis and upper femur, spine, skull, upper tibia and proximal humerus. Paget disease is often asymptomatic and seen as an incidental finding on radiographs performed for other reasons. The clinical presentation may otherwise be quite variable and falls into three broad categories:

- General symptoms: pain and fatigue
- Symptoms related to specific sites:
   (i) Cranial nerve pressure; blindness, deafness;
   (ii) Increased hat size;
   (iii) Local hyperthermia of overlying skin.
- Complications:
   (i) Pathological fracture;
   (ii) Secondary osteoarthritis;
   (iii) Sarcoma formation (rare).

Radiographic changes of Paget disease reflect an early active phase of bone resorption, an inactive phase of sclerosis and cortical thickening, and, most commonly, a mixed lytic and sclerotic phase. These changes include:

- Well-defined reduction in density of the anterior skull: osteoporosis circumscripta.
- V-shaped lytic defect in long bones extending into the shaft of the bone from the subarticular region.
- Thick cortex and coarse trabeculae with enlarged bone (Fig. 12.11).
- Bowing of long bones.

OSTEOPOROSIS

Osteoporosis may be defined as a condition in which the quantity of bone per unit volume or bone mineral density (BMD) is decreased in amount. Osteoporosis is increasing in incidence with gradual aging of the

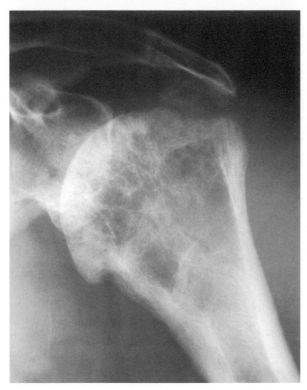

Fig. 12.11 *Paget disease of the humerus. Note the coarse trabecular pattern in the humeral head and thickening of the bony cortex.*

population. It leads to fragility of bone with an increased incidence of fracture, particularly crush fractures of the vertebral bodies, and hip and wrist fractures. There is now compelling evidence that treatment of osteoporosis can help to reduce the incidence of fragility fractures. The three most important factors in the decision to treat osteoporosis are the age of the patient, the presence of a previous fragility fracture and the BMD. Accurate measurement of BMD is the key to the diagnosis of osteoporosis and the decision to institute treatment.

The radiographic signs of osteoporosis relate to fragility fractures, particularly of the spine. These signs include concavity of vertebral end plates as well as crush fractures. Other signs of osteoporosis that have been described include thinning of the bone cortex and trabeculae; however, these are not reliable.

Dual X-ray absorptiometry (DEXA) is widely accepted as a highly accurate, low radiation dose technique for measuring BMD. It uses an X-ray source, which produces X-rays of two different energies. The lower of these energies is absorbed almost exclusively by soft tissue. The higher energy is absorbed by bone and soft tissue. Calculation of the two absorption patterns gives an attenuation profile of the bone component from which BMD may be estimated. Measurements are usually taken from the lumbar spine (L2–L4) and the femoral neck. The DEXA report gives an absolute measurement of BMD expressed as grams per square centimetre (g/cm^2). This value is compared with a normal young adult population to give a T score. The T score is expressed as the number of standard deviations from the mean for the normal young population. Osteoporosis is defined as a BMD of 2.5 standard deviations below the young normal adult mean (i.e. a T score of equal to or less than −2.5). A T score of −1 to −2.5 is defined as osteopenia, with normal being a T score of more than −1.

Treatment of osteoporosis includes drug regimes (including biphosphonates), hormone replacement therapy and weight-bearing exercise. There is good evidence for the following treatment guidelines based on BMD as calculated with DEXA:

- T score > −1: no treatment.
- T score −1 to −2.5: treatment if there is a previous fragility fracture.
- T score < −2.5: treatment recommended whether there is a previous fracture or not.

OSTEOMYELITIS

Osteomyelitis may have various causes. In infants and children osteomyelitis is mainly caused by haematogenous spread with multisite involvement common. The most common infective organism in children is *Staphylococcus aureus*, with group B *Streptococcus* common in neonates. The vascular anatomy is crucial to the distribution of bone infection in children. In infants metaphyseal infection with epiphyseal extension occurs. In children older than 18 months metaphyseal infection predominates. In adults, osteomyelitis may occur from a number of causes including trauma, especially compound fractures, adjacent soft-tissue infection, diabetes and intravenous drug use.

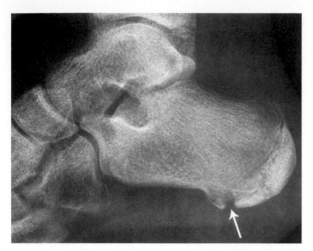

Fig. 12.12 *Osteomyelitis seen as a small focus of destruction of the bony cortex (arrow) on the under-surface of the calcaneus in a 12-year-old boy.*

Radiographs of the affected bone are usually normal for up to 7–14 days following infection. Radiographic signs, when they do occur, include metaphyseal destruction and periosteal reaction, soft-tissue swelling, and epiphyseal lucency in infants (Fig. 12.12). Brodie abscess is a type of chronic circumscribed osteomyelitis. It is most common in the lower extremity and may be seen radiographically as a focal lucency with marginal sclerosis.

Bone scintigraphy with ^{99m}Tc-MDP will be positive within 24–72 hours of infection. Gallium (^{67}Ga) scintigraphy may help to confirm bone infection and is particularly useful in confirming chronic osteomyelitis as a cause of persistent bone pain in the appropriate clinical setting, such as diabetes or non-union of a fracture. Ultrasound may be useful for the diagnosis of acute osteomyelitis in children, prior to radiographic changes becoming evident.

LANGERHANS CELL HISTIOCYTOSIS

What used to be referred to as the three forms of histiocytosis X (eosinophilic granuloma, Hand–Christian–Schuller disease and Letterer–Siwe disease) are now classified under the single entity of Langerhans cell histiocytosis (LCH). This describes a spectrum of disorders, the common feature being histiocytic infiltration of tissues and aggressive bone lesions. Langerhans cell histiocytosis (LCH) may be subclassified as restricted

or extensive LCH. Extensive LCH refers to visceral organ involvement with or without bone lesions. Visceral involvement may produce organ dysfunction and failure. Skin rash and diabetes insipidus are common.

Restricted LCH refers to monostotic bone or polyostotic bone lesions, or isolated skin lesions. The monostotic bone lesion of LCH occurs with a peak age of incidence of 5–10 years, though it may be seen in older patients. Langerhans cell histiocytosis produces focal skeletal lesions in the skull, spine and long bones. Presentation may be with local pain or pathological fracture (Fig. 11.9, page 162). Radiographically, LCH is usually seen as a well-defined lytic lesion with periosteal reaction.

FIBROUS DYSPLASIA

Fibrous dysplasia refers to a common condition characterized by single or multiple benign bone lesions composed of a fibrous stroma with islands of osteoid and woven bone. It may occur up to the age of 70 years, though is more usually seen from 10 to 30 years. Bone lesions are solitary in 75 per cent of cases. Fibrous dysplasia most commonly involves the lower extremity or skull. It usually presents with local swelling, pain, or pathological fracture. Two common radiographic patterns are seen with fibrous dysplasia:

- Expansile lytic lesion with cortical thinning (Fig. 12.13).
- Bone expansion with a homogeneously dense 'ground glass' matrix (Fig. 12.14).

Associated syndromes may also occur:

- McCune–Albright syndrome: polyostotic fibrous dysplasia, patchy cutaneous pigmentation, and sexual precocity.
- Leontiasis ossea ('lion's face'): asymmetric sclerosis and thickening of skull and facial bones.
- Cherubism: expansile lesions of the jaws in children under 4 years old.

OSTEOCHONDRITIS DISSECANS

Osteochondritis dissecans is a traumatic bone lesion that affects males more than females, most commonly

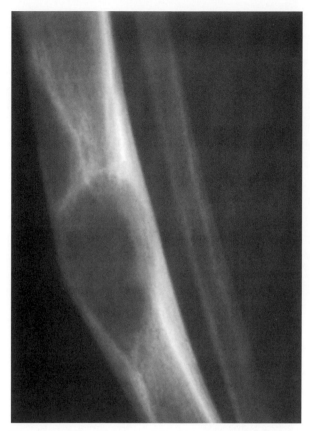

Fig. 12.13 *Fibrous dysplasia of the tibia seen as a well-defined lucent lesion expanding the midshaft of the tibia.*

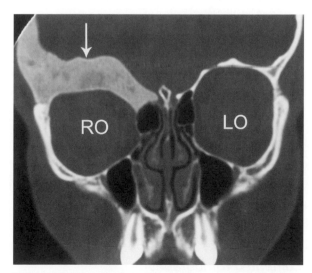

Fig. 12.14 *Fibrous dysplasia of the skull: computed tomography (CT). A coronal CT shows the right and left orbits (RO, LO). The roof of the right orbit is thickened and diffusely sclerotic (arrow), a pattern typical of fibrous dysplasia in the skull and face*

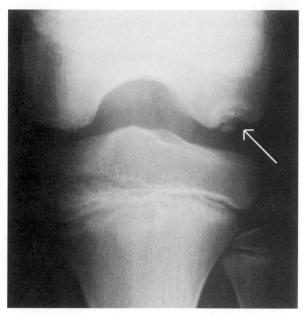

Fig. 12.15 *Osteochondritis dissecans of the lateral femoral condyle seen as a round lucent defect in the cortical surface with a loose bone fragment (arrow).*

in the 10- to 20-year age-group. The knee is most often affected with other sites including the dome of the talus and the capitulum. In the knee the lateral aspect of the medial femoral condyle is involved in 75–80 per cent of cases, with the lateral femoral condyle in 15–20 per cent and the patella in 5 per cent. Trauma is thought to be the underlying cause in most cases. Subchondral bone is first affected, then overlying articular cartilage. Subsequent revascularization and healing occur, though a necrotic bone fragment may persist. This may become separated and displaced as a loose body in the joint.

Radiographs show a lucent defect on the cortical surface of the femoral condyle, often with a separate bone fragment (Fig. 12.15). This needs to be differentiated from normal cortical irregularities of the posterior femoral condyles that are seen as normal variations in children.

Magnetic resonance imaging is usually performed to further define the bone and cartilage abnormality. It helps to establish prognosis, guide management and confirm healing.

AN APPROACH TO PRIMARY BONE TUMOURS

Primary bone tumours are relatively rare, representing less than 1 per cent of all malignancies. Imaging, particularly radiographic assessment is vital to the diagnosis and delineation of bone tumours and a basic approach is outlined here, along with a summary of the roles of the various modalities. In the analysis of a solitary bone lesion, a couple of things need to be borne in mind:

- In adult patients, a solitary bone lesion is more likely to be a metastasis than a primary bone tumour.
- A number of conditions may mimic bone tumour in children and adults including:
   (i) Osteomyelitis;
   (ii) Fibrous dysplasia;
   (iii) Bone cyst;
   (iv) Histiocytosis;
   (v) Intraosseous ganglion;
   (vi) Stress fracture.

A few very basic features of the clinical history may be extremely helpful. First, it is vital to know the age of the patient. For example, osteogenic sarcoma and Ewing sarcoma occur in the second to third decades while chondrosarcoma and multiple myeloma occur in older patients. Next, it is important to know which bone is involved. Chondrosarcoma and Ewing sarcoma tend to involve flat bones such as the pelvis, while osteogenic sarcoma most commonly involves the metaphysis of long bones. Chondroblastoma and giant cell tumour arise in the epiphyses of long bones.

   On examination of the radiograph a number of parameters are assessed:
- Type of bone lesion:
   (i) Lytic i.e. lucent or dark;
   (ii) Sclerotic, i.e. dense or white;
- Zone of transition:
   (i) The part of bone between the lesion itself and normal bone;
   (ii) May be wide and irregular, or narrow;

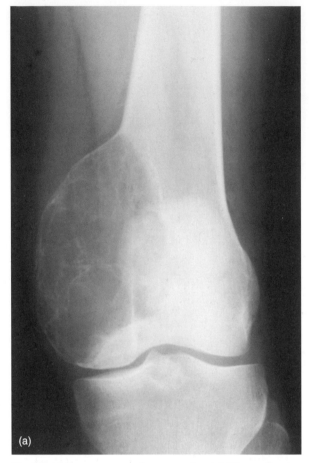

(a)

Fig. 12.16 *Bone tumours: three examples. (a) Giant cell tumour of the distal femur seen as an eccentric lytic expanded lesion with a well-defined margin.*

- Effect on surrounding bone:
   (i) Penetration of cortex;
   (ii) Periosteal reaction and new bone formation;
- Associated features:
   (i) Soft-tissue mass;
   (ii) Pathological fracture.

Most diagnostic information as to tumour type comes from clinical assessment plus the plain film (Fig. 12.16). The other imaging modalities add further, often complementary information on staging and complications.

Computed tomography

Computed tomography provides accurate localization and is sensitive for cortical destruction and soft-tissue

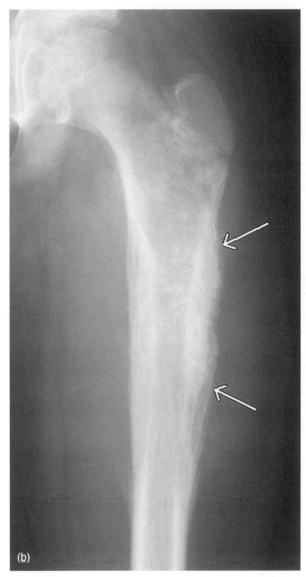

(b)

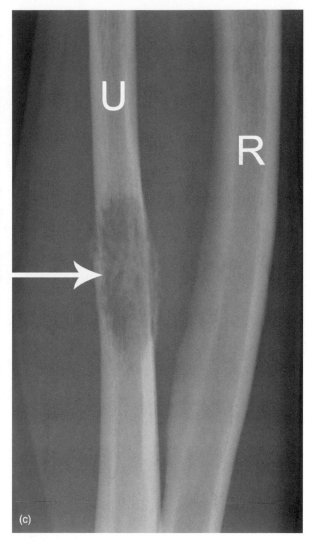

(c)

Fig. 12.16 (c) *Metastasis (from non-small cell carcinoma of the lung) in the ulna (arrow) seen as a lytic lesion with irregular margins. Compare this with the sclerotic metastases shown in Fig. 9.15.*

Fig. 12.16 (b) *Osteosarcoma of the upper femur. Note irregular cortical thickening with new bone formation beneath elevated periosteum (arrows).*

Magnetic resonance imaging

Magnetic resonance imaging provides accurate definition of tumour extent within the marrow cavity of the bone, and beyond into soft tissues (Fig. 12.17).

SKELETAL METASTASES

Almost any primary tumour may metastasize to bone. The most common primary sites are:
- Breast.
- Prostate.

mass. It may also be useful for biopsy guidance and for staging in the detection of distant metastases, for example to the lung.

Scintigraphy

Scintigraphy with ^{99m}Tc-MDP is used to assess the activity of the primary bone lesion and to detect multiple lesions.

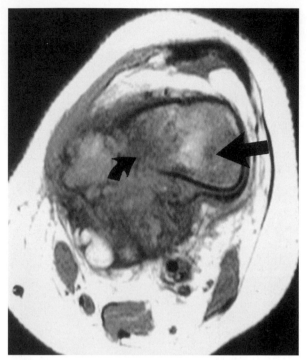

Fig. 12.17 *Osteosarcoma of the distal femur: magnetic resonance imaging, transverse plane. Note the low-signal tumour replacing fatty marrow in the medullary cavity of the femur (straight arrow), plus a focal area of cortical destruction (curved arrow) with soft tissue extension.*

- Kidney.
- Lung.
- Gastrointestinal tract.
- Thyroid.
- Melanoma.

Bone metastases are often clinically occult, or they may present with bone pain, pathological fracture, or hypercalcaemia. Radiographically, skeletal metastases are most commonly lytic, with focal lesions of bone destruction seen (Fig. 12.16c). Sclerotic metastases occur with prostate (Fig. 9.15, page 140), stomach, and carcinoid tumour. The most common sites are spine, pelvis, ribs, proximal femur and proximal humerus. Skeletal metastases are uncommon distal to the knee and elbow.

Scintigraphy with ^{99m}Tc-MDP usually shows multiple areas of increased uptake (Fig. 12.18). Given that a large percentage of skeletal metastases are clinically occult at the time of diagnosis of the primary tumour, scintigraphy is often used for staging. This is especially true for tumours that have a high incidence of metastasizing to bone, such as prostate, breast and lung.

MULTIPLE MYELOMA

Multiple myeloma is a common malignancy of plasma cells characterized by diffuse infiltration or multiple nodules in bone. It occurs in elderly patients, being rare below the age of 40 years. Multiple myeloma may present in a number of non-specific ways, including bone pain, anaemia, hypercalcaemia or renal failure. Unlike most other bone malignancies, bone scintigraphy is relatively insensitive so that it is particularly important to recognize the plain film findings. Common sites of involvement include spine, ribs, skull (Fig. 12.19), pelvis and long bones. Several different radiographic patterns may be seen with multiple myeloma including:

- Generalized severe osteoporosis.
- Multiple lytic, punched-out defects (Fig. 12.19).
- Multiple destructive and expansile lesions.

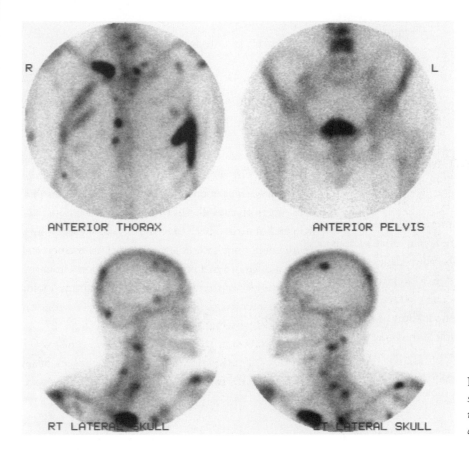

R · L

ANTERIOR THORAX   ANTERIOR PELVIS

RT LATERAL SKULL   LT LATERAL SKULL

Fig. 12.18 *Skeletal metastases, seen on scintigraphy as multiple areas of increased activity.*

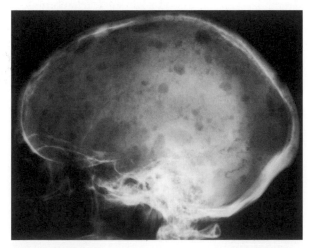

Fig. 12.19 *Multiple myeloma. Note the presence of multiple lucent 'punched-out' defects throughout the skull.*

Spine

RADIOGRAPHIC ANATOMY (FIGS 13.1–13.3)

Each vertebra consists of an anterior vertebral body, a posterior bony arch forming the spinal canal, various processes and intervertebral joints. The pedicles are posterior bony projections from the posterolateral corners of the vertebral body. The laminae curve posteromedially from the pedicle. They join at the midline at the base of the spinous process and complete the bony arch of the spinal canal. The spinous process projects posteriorly and often inferiorly. Transverse processes project laterally from the junction of pedicle and lamina.

There are multiple articulations between adjoining vertebrae. The intervertebral disc takes up the space between each vertebral body. Articular processes project superiorly and inferiorly from the junction of pedicle and lamina. These form the zygapophyseal joints, more commonly known as facet joints. In the cervical spine a ridge or lip of bone projects superiorly from the lateral surface of the vertebral body. This forms a joint with the lateral edge of the vertebral body above known as the uncovertebral joint.

The exception to the above pattern occurs at C1 and C2. C1, also known as the atlas, consists of an anterior arch, two lateral masses, and a posterior

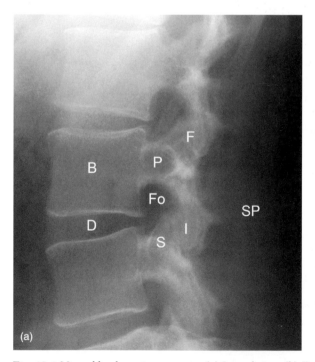

(a)

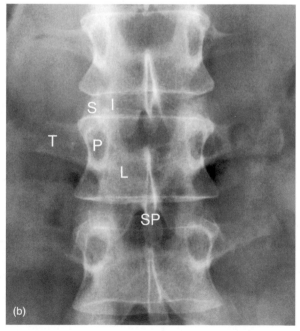

(b)

Fig. 13.1 *Normal lumbar spine anatomy. (a) Lateral view. (b) Frontal view. Note the following features: vertebral body (B), intervertebral disc (D), pedicle (P), facet joint (F), intervertebral foramen (Fo), inferior articular process (I), superior articular process (S), transverse process (T), lamina (L) and spinous process (SP).*

arch. The lateral masses articulate superiorly with the occiput (atlanto-occipital joints) and inferiorly with superior articular processes of C2. A vertical projection of bone extends superiorly from the body of C2. Known as the odontoid peg or dens, this articulates with the anterior arch of C1.

SPINE TRAUMA

The roles of imaging in the assessment of spinal trauma are:

- Diagnosis of fractures/dislocation.
- Assessment of stability/instability.

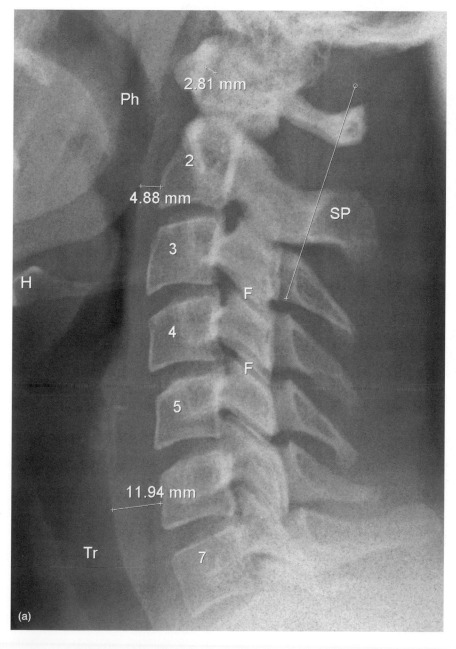

Fig. 13.2 *Normal cervical spine anatomy. (a) Lateral view. Note the following: facet joint (F), spinous process (SP), pharynx (Ph), hyoid bone (H), trachea (Tr) and posterior cervical line from C1 to C3. Note also measurements of predental space (between anterior arch of C1 and the odontoid peg), retropharyngeal space at C2 and retrotracheal space at C6.*

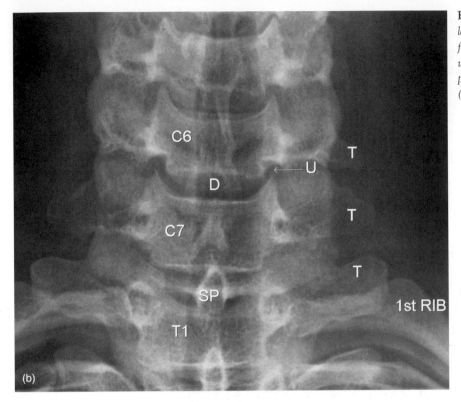

Fig. 13.2 (b) *Frontal view of lower cervical spine. Note the following: intervertebral disc (D), uncovertebral joint (U), transverse process (T) and spinous process (SP).*

- Diagnosis of damage to, or impingement on, neurological structures.
- Follow-up:
  (i) Assessment of treatment;
  (ii) Diagnosis of long-term complications such as post-traumatic syrinx or cyst formation.

CERVICAL SPINE RADIOGRAPHS

Radiographic assessment of the cervical spine should be performed in all trauma patients with neck pain or tenderness, other signs of direct neck injury or abnormal findings on neurological examination. Cervical spine films should also be performed in all patients with severe head or facial injury, or following high-velocity blunt trauma or near-drowning.

The following radiographs should be performed:
- Lateral view with patient supine showing all seven cervical vertebrae:
  (i) Traction on the shoulders may be used;
  (ii) Traction on the head must never be used.
- Anteroposterior (AP) view of the cervical spine.
- AP open mouth view to show the odontoid peg.

Oblique views to show the facet joints and intervertebral foramina may also be performed where facet joint dislocation or locking is suspected.

Functional views may be performed where no fractures are seen on the neutral views to diagnose posterior or anterior ligament damage. Functional views consist of lateral views in flexion and extension with the patient erect. The patient must be conscious and co-operative and must themselves perform flexion and extension; the head must not be moved passively by doctor or radiographer.

Cervical spine radiographs should be checked in a logical fashion for the following factors:
1 Vertebral alignment:
  – Disruption of anterior and posterior vertebral body lines: lines joining the anterior and

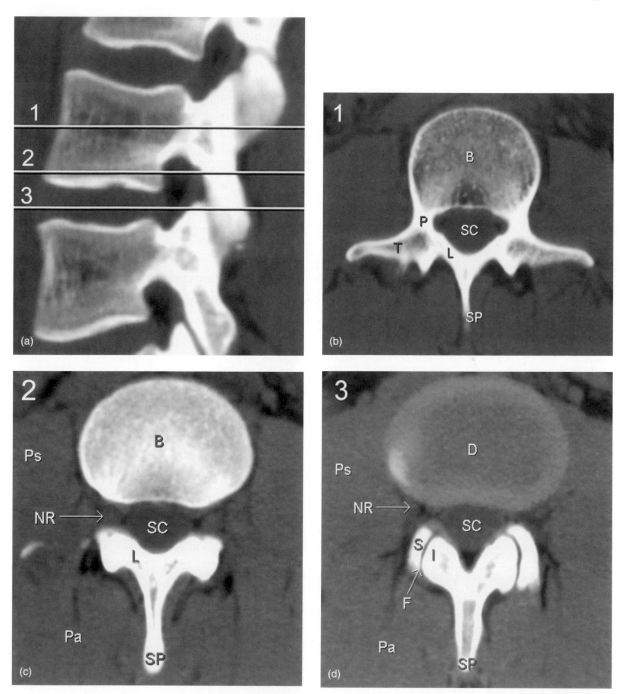

Fig. 13.3 *Normal lumbar spine anatomy: computed tomography. (a) Reconstructed image in the sagittal plane showing the levels of the three following transverse sections. (b) Transverse section at level of pedicles. (c) Transverse section at level of intervertebral foramina. (d) Transverse section at level of intervertebral disc. In images (b–d) note the following: vertebral body (B), pedicle (P), facet joint (F), inferior articular process (I), superior articular process (S), transverse process (T), lamina (L), spinous process (SP), nerve root (NR), spinal canal (SC), psoas muscle (Ps), intervertebral disc (D) and paraspinal muscle (Pa).*

posterior margins of the vertebral bodies on the lateral view;
- Disruption of the posterior cervical line: a line joining the anterior aspect of the spinous processes of C1, C2 and C3; disruption of this line may indicate upper cervical spine fractures, especially of C2 (Fig. 13.2);
- Facet joint alignment at all levels; abrupt disruption at one level may indicate locked facets;
- Widening of the space between spinous processes on the lateral film;
- Rotation of spinous processes on the AP film;
- Widening of the predental space: >5 mm in children; >3 mm in adults.
2 Bone integrity:
- Vertebral body fractures;
- Fractures of posterior elements, i.e. pedicles, laminae and spinous processes;
- Integrity of odontoid peg: anterior/posterior/lateral displacement
3 Disc spaces: narrowing or widening.
4 Prevertebral swelling:
- Widening of the retrotracheal space: posterior aspect of trachea to C6: >14 mm in children; >22 mm in adults;
- Widening of the retropharyngeal space: posterior aspect of pharynx to C2: >7 mm in adults and children.

COMMON PATTERNS OF CERVICAL SPINE INJURY

Flexion: anterior compression with posterior distraction (Fig. 13.4)

- Vertebral body compression fracture.
- 'Teardrop' fracture, i.e. small triangular fragment at lower anterior margin of vertebral body.

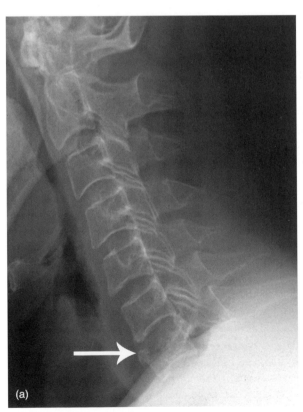

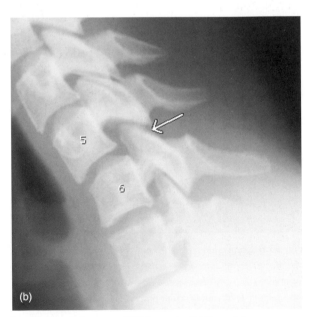

Fig. 13.4 *Flexion injuries of the cervical spine: three separate examples. (a) Crush fracture of C7 (arrow). (b) Facet joint subluxation. The space between the spinous processes of C5 and C6 is widened. The inferior articular processes of C5 are shifted forwards on the superior articular processes of C6 (arrow) indicating facet joint subluxation.*

- Disruption of posterior vertebral line.
- Disc space narrowing.
- Widening of facet joints.
- Facet joint dislocation and locking.
- Widening of space between spinous processes.

Extension: posterior compression with anterior distraction (Fig. 13.5)

- 'Teardrop' fracture of upper anterior margin of vertebral body: indicates severe anterior ligament damage.
- Disc space widening.
- Retrolisthesis (posterior shift of vertebral body) with disruption of anterior and posterior vertebral lines.
- Fractures of posterior elements: pedicles, spinous processes, facets.
- 'Hangman's' fracture: bilateral C2 pedicle fracture (Fig. 13.6).

Rotation (Fig. 13.7)

- Anterolisthesis (anterior shift of vertebral body) with disruption of posterior vertebral line.
- Lateral displacement of upper vertebral body on AP view.
- Abrupt disruption of alignment of facet joints: locked facets.

Stability

As well as diagnosing and classifying cervical spine injuries, it is important to decide if the injury is stable or not. Instability implies the possibility of increased spinal deformity or neurological damage occurring with continued stress.

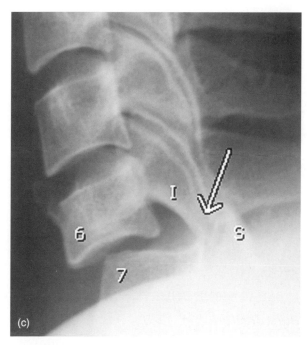

Fig. 13.4 (continued) (c) Bilateral locked facets. Both facet joints at C6/7 are dislocated. The posterior corners of the inferior articular processes (I) of C6 are locked anterior to the superior articular processes (S) of C7 (arrow).

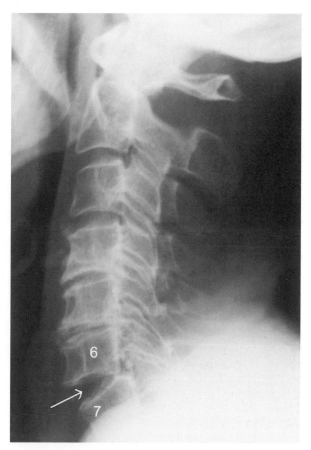

Fig. 13.5 Extension injury cervical spine. Note widening of the anterior disc space at C6/7 (arrow).

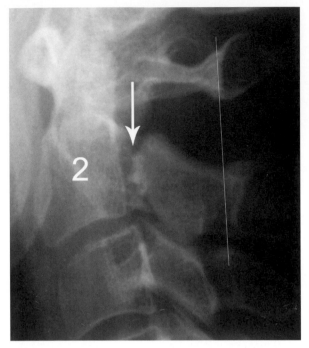

Fig. 13.6 *Hangman's fracture. Fracture of the pedicles of C2 (arrow) with loss of continuity of the posterior cervical line.*

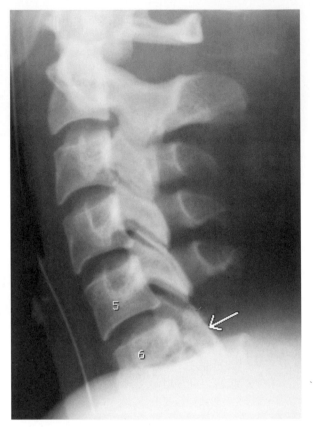

Fig. 13.7 *Flexion and rotation injury of the cervical spine: unilateral locked facet. There is widening of the space between the spinous processes of C5 and C6. Only one normally aligned facet joint is seen at C5/6. Compare this with the levels above where two normally aligned facet joints can be seen. Note the bare articular surface of one of the superior articular processes of C6 (arrow) as a result of dislocation of this facet joint.*

Radiographic signs of instability include:
- Displacement of vertebral body.
- 'Teardrop' fractures of vertebral body.
- Odontoid peg fracture.
- Widening or disruption of alignment of facet joints including locked facets.
- Widening of space between spinous processes.
- Fractures at multiple levels.

THORACIC AND LUMBAR SPINE RADIOGRAPHS

Assessment of plain films of the thoracic and lumbar spine following trauma is similar to that outlined for the cervical spine with particular attention to the following factors:
- Vertebral alignment.
- Vertebral body height.
- Disc space height.
- Facet joint alignment.

- Space between pedicles on AP film: widening at one level may indicate a burst fracture of the vertebral body.

COMMON PATTERNS OF THORACIC AND LUMBAR SPINE INJURY

Burst fracture (Fig. 13.8)

- Complex fractures of the vertebral body with a fragment pushed posteriorly into the spinal canal.
- Multiple fracture lines through vertebral end plates.

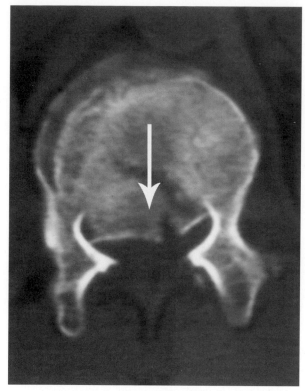

Fig. 13.8 *Burst fracture lumbar spine. CT in the transverse plane shows a fracture of the vertebral body with a retropulsed bone fragment (arrow) extending into the spinal canal.*

Compression (crush) fracture (Fig. 13.9)

* Common in osteoporosis.
* Loss of height of vertebral body most marked anteriorly giving a wedge-like configuration.

Fracture/dislocation

* Vertebral body displacement.
* Disc space narrowing or widening.
* Fractures of neural arches, including facet joints.
* Widening of facet joints or space between spinous processes.

Chance fracture (seatbelt fracture) (Fig. 13.10)

* Fracture of posterior vertebral body.
* Horizontal fracture line through spinous process, laminae, pedicles and transverse processes.
* Most occur at thoracolumbar junction.

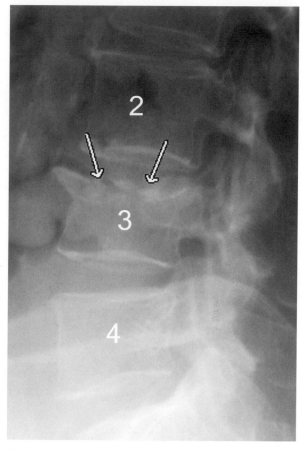

Fig. 13.9 *Crush fracture lumbar spine. Lateral view showing a crush fracture of the upper body of L3 (arrows).*

* High association with abdominal injury, i.e. solid organ damage, intestinal perforation, duodenal haematoma.

OTHER IMAGING MODALITIES IN SPINE TRAUMA

Computed tomography

Computed tomography (CT) is used for further delineation of fractures and associated deformity. It provides more accurate assessment of bony injuries, especially those of the neural arches and facet joints, as well as an accurate estimation of the dimensions of the spinal canal. Retropulsed bone fragments projecting into the spinal canal and compressing neural structures are well seen (Fig. 13.8). With multislice CT, multiplanar and three-dimensional (3D) images greatly assist in

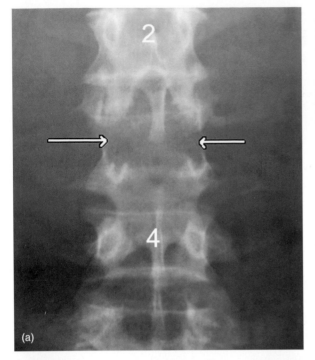

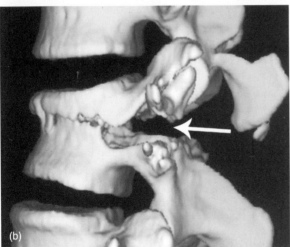

Fig. 13.10 *Chance fracture (seatbelt fracture) lumbar spine. (a) Frontal view showing a transverse fracture at L3 including horizontal splitting of the pedicles (arrows). (b) Three-dimensional computed tomography reconstructed image showing the transverse fracture of the pedicles and posterior vertebral body (arrow).*

delineation of both subtle fractures and complex injuries (Fig. 13.10). It is not unreasonable to perform a CT examination of the cervical spine at the same time as a head CT in the setting of major trauma or an unconscious patient, unable to be assessed clinically.

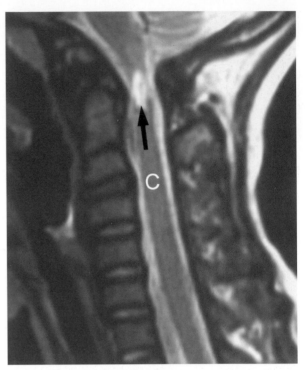

Fig. 13.11 *Spinal cord injury: magnetic resonance imaging, sagittal plane. The spinal cord (C) is well shown in the sagittal plane. Note a focal cystic lesion associated with focal thinning of the spinal cord at C2 indicating myelomalacia (arrow).*

In patients receiving a chest CT for chest trauma, a diagnostically adequate study of the thoracic spine can be obtained from reconstruction of multislice CT data on a workstation, without further irradiation of the patient. The same comment can be made for images of the lumbar spine reconstructed from abdominal CT.

Magnetic resonance imaging

Magnetic resonance imaging (MRI) is the investigation of choice for assessment of spinal cord damage (Fig. 13.11). Signs of cord trauma that may be appreciated on MRI include cord transection, cord oedema and haemorrhage, plus late sequelae such as cyst and syrinx formation. Soft-tissue changes such as post-traumatic disc protrusion and spinal canal haematoma are also seen on MRI.

Because MRI is able to show bone marrow oedema it is used to assess crush fractures of the thoracic and lumbar spine. Specifically, MRI may be used to differentiate acute crush fractures from older, healed injuries. This is now a common indication given the widespread acceptance of vertebroplasty for treatment of osteoporotic crush fractures (see below).

NECK PAIN

Neck pain is an extremely common complaint. Most cases of neck pain result from musculoligamentous strain or injury. About 70 per cent of episodes of neck pain resolve within 1 month. Most of the remaining 30 per cent resolve over the longer term, with a small minority going on to have chronic neck problems. In the clinical assessment of neck pain there are three major sources of diagnostic difficulty. First, many structures in the neck are capable of producing pain. These include vertebral bodies, ligaments, muscles, intervertebral discs, vascular and neural structures. Second, pain may be referred to the neck from other areas such as shoulder, heart, diaphragm, mandible and temporomandibular joints. Finally, pain from the neck may be referred to the shoulders and arms.

OSTEOARTHRITIS (DEGENERATIVE ARTHROPATHY) OF THE CERVICAL SPINE

Osteoarthritis (OA) is a major cause of neck pain. Intervertebral disc degeneration is most common at C5/6 and C6/7, with increasing incidence in old age. Degenerate discs may herniate into the spinal canal or intervertebral foramina, with direct compression of the spinal cord or nerve roots. More commonly, disc degeneration leads to abnormal stresses on the vertebral bodies and on the facet and uncovertebral joints. These abnormal stresses lead to formation of bone spurs or osteophytes. These osteophytes may project into the spinal canal causing compression of the cervical cord, or into the intervertebral foramina causing nerve root compression. Osteoarthritis uncomplicated by compression of neural structures may cause episodic neck pain. This pain tends to be increased by activity, may be associated with shoulder pain or headache and usually resolves over 7–10 days.

Cervical cord compression presents clinically with neck pain associated with a stiff gait and brisk lower limb reflexes. As stated above, OA is the most common cause of cervical spinal cord compression. Other less common causes may occur as follows:
- Syrinx.
- Spinal cord tumours: ependymoma, glioma, neurofibroma, meningioma.
- Vertebral body tumours: metastases, giant cell tumour, chordoma.

Nerve root compression produces local neck pain plus pain in the distribution of the compressed nerve.

IMAGING OF THE PATIENT WITH NECK PAIN

The goals of imaging of the patient with neck pain should be to exclude conditions requiring urgent attention, to diagnose a treatable condition and to direct management.

With these goals in mind, and given the fact that most neck pain resolves spontaneously, it follows that the majority of patients do not require imaging. Imaging should be reserved for those cases where symptoms are severe and persistent, or where there are other relevant factors on history or examination such as trauma or a known primary tumour.

Initial imaging in the majority of cases will be a plain film examination of the cervical spine. This should include oblique views to assess the intervertebral foramina.

Radiographic signs of osteoarthritis include:
- Disc space narrowing, most common at C5/6 and C6/7 (Fig. 13.12).
- Osteophyte formation on the vertebral bodies and facet joints.
- Osteophytes projecting into the intervertebral foramina.

Magnetic resonance imaging is the investigation of choice where further imaging is required for persistent nerve root pain, or for assessment of a possible spinal cord abnormality. Computed tomography is used in the investigation of neck pain where fine bone detail

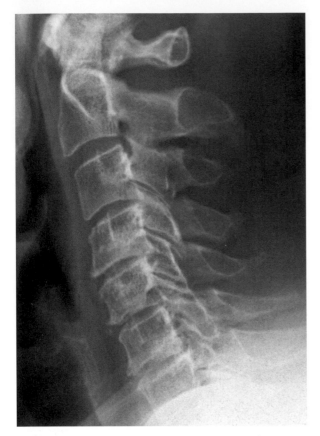

Fig. 13.12 *Osteoarthritis of the cervical spine. Note disc space narrowing at multiple levels.*

is required such as in the assessment of vertebral body tumour.

LOW BACK PAIN

Low back pain refers to back pain that does not extend below the iliac crests. Pain extending to the buttocks or legs is referred to as sciatica. This is a separate clinical problem from back pain and is considered below.

Low back pain may be classified into acute or chronic, with the term 'acute back pain' usually referring to pain of less than 12 weeks duration. There are now well-developed evidence-based guidelines for the management and investigation of acute back pain. There are some variations to guidelines in different parts of the world; however, a number of consistent recommendations can be identified. Primary among

these is the need for diagnostic triage of patients into three major groups:

1 Non-specific low back pain;
2 Specific low back pain;
3 Sciatica or radicular pain, with neurological changes and positive straight-leg raise test.

As will be discussed below, sciatica is best investigated with MRI or CT. Specific low back pain refers to back pain with associated clinical symptoms or signs, known as 'red flags', that may indicate an underlying problem. Examples of these 'red flags', some of which will be discussed below include:

- Known primary tumour such as prostate or breast.
- Systemic symptoms: unexplained fever or weight loss.
- Recent trauma.
- Known osteoporosis or prolonged steroid use.
- Age at onset of pain: <20 years or >55 years.
- Thoracic pain.
- Neurological changes.

NON-SPECIFIC LOW BACK PAIN

Acute low back pain

All of the evidence-based guidelines on acute back pain agree that imaging assessment, including radiographs of the lumbar spine, is not indicated in patients with non-specific acute back pain. This reflects the fact that most cases of non-specific low back pain are caused by musculoligamentous injury or exacerbation of degenerative arthropathy and will resolve, usually within a few weeks. Most guidelines emphasize the importance of reassurance, discouragement of bed rest and the recognition of psychosocial risk factors leading to chronic back pain.

Chronic low back pain

In most cases, guidelines on low back pain deal with acute back pain only. There are no actual guidelines dealing with the management and investigation of chronic back pain. There is, however, a wealth of evidence in the literature that may be helpful. Most of this evidence points to the exclusion of 'red flag' conditions. In most cases a multidisciplinary approach to therapy is required, including exercise, education and

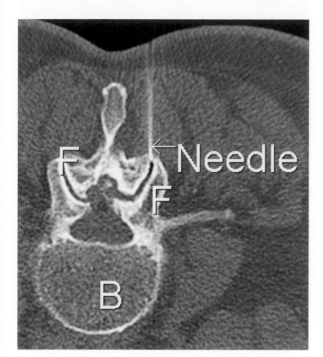

Fig. 13.13 *Facet joint block: computed tomography guidance. The patient is lying prone with the vertebral body (B) toward the bottom of the image. A fine needle is inserted into the facet joint (F) for injection of local anaesthetic and steroid.*

counselling. Although it may sound strange, in most cases a specific diagnosis as to the cause of pain is not required. In some cases, however, particularly when pain is severe and debilitating, or causing other problems such as loss of employment or depression, a specific diagnosis may be required as a guide to therapy.

It can be shown that most cases of chronic back pain result from facet joint pain, sacroiliac joint pain or internal disruption of intervertebral discs. In the majority of cases, imaging techniques such as radiography, CT and MRI are unable to pinpoint the cause of pain. Again, this may sound strange, as these techniques certainly show changes of degenerative arthropathy in a large percentage of patients examined. The trouble is that imaging findings are very non-specific. For example, radiographs may show a narrowed disc space; this does not mean that this is definitely the cause of the patient's pain. The only way to prove that a certain structure, such as a facet joint, is the cause of pain is to inject local anaesthetic into that structure and assess the response.

Such injections are now commonplace in the management of chronic back pain and are performed under CT or fluoroscopic guidance (Fig. 13.13). These procedures include facet joint blocks and sacroiliac joint blocks. If a facet joint is found to be the cause of pain, the nerves supplying that joint may be permanently blocked with radiofrequency ablation.

Discography is used to prove that pain is arising from one or more intervertebral discs. Under fluoroscopic guidance, a fine needle is positioned in the centre of the intervertebral disc. A small amount of dilute contrast material is injected to 'stress' the disc. The patient's pain response is recorded. Contrast material is used to assess the actual morphology of the disc and to diagnose annular tears.

SPECIFIC BACK PAIN SYNDROMES: IMAGING FINDINGS

As discussed above, imaging is not required for the management of most people with acute or chronic back pain. Imaging may be required for assessment of back pain associated with 'red flags' as listed above. An initial radiographic examination of the lumbar spine is reasonable in these patients (Fig. 13.14). This will help exclude obvious bony causes of pain as well as delineate any other relevant factors such as scoliosis. The major limitation of radiographs of the lumbar spine is that soft-tissue structures such as ligaments, muscles and nerve roots are not imaged. Radiographs are relatively insensitive for many painful bone conditions such as infection. Furthermore, the cross-sectional dimensions of the spinal canal are not assessed.

Scintigraphy with ^{99m}Tc-methylene diphosphonate (MDP) is used where a bony cause of back pain is to be excluded. It is particularly useful for the following:

- Infection.
- Suspected neoplasm, especially to exclude spinal metastases where there is a known primary tumour.
- Pars interarticularis fractures; these may be difficult to see on plain films, particularly in young patients with subtle stress fractures.

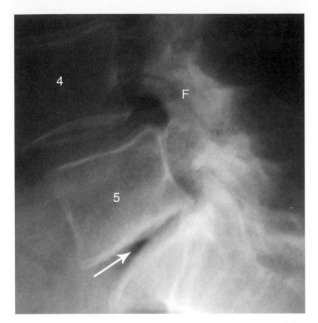

Fig. 13.14 *Osteoarthritis of the lumbar spine. Narrowing of the intervertebral disc space between L5 and S1 (arrow). Sclerosis of the facet joints at L4/5 (F) with degenerative spondylolisthesis at this level.*

Cross-sectional imaging techniques, MRI and CT, are recommended for assessment of sciatica syndromes, as outlined below. Depending on findings on radiographs or scintigraphy, MRI or CT may be indicated for further assessment. In many conditions such as suspected infection or suspected acute osteoporotic crush fracture, MRI is the investigation of choice. Computed tomography is highly accurate for assessment of bony lesions such as suspected tumours or pars interarticularis defects.

PARS INTERARTICULARIS DEFECTS AND SPONDYLOLISTHESIS

The pars interarticularis represents a mass of bone between the superior and inferior articular processes of the vertebral body. It is best seen radiographically on oblique views of the lumbar spine. Defect of the pars interarticularis, also known as spondylolysis, may be congenital or caused by trauma. Congenital pars interarticularis defects are often associated with other developmental anomalies of the lumbar spine, especially spina bifida occulta. Acute trauma may produce an acute

fracture through the pars interarticularis, and stress fractures may occur associated with sports such as gymnastics and fast bowling (cricket). Regardless of aetiology, pars interarticularis defects are most common at L5, though may occur at other levels. Bilateral pars defects may be associated with spondylolisthesis (i.e. anterior shift of L5 on S1).

In spondylolysis and spondylolisthesis back pain may be caused by a number of factors. These include the bony defects themselves, segmental instability and degenerative changes in the intervertebral disc. Spondylolysis is suspected in back pain presenting in otherwise healthy young adults, particularly those participating in typical sporting activities. Spondylolisthesis also causes narrowing of the intervertebral foramina between L5 and S1 with compression of the exiting L5 nerve roots producing bilateral posterior leg pain and a sensation of hamstring tightness.

Spondylolysis and spondylolisthesis may be investigated with plain films, scintigraphy, and CT. Radiographically, pars interarticularis defects are best seen on oblique views of the lower lumbar spine. The complex of overlapping shadows from the superior and inferior articular processes, the pars interarticularis and the transverse process forms an outline resembling that of a Scottish terrier dog. A pars defect is seen as a line across the neck of the 'dog' (Fig. 13.15).

Scintigraphy with ^{99m}Tc-MDP may be used to diagnose subtle stress fractures not able to be visualized radiographically. Pars interarticularis defects are also well shown on CT, particularly with multidetector CT, which allows multiplanar reconstructions. The choice between CT and scintigraphy depends largely on local preferences. Scintigraphy imposes a slightly lower radiation dose than CT, and this is a significant factor in a young adult population. However, scintigraphy supplies less anatomical information and many patients with a positive bone scan will proceed to CT anyway. Magnetic resonance imaging is often used when there is frank spondylolisthesis on the lumbar spine radiographs. It provides more information on the state of the intervertebral disc and is also the best method for assessing the degree of narrowing of the intervertebral foramina and associated nerve root compression.

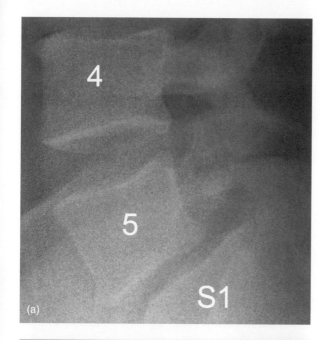

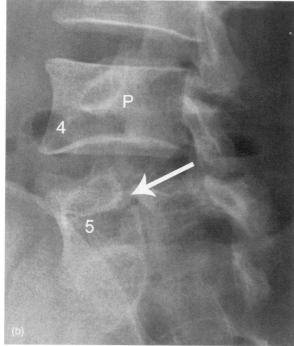

Fig. 13.15 *Pars interarticularis defect. (a) Lateral view of the lower lumbar spine shows spondylolisthesis of L5 on S1. (b) Oblique view of the lower lumbar spine showing a pars interarticularis defect at L5 (arrow). Note also the intact pars interarticularis at L4 (P) and the facet joints.*

VERTEBRAL INFECTION

Most vertebral infection commences in the intervertebral disc. This may spread to involve the vertebral body giving vertebral osteomyelitis, or may invade the spinal canal to produce an epidural abscess. Discitis may occur in children or adults and is more common in the lower spine. It is usually caused by blood-borne infection. In adults there may be a history of recent surgery and vertebral infection is common in intravenous drug users. Clinical features include rapid onset of back pain accompanied by fever and malaise. In young children there may be less-specific symptoms such as limp or failure to weight bear.

Radiographic findings occur late in the disease process and include narrowing of the intervertebral disc, with blurring of the vertebral endplates (Fig. 13.16). Magnetic resonance imaging is now the investigation of choice for the diagnosis of vertebral infection. This should include scans with contrast material injection (gadolinium). Magnetic resonance imaging will be positive before radiographic signs are evident. It is also the best imaging method for showing epidural abscess.

VERTEBRAL METASTASES

Vertebral metastatic disease is suspected when back pain occurs in a patient with a known primary tumour. Other suspicious clinical factors include weight loss and raised prostate-specific antigen (PSA). Tumours with a high incidence of vertebral metastases include prostate, breast, lung, kidney and melanoma. Lymphoma and multiple myeloma may also involve the spine.

Radiographs of the lumbar spine may show focal sclerotic (dense) lesions throughout the vertebral bodies in metastases from prostatic primary (Fig. 9.15, page 140). Other primary tumours tend to produce lytic or destructive metastases that may be difficult to appreciate on radiographs. Scintigraphy with ^{99m}Tc-MDP is generally the investigation of choice in screening for skeletal metastases, including the spine (Fig. 12.18, page 195).

Occasionally, a vertebral metastasis may expand into the spinal canal and compress the spinal cord, causing an acute myelopathy. This is most common in

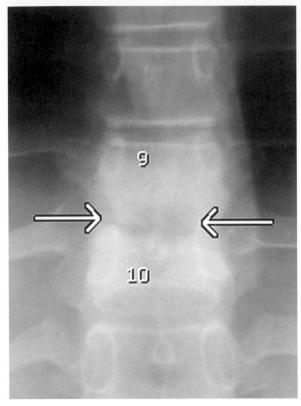

Fig. 13.16 *Discitis. Anteroposterior view of the thoracic spine showing narrowing of the disc space between T9 and T10 with blurring of the vertebral endplates (arrows). Compare this with the normal disc spaces above and below.*

the thoracic region and may require acute surgical decompression or radiotherapy. With spinal cord compression there are usually motor problems in the legs leading to difficulty in walking. This may be accompanied by sensory disturbances, a band-like sensation around the abdomen and voiding difficulties. Magnetic resonance imaging is the investigation of choice for suspected spinal cord compression.

ACUTE OSTEOPOROTIC CRUSH FRACTURE

Individuals with osteoporosis are at an increased risk for the development of a crush fracture of the spine. These occur most commonly in the lower thoracic and lumbar spine. The patient usually presents with acute back pain that is mechanical in type (i.e. worsened by movement or activity). There may be an associated

band-like distribution of pain around the chest wall or abdomen, depending on the level involved. The pain associated with osteoporotic crush fracture usually settles in a matter of weeks. In some patients, however, the pain persists and may become quite disabling. There may be inhibition of respiration and difficulty sleeping. In elderly patients there is a significant mortality and morbidity associated with osteoporotic crush fractures. Percutaneous vertebroplasty is now a widely accepted technique for the treatment of the pain associated with acute osteoporotic crush fractures.

Radiographs of the spine will usually diagnose the crush fracture (Fig. 13.9, page 203). A major limitation of radiography is that there is no reliable way to distinguish an acute crush fracture from an older, healed injury. This becomes relevant in particular where percutaneous vertebroplasty is being considered and multiple crush fractures are seen on radiography. Magnetic resonance imaging is used to define the acute level(s). It is able to show bone marrow oedema in acutely crushed vertebral bodies (see Fig. 1.34, page 23). Older, healed crush fractures show normal bone marrow signal with no evidence of oedema.

Vertebroplasty involves the insertion of a large-bore needle (11 or 13 gauge) into the vertebral body followed by injection of bone cement. The bone cement is mixed with barium powder so it can be visualized radiographically. Needle placement and cement injection are performed under direct fluoroscopic guidance to avoid injury to neurological structures (Fig. 13.17). Vertebroplasty is a highly effective technique for reducing pain, restoring mobility and reducing dependence on analgesics. It does not restore vertebral body height. An extension of vertebroplasty known as kyphoplasty may be used to restore vertebral body height. In kyphoplasty, a balloon is inflated in the vertebral body creating a cavity into which bone cement is injected.

SCOLIOSIS

Scoliosis refers to abnormal curvature of the spine. Scoliosis may be congenital and is caused by abnormal vertebral segmentation. Scoliosis may also be seen as

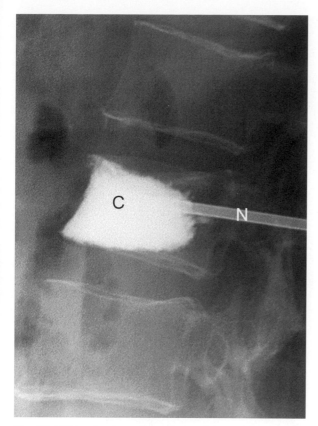

Fig. 13.17 *Vertebroplasty. Lateral view showing radio-opaque bone cement (C) being injected into the vertebral body via a large bone biopsy needle (N).*

part of a syndrome such as neurofibromatosis. An acute painful scoliosis may indicate the presence of vertebral infection or a tumour such as osteoid osteoma. Most commonly, scoliosis is idiopathic. Idiopathic scoliosis is classified according to the age of onset with three major groups described:

• Infantile: birth to 3 years.
• Juvenile: 4–9 years.
• Adolescent: 10 years or later.

Adolescent idiopathic scoliosis (AIS) accounts for 90 per cent of patients with scoliosis. The key clinical test for the diagnosis of AIS is the forward bend test. With a positive forward bend test there is convex bulging of the contour of the back on the side of the convexity of the spinal curve. This is caused by rotation of the spine producing prominence of the posterior ribs on the convex side.

Patients with suspected scoliosis should be assessed radiographically. This consists of a single AP long film of the thoracic and lumbar spine taken with the patient standing erect. The key to radiographic diagnosis is measurement of the Cobb angle. To measure the Cobb angle a line is drawn parallel to the superior vertebral endplate of the most tilted vertebral body at the upper end of the curve. A similar line is drawn parallel to the lower vertebral endplate of the lower most tilted vertebral body. The angle between these lines is the Cobb angle. With computed radiography, the Cobb angle can be measured electronically, improving its accuracy (Fig. 13.18). A Cobb angle of 10° or greater is considered abnormal.

Curves are described by their region, thoracic or lumbar, and by the direction of convexity. A right curve is convex to the right. The largest curve is termed the 'major' or 'primary' curve. Compensatory or secondary curves occur above and below the primary curve; these usually have smaller Cobb angles than the primary curve. The most common pattern in AIS is a right thoracic primary curve with a left lumbar or thoracolumbar secondary curve.

A single erect radiograph is usually sufficient for the imaging assessment of AIS. Further imaging with MRI may be indicated by visible abnormalities on the plain film of the spine or by atypical curves. In particular, a left thoracic primary curve is associated with a central cyst of the cord (syrinx) and other anomalies and MRI is indicated in such cases.

SCIATICA

DEGENERATIVE DISC DISEASE AND SPINAL CANAL STENOSIS

The two major risk factors for degenerative disc disease of the lumbar spine are increasing age and trauma. Each intervertebral disc is composed of a tough outer layer, the annulus fibrosis, and a softer semi-fluid centre, the nucleus pulposus. With degeneration of the disc, small microtears appear in the annulus fibrosis allowing

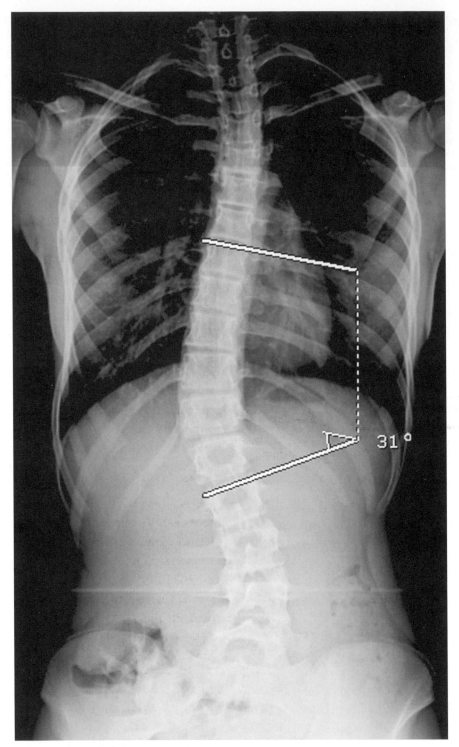

Fig. 13.18 *Adolescent idiopathic scoliosis. Frontal 'long film' showing a primary thoracic scoliosis convex to the right and a secondary lumbar scoliosis convex to the left. Note the method of Cobb angle measurement.*

generalized bulging of the nucleus pulposus. This causes the disc to bulge beyond the margins of the vertebral bodies causing narrowing of the spinal canal. Secondary effects of degenerative disc disease include abnormal stresses on the vertebral bodies leading to osteophyte formation, as well as facet joint sclerosis and hypertrophy. These changes may lead to further narrowing of the spinal canal producing spinal canal stenosis.

The next step in disc degeneration is a localized tear in the annulus fibrosis through which the nucleus pulposus may herniate. This produces a focal protrusion of disc material that may project centrally into the spinal canal or posterolaterally into the intervertebral foramen. A disc herniation that penetrates the posterior longitudinal ligament is referred to as an extruded disc. Extruded discs may separate from the parent disc and migrate superiorly or inferiorly in the spinal canal. This is referred to as a free fragment or sequestration. The use of the terms 'annular bulge', 'protrusion', 'extrusion' and 'sequestration' to describe the various stages and types of intervertebral disc pathology is to be encouraged as the use of a standard terminology will assist in the understanding and management of degenerative disc disease.

SCIATICA SYNDROMES

Sciatica or leg pain syndromes are classified based on whether the pain is acute or chronic, unilateral or bilateral.

Unilateral acute nerve root compression: sciatica

Sciatica refers to pain confined to a nerve root distribution with the leg pain being more severe than back pain. It is accompanied by other neurological symptoms such as paraesthesia, and by signs of nerve root irritation such as positive straight-leg raise test. Sciatica is usually caused by a focal disc protrusion or spondylolisthesis.

Bilateral acute nerve root compression: cauda equina syndrome

Cauda equina syndrome refers to the sudden onset of bilateral leg pain accompanied by bladder and/or bowel dysfunction. It is usually caused by a massive disc protrusion or sequestration.

Unilateral chronic nerve root compression: sciatica lasting for months

Unilateral chronic sciatica is usually caused by disc protrusion or spinal stenosis.

Bilateral chronic nerve root compression

Bilateral chronic nerve root compression refers to vague bilateral leg pain aggravated by walking and slowly relieved by rest. The usual cause is spinal canal stenosis. A common difficulty is differentiating neural compression from vascular claudication. Helpful clinical pointers to a vascular cause include absent peripheral pulses and pain in the exercised muscles; pain relief with rest is usually rapid.

IMAGING OF SCIATICA

Magnetic resonance imaging

For a number of reasons MRI is the investigation of choice for most neurological disorders of the spine. It has better soft-tissue contrast resolution than CT. Nerve roots and the distal spinal cord and conus can be imaged without the use of contrast material. Magnetic resonance imaging is able to outline the anatomy of the spinal canal and the intervertebral discs. It is highly sensitive for the detection of spinal canal stenosis, disc herniation and narrowing of the intervertebral foramina (Fig. 13.19).

Computed tomography

Computed tomography is a reasonable alternative for investigation of sciatica where MRI is not available.

Selective nerve root block

Selective nerve root block is a relatively simple procedure in which a small volume of steroid and local anaesthetic is injected immediately adjacent to a nerve root. A fine needle is positioned adjacent to the nerve root under CT or fluoroscopic guidance. Selective

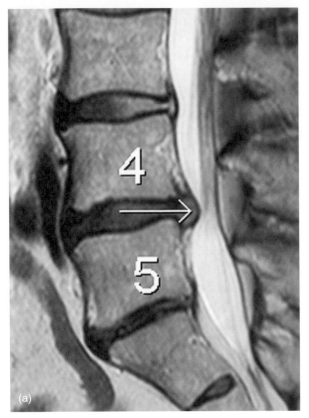

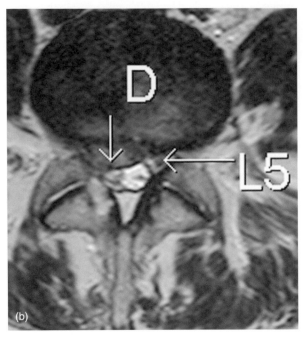

Fig. 13.19 *Intervertebral disc protrusion: magnetic resonance imaging. (a) Sagittal image showing posterior protrusion of the L4/5 disc (arrow). (b) Transverse image through the intervertebral disc (D) showing protrusion into the right side of the spinal canal (arrow). Note the normal left L5 nerve root. The right L5 nerve root is compressed and cannot be visualized.*

nerve root block is both a diagnostic tool and a means of giving temporary pain relief.

In terms of diagnosis, it is not unusual for patients with sciatica to present with imaging findings of nerve root compression at multiple levels. Alternatively, there may be no imaging evidence on CT or MRI of nerve root compression, despite a convincing clinical presentation. In these cases selective nerve root block may be extremely helpful in confirming the source of the patient's pain.

Selective nerve root block may also be used for therapy. It is an excellent procedure for providing temporary pain relief from sciatica while surgery is planned. In some patients the effects of selective nerve root block may be long-lasting. This is particularly useful where surgery is contraindicated because of anaesthetic risk or other factors.

Central nervous system

IMAGING INVESTIGATION OF BRAIN DISORDERS

Computed tomography (CT) and magnetic resonance imaging (MRI) are by far the most common imaging investigations performed for assessment of brain disorders (Fig. 14.1). In modern clinical practice, MRI is the investigation of choice for most indications. The two most common exceptions are acute trauma and suspected acute subarachnoid haemorrhage. The accuracy of CT in certain pathologies such as tumour and infection is increased with the use of intravenous injection of contrast material. With the widespread availability of MRI, CT of the brain is increasingly used as an initial screening test, particularly in more non-specific clinical presentations such as headache. For these purposes, a non-contrast enhanced CT is adequate in the majority of cases. The reasoning for this is that if an abnormality is found that cannot be characterized on a non-contrast CT then further assessment with MRI will usually be performed. Also, MRI will usually be performed if the CT is negative and there is ongoing clinical suspicion of an abnormality.

Skull X-ray may occasionally be performed as part of a skeletal survey, for example in multiple myeloma (see Fig. 12.19, page 195) or suspected nonaccidental injury in children. It may also be performed for a few uncommon skull vault disorders such as craniosynostosis (premature fusion of cranial sutures in infants).

Cranial ultrasound is a useful investigation in infants where the anterior fontanelle is open. The commonest indication for cranial ultrasound (US) is the diagnosis and monitoring of cerebral haemorrhage in premature infants. Cranial US is also a useful screening test in older infants for assessment of increasing head circumference. In adults, US may occasionally be used to assist in neurosurgery, specifically in the localization of small peripheral tumours, where an US probe is directly applied to the surface of the brain at craniotomy. Otherwise, US cannot be performed in adults because of the inability of sound waves to penetrate the skull vault.

HEAD TRAUMA

Computed tomography is the investigation of choice for the patient with head trauma. It is able to identify rapidly cranial trauma that require urgent neurosurgical intervention, and most other traumatic lesions that may require observation and further follow-up. Indications for head CT in the setting of trauma vary from centre to centre and include:

- Confusion/drowsiness not improved at 4 hours.
- New focal neurological signs.
- Deterioration in level of consciousness.
- Fully conscious with:
  (i) Fitting;
  (ii) Nausea and vomiting;
  (iii) New and persisting headache.
- Glasgow Coma Scale (GCS) <15.
- Clinically obvious compound or depressed skull fracture.
- Suspected fractured skull: scalp laceration to bone; boggy scalp haematoma.
- Signs of fractured base of skull: discharge of blood or cerebrospinal fluid (CSF) from nose or ear.
- Penetrating head injuries.
- Suspected intracranial foreign body.

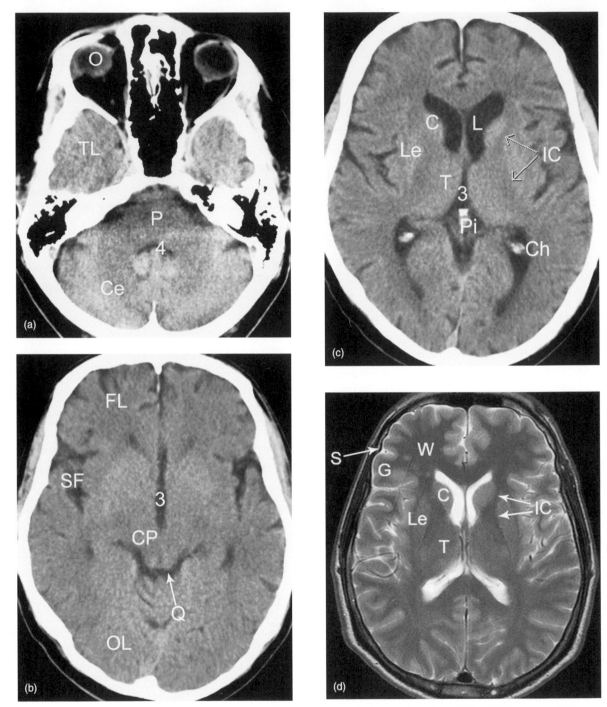

Fig. 14.1 *Normal brain anatomy: computed tomography (CT) and magnetic resonance imaging (MRI). (a) Transverse CT scan through the posterior fossa. (b) Transverse CT scan through the cerebral peduncles. (c) Transverse CT scan through the basal ganglia. (d) Transverse T2-weighted MRI scan through the basal ganglia. Note the following: orbit (O), frontal lobe (FL), temporal lobe (TL), occipital lobe (OL), lateral ventricles (L), third ventricle (3), fourth ventricle (4), cerebellum (Ce), pons (P), cerebral peduncles (CP), quadrigeminal plate cistern (Q), Sylvian fissure (FS), sulcus (S), gyrus (G), white matter (WM), caudate nucleus (C), lentiform nucleus (Le), thalamus (T), internal capsule (IC), pineal gland (Pi) and choroid plexus in lateral ventricle (Ch).*

COMMON COMPUTED TOMOGRAPHY FINDINGS OF HEAD TRAUMA

Acute intracranial haematoma

Acute intracranial haematoma is of high attenuation on CT (white). Over 7–10 days the attenuation gradually decreases to approximately that of adjacent brain tissue. A subdural haematoma of this age is the same attenuation as brain and may therefore be difficult to see. Over the ensuing couple of weeks the attenuation decreases further to approximately that of CSF (black).

Extradural haematoma is usually associated with a skull fracture and is the result of tearing of meningeal blood vessels. It shows on CT as a high-attenuation peripheral lesion with a convex inner margin (Fig. 14.2). Subdural haematoma is associated with underlying brain swelling and is caused by bleeding from peripheral cerebral veins. Subdural haematoma is seen on CT as a high-attenuation peripheral lesion with a concave inner margin, and often spreading over much of the cerebral hemisphere (Fig. 14.3). There is usually associated mass effect due to swelling of the underlying damaged brain. Subdural haematoma decreases in density with time, so that after 2–3 weeks it is of lower attenuation than underlying brain.

Although more commonly caused by rupture of a cerebral aneurysm, subarachnoid haemorrhage may occur with trauma. As with the more common non-traumatic subarachnoid haemorrhage it shows on CT as high-attenuation material in the basal cisterns, sylvian fissures, cerebral sulci and ventricles. Intracerebral haematoma shows on CT as a high-attenuation area in the brain tissue, usually surrounded by a low-attenuation rim of oedema. With resolution, intracerebral haematoma decreases in density to be of lower attenuation than the surrounding brain after about 4 weeks.

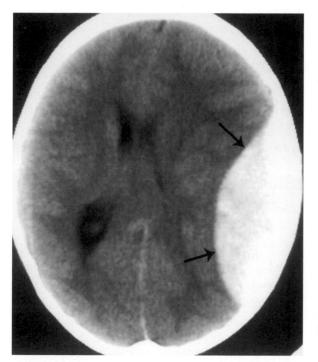

Fig. 14.2 *Extradural haematoma. Acute blood is of high attenuation on computed tomography. Note the convex inner margin (arrows).*

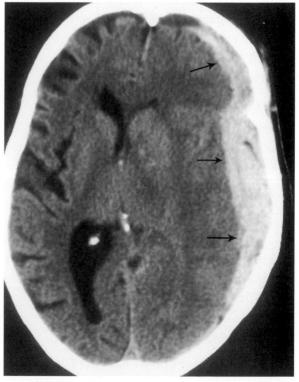

Fig. 14.3 *Subdural haematoma. Note the concave inner margin of the haematoma (arrows).*

Other computed tomography signs of brain damage

Cerebral oedema produces low-attenuation areas that may be focal, multifocal, or diffuse. There is associated mass effect with compression and distortion of cerebral ventricles and basal cisterns. Cerebral contusion is seen as areas of mixed high and low attenuation, which may be focal or multifocal. With time the haemorrhagic component resolves leaving irregular areas of low attenuation. Diffuse axonal (shearing) injuries may be seen as small haemorrhagic areas at the grey–white matter junctions, brainstem and corpus callosum.

Other computed tomography signs of head trauma

As well as brain injury, CT may reveal fractures, scalp swelling, intracranial air (pneumocephalus) resulting from penetrating injury or fractures through paranasal sinuses or skull base, fluid levels in paranasal sinuses and foreign bodies. Computed tomography is especially useful for defining base-of-skull fractures (see Chapter 15).

OTHER INVESTIGATIONS IN HEAD TRAUMA

Magnetic resonance imaging

Owing to relatively poor visualization of acute haemorrhage, time taken for performance of examination and logistical problems with monitoring equipment, MRI has not been recommended for initial screening of acute head trauma. It is most useful in the non-acute situation of an otherwise stable patient with an ongoing neurological or cognitive deficit. In particular, MRI is highly sensitive for the detection of diffuse axonal injury. This potentially serious injury may be difficult to detect with CT.

Cervical spine radiographs

In all major trauma and head injury cases radiographs of the cervical spine should be obtained (see Chapter 13). This must include a lateral cervical spine view showing all seven cervical vertebrae.

SUBARACHNOID HAEMORRHAGE

Patients with non-traumatic (spontaneous) subarachnoid haemorrhage (SAH) present with sudden onset of severe headache, usually described as the worst headache of their lives. This may be accompanied by neck pain and stiffness. The most common causes of spontaneous SAH are ruptured cerebral artery aneurysm in 80–90 per cent and cranial arteriovenous malformation (AVM) in 5 per cent. Less common causes include spinal AVM, coagulopathy, tumour and venous or capillary bleeding.

The vast majority of cerebral aneurysms are congenital 'berry' aneurysms. They occur in 2 per cent of the population and are multiple in 10 per cent of cases. There is an increased incidence of berry aneurysms in association with coarctation of the aorta and autosomal dominant polycystic kidney disease. The majority of berry aneurysms occur around the circle of Willis, the most common sites being:

- Anterior communicating artery.
- Posterior communicating artery.
- Middle cerebral artery.
- Bifurcation of internal carotid artery.
- Tip of basilar artery.

The imaging investigation of suspected SAH consists of CT to confirm the diagnosis, followed by angiography to define the cause and direct subsequent management.

Computed tomography

Computed tomography is the primary imaging investigation of choice in suspected subarachnoid haemorrhage. The roles of CT are to confirm the diagnosis, to suggest a possible site of bleeding and/or cause, and to diagnose complications. Acute SAH shows on CT as high-attenuation material (fresh blood) in the basal cisterns, sylvian fissures, ventricles and cerebral sulci (Fig. 14.4). By localizing the greatest concentration of blood a possible site of haemorrhage can be suggested. For example, blood concentrated in a sylvian fissure indicates bleeding from the ipsilateral middle cerebral artery. Occasionally, the cause of SAH may be seen on

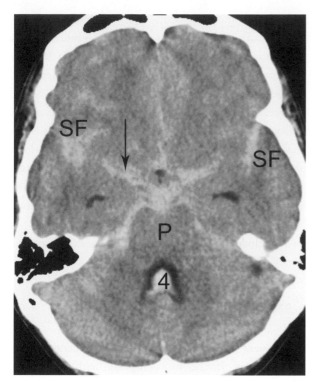

Fig. 14.4 *Subarachnoid haemorrhage. Acute blood is seen as high-density material in the basal cisterns (arrow), anterior to the pons (P), in the Sylvian fissures (SF) and fourth ventricle (4).*

CT. Examples of this would include a large aneurysm, AVM or tumour. Large aneurysms show as well-defined high-attenuation lesions that show intense enhancement with contrast material. Arteriovenous malformation accounts for 5 per cent of SAH.

The CT signs of AVM include poorly defined, irregular areas of mixed attenuation, often with calcification, intense enhancement with contrast material and visualization of feeding arteries and tortuous draining veins. Complications of SAH visible on CT include hydrocephalus and vasospasm. Hydrocephalus is a common finding because of obstruction of CSF pathways with blood. It may occur within hours of the haemorrhage. Vasospasm may lead to ischaemia and infarction seen on CT as areas of low attenuation.

A normal CT does not exclude a small SAH. Up to 5 per cent of patients with a proven SAH have a normal CT, though this figure is probably smaller with modern scanners. In cases of negative CT, diagnostic lumbar puncture is usually performed to look for fresh blood in the CSF, or xanthochromia. This is not a perfect test. A blood-stained tap may occur, and there may be problems with interpretation of xanthochromia. Given more widespread availability of multislice CT scanners, the modern trend is to dispense with the lumbar puncture and instead perform a CT angiogram to try to demonstrate a berry aneurysm.

Computed tomography angiography and magnetic resonance angiography

Computed tomography angiography (CTA) and magnetic resonance angiography (MRA) may be used to image the cerebral vessels. Both techniques are of comparable sensitivity to catheter angiography for displaying aneurysms of 3 mm or greater. Both CTA and MRA produce three-dimensional (3D) images that may be rotated and manipulated on a viewing workstation, allowing a highly detailed examination. The choice of whether to perform CTA or MRA largely depends on local expertise and availability. Also, CTA and MRA each have relative advantages and disadvantages that may influence selection of technique in individual patients.

Magnetic resonance angiography is non-invasive and contrast material injection is not required. It has relatively long scan times that may be a problem in restless or claustrophobic patients. It is contraindicated in patients with pacemakers, ferromagnetic clips and implants, and ocular metal foreign bodies. Computed tomography angiography has shorter scan times of the order of 20–30 seconds, and is therefore better tolerated in restless patients. The main disadvantage of CTA is that it requires the use of iodinated contrast material.

Whichever technique is used, the aims of CTA or MRA are to show the aneurysm (Fig. 14.5), demonstrate the relationship of the neck of the aneurysm to the vessel of origin, and to diagnose multiple aneurysms, if present (10 per cent of cases). Computed tomography angiography and MRA may also be used for screening purposes for individuals with a history of SAH or cerebral aneurysm in a first-degree relative. Screening may also be used for patients with a condition known to be associated with berry aneurysm, including coarctation of

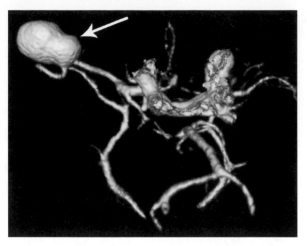

Fig. 14.5 *Cerebral aneurysm: computed tomography (CT) angiogram. Three-dimensional reconstructed image from a CT angiogram shows an aneurysm of the right middle cerebral artery (arrow).*

the aorta and autosomal dominant polycystic kidney disease. Computed tomography angiography and MRA may also be useful in certain clinical presentations with a high probability of cerebral aneurysm. A common example is isolated third cranial nerve palsy, which may be caused by an aneurysm of the posterior communicating artery.

Catheter angiography

Angiography with selective catheterization of the carotid and vertebral arteries remains the 'gold standard' for the diagnosis of cerebral aneurysms in the setting of SAH. In many centres, however, it has been replaced by CTA or MRA for diagnosis and is reserved for use with interventional therapy. Negative angiograms occur in up to 15 per cent of SAH and these may be due to clotting of the aneurysm or non-filling because of severe local vasospasm. In these cases a repeat angiogram may be worthwhile. If the repeat angiogram is negative, a spinal site of bleeding should be considered and MRI of the spine performed.

Interventional radiology

Interventional radiology is now commonly used to treat aneurysms and AVMs. The basic tool of neurointervention is the microcatheter. Microcatheters

can be advanced coaxially through larger conventional catheters deep into the intracerebral arteries. Relevant techniques in the setting of SAH include coil embolization of aneurysms and glue occlusion of intracerebral AVMs (Fig. 14.6).

Neurointerventional procedures are often done under general anaesthetic. Adequate informed consent is mandatory. Complications, though uncommon, include stroke and death from inadvertent embolization or rupture. Post procedure care often requires close observation in an intensive care unit (ICU) or high-dependency unit. Contraindications to neurointerventional procedures include bleeding disorder and lack of vascular access due to unsuitable arterial anatomy.

STROKE

A transient ischaemic attack (TIA) is an acute neurological deficit that resolves completely within 24 hours. These attacks are thought to be caused by transient reduction of blood flow to the brain or eye as a result of emboli, and are associated with underlying stenosis of the internal carotid or cerebral arteries.

The generic term 'stroke' refers to an acute event leading to a focal neurological deficit that lasts for more than 24 hours. Broadly speaking, stroke may be caused by either decreased blood flow to the brain (ischaemia and infarction) or by intracranial haemorrhage. The common aetiologies of stroke are as follows:

- Cerebral ischaemia and infarction (acute ischaemic stroke): 80 per cent.
- Parenchymal (primary intracerebral) haemorrhage: 15 per cent.
  - (i) Usually caused by hypertension;
  - (ii) Common sites: basal ganglia, brainstem, cerebellum, and deep white matter of the cerebral hemispheres.
- Spontaneous subarachnoid haemorrhage: 5 per cent (see above).
- Cerebral venous occlusion: <1 per cent.

Most acute ischaemic strokes are caused by acute thromboembolic occlusion of cerebral arteries. Haemorrhagic

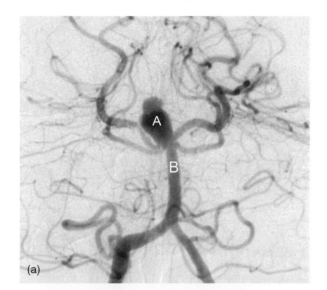

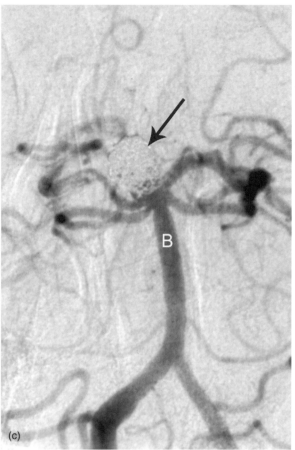

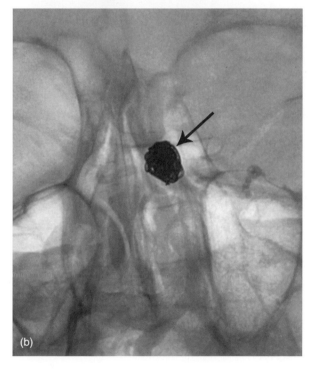

Fig. 14.6 *Treatment of cerebral aneurysm: coil embolization. (a) Diagnostic angiogram showing an aneurysm (A) arising from the distal tip of the basilar artery (B). (b) Non-subtracted images showing dense coils (arrow), which have been inserted into the aneurysm via microcatheter. (c) Post-procedure subtracted angiogram image shows no blood flow into the aneurysm (arrow), indicating successful treatment.*

infarction refers to haemorrhage into a region of infarcted brain. Haemorrhagic infarction may occur following clearing of an arterial occlusion with restoration of blood flow to damaged brain.

An acute arterial occlusion produces a central region of infarcted brain tissue with a surrounding zone of hypoxic tissue. This hypoxic tissue is potentially salvageable and is termed the ischaemic penumbra.

There have been recent advances in the treatment of acute ischaemic stroke, particularly infusion of the thrombolytic agent tissue plasminogen activator (tPA). Studies have suggested that the use of tPA within the first 3–6 hours following stroke onset may salvage reversibly damaged brain tissue in the ischaemic penumbra. It may be given by intravenous or intra-arterial infusion. Intra-arterial infusion has the theoretical advantage of achieving recanalization of thrombosed arteries with the use of a lower dose and therefore potentially fewer complications. The main disadvantage of intra-arterial infusion is the requirement for selective cerebral artery catheterization, performed by a specialist neurointerventionist. Thrombolytic agents are contraindicated in the presence of haemorrhage.

Based on the above principles, it can be seen that the main, often overlapping roles of imaging in the investigation and management of stroke/TIA are:

- To diagnose the type of stroke, in particular to exclude haemorrhage in the acute situation.
- To accurately delineate the anatomy and early changes of acute ischaemic stroke.
- Selection of patients suitable for treatment with tPA.
- Identification of arterial stenosis and occlusion.
- Identification of the source of emboli.
- Identification of asymptomatic patients who may be at risk of stroke.

INITIAL IMAGING ASSESSMENT OF STROKE

Computed tomography remains the investigation of choice in most centres for the initial assessment of the patient with symptoms of stroke or TIA. It will diagnose haemorrhagic causes of stroke such as parenchymal haemorrhage and subarachnoid haemorrhage. Acute parenchymal haemorrhage shows as an area of increased attenuation within the brain substance (Fig. 14.7). Parenchymal haemorrhage may rupture into the cerebral ventricles, producing secondary subarachnoid haemorrhage. Although usually caused by hypertension, parenchymal haemorrhage in younger patients or in atypical locations should raise the suspicion of an underlying vascular lesion, such as an aneurysm or AVM. In such cases, follow-up with MRI and MRA is indicated. Haemorrhagic infarct can usually be distinguished from primary intracerebral haemorrhage in that it is normally wedge-shaped, conforms to a vascular territory and involves the cerebral cortex (Fig. 14.8).

With improvements in CT technology and expertise, early changes of acute ischaemic stroke are increasingly

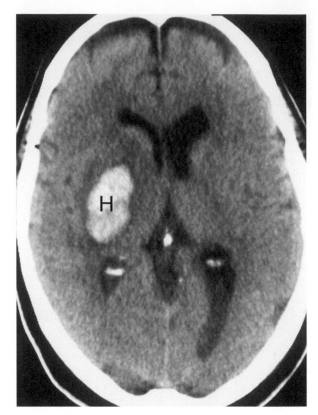

Fig. 14.7 *Primary hypertensive haemorrhage seen as an oval-shaped high-attenuation lesion in the right basal ganglia (H).*

recognized. These subtle CT changes result from mild cerebral swelling and mass effect, decreased attenuation of affected brain tissue and increased density of cerebral arteries due to thrombosis and vascular stasis (Fig. 14.9). Such signs may be appreciated on modern scanners within 3–6 hours of the onset of symptoms. From 12 to 24 hours and over the next 3 days there is increased oedema with more obvious flattening of cerebral gyri and mass effect.

SELECTION OF PATIENTS FOR ANTICOAGULANT THERAPY

Indications for tPA therapy are acute ischaemic stroke, within 3–6 hours of onset of symptoms, and with an identified area of potentially salvageable brain tissue, the ischaemic penumbra. Contraindications to treatment with tPA include duration of symptoms for more than

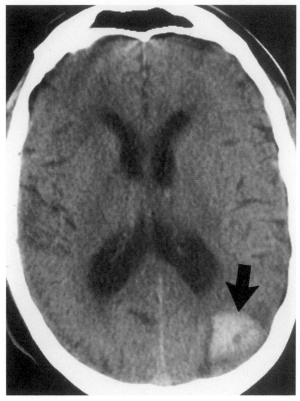

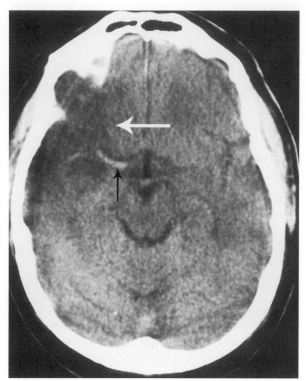

Fig. 14.8 *Haemorrhagic infarct seen as a peripheral wedge-shaped lesion in the left parieto-occipital region (arrow).*

Fig. 14.9 *Early infarct seen on computed tomography as an area of vague low attenuation (white arrow). Note also high attenuation in the right middle cerebral artery due to thrombosis (black arrow).*

3–6 hours, presence of haemorrhage and significant oedema. In this context, significant oedema is defined as low attenuation of more than one-third of the middle cerebral artery territory on CT.

As described above, CT is increasingly able to identify changes of early acute ischaemic stroke. It can also accurately exclude haemorrhage. The main limitation of CT is in the delineation of very subtle changes of ischaemia and in the identification of the ischaemic penumbra. Magnetic resonance imaging with diffusion-weighted imaging and perfusion-weighted imaging now has an important role in the identification of hyperacute infarction and ischaemia.

Diffusion-weighted imaging (DWI) is sensitive to the random Brownian motion (diffusion) of water molecules within tissue. The greater the amount of diffusion, the greater the signal loss on DWI. Areas of reduced water molecule diffusion show on DWI as

high signal. With the onset of acute ischaemia and cell death there is increased intracellular water (cytotoxic oedema) with restricted diffusion of water molecules. An acute infarct therefore shows on DWI as an area of relatively high signal (Fig. 14.10). Diffusion-weighted imaging is the most sensitive imaging test available for the diagnosis of hyperacute infarction.

Perfusion-weighted imaging (PWI) can also be used to calculate the relative blood supply of a particular volume of brain. For PWI the brain is rapidly scanned following injection of a bolus of contrast material (gadolinium). The data obtained may be represented in a number of ways, including maps of regional cerebral blood volume and mean transit time.

Studies have shown that, in general, the perfusion defects identified with PWI are larger than the diffusion abnormalities shown on DWI. The difference between these areas represents the ischaemic penumbra.

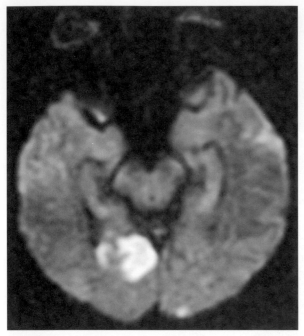

Fig. 14.10 *Infarct: diffusion-weighted magnetic resonance imaging. Acute infarct in the right occipital lobe seen as an area of high signal indicating restricted diffusion of water molecules.*

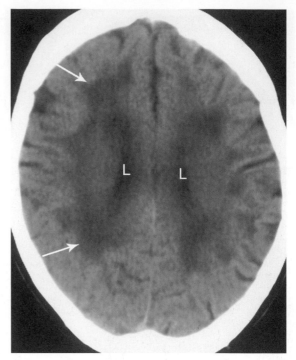

Fig. 14.11 *Chronic brain ischaemia: computed tomography (CT). A CT section at the level of the superior surfaces of the lateral ventricles (L) shows multiple bilateral areas of low attenuation in the white matter (arrows).*

Magnetic resonance imaging using the above sequences is therefore able to accurately diagnose hyperacute infarction and identify the ischemic penumbra. The main limitation is availability of MRI within the time-frame of 3–6 hours of onset of symptoms. This may not be a problem in large tertiary referral centres, but in many institutions CT remains the investigation of choice for patient selection.

IDENTIFICATION OF ARTERIAL STENOSIS AND OCCLUSION

Both CTA and MRA are able to diagnose stenosis or occlusion of carotid and cerebral vessels (see Fig. 1.15, page 12). Choice of technique is largely dictated by local expertise and availability. Each technique has relative advantages and disadvantages, as outlined in the previous section on subarachnoid haemorrhage. Carotid ultrasound is able to diagnose and quantify atheromatous disease of the carotid arteries in the neck (see below) but is unable to image cerebral vessels.

IDENTIFICATION OF ASYMPTOMATIC 'AT RISK' PATIENTS

Identification of patients at risk for developing stroke involves identification of risk factors plus the diagnosis of structural abnormalities. Risk factors for stroke include hypertension, diabetes and hypercholesterolaemia. Approximately 30 per cent of patients with TIA will develop a subsequent infarct. Miscellaneous indications of risk include coronary artery disease and severe peripheral artery disease. Clinical findings may include a bruit in the neck or retinal emboli.

Relevant structural abnormalities include previous 'silent' brain infarcts, white matter ischaemic change and atheromatous disease of the internal carotid arteries. Computed tomography or MRI may be used to diagnose ischaemic changes in the brain. On CT these changes may include generalized low attenuation in the periventricular tissues and deep white matter, with high signal in these areas seen on MRI (Fig. 14.11).

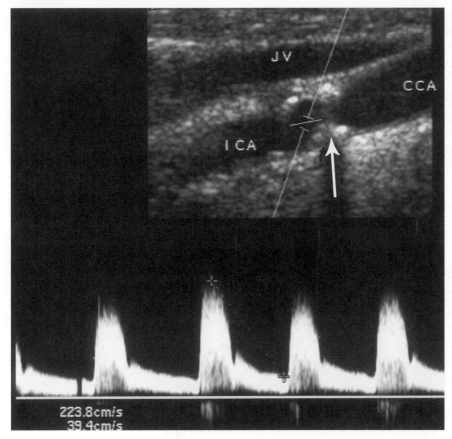

Fig. 14.12 *Internal carotid artery stenosis: duplex ultrasound. This shows a large calcified plaque (arrow) at the origin of the internal carotid artery (ICA). Velocity measurements indicate stenosis in the range of 50–69 per cent. Note also the common carotid artery (CCA) and internal jugular vein (JV).*

Old infarcts are seen on CT as well-defined peripheral areas of low attenuation associated with shrinkage, and lacunar infarcts as small well-defined low attenuation lesions in the basal ganglia and deep white matter.

Ultrasound examination of the carotid arteries is a useful screening test able to diagnose atheromatous disease causing stenosis and occlusion of the internal carotid artery. The arteries are directly visualized with ultrasound and the arterial lumen examined with colour Doppler. Blood flow velocity is measured in the common carotid artery and internal carotid artery. This includes measurements of peak systolic velocity (PSV) and end-diastolic velocity (EDV) given in centimetres per second. Comparison of PSV for the internal carotid artery and common carotid artery gives the ICA/CCA ratio. A stenosis will be indicated by direct visualization of arterial narrowing plus increased measured flow rate in the internal carotid artery (Fig. 14.12). Based on the

ultrasound appearance of the carotid arteries plus the measured blood flow velocities, the degree of internal carotid artery disease may be classified as follows:

- Normal: no plaque visualized; internal carotid artery PSV <125 cm/s.
- <50 per cent stenosis: plaque visualized; internal carotid artery PSV <125 cm/s.
- 50–69 per cent stenosis: plaque visualized; internal carotid artery PSV 125–230 cm/s.
- 70 per cent – near occlusion: plaque visualized; internal carotid artery PSV >230 cm/s.
- Near occlusion: markedly narrowed lumen visualized by colour Doppler.
- Complete occlusion: no blood flow visualized by colour Doppler.

This classification is clinically relevant as carotid endarterectomy is beneficial in stenosis of 70 per cent to near occlusion, with no definite benefit shown for stenosis of <70 per cent. Complete occlusion is considered to be inoperable.

HEADACHE

Headache is a very common symptom. Common causes include stress or tension headache and migraine. Headache may also be a non-specific symptom of generalized malaise such as may occur in common viral or bacterial infections. Most patients with headache can

be diagnosed and treated on clinical grounds, without any need for imaging assessment. There are, however, certain specific types of headache and associated clinical scenarios that do warrant imaging assessment and several examples of these are outlined below.

Suspected subarachnoid haemorrhage (see above)

- Sudden onset of severe headache.
- 'Worst headache of my life'.
- Associated neck pain and stiffness.
- Investigation of choice: CT.

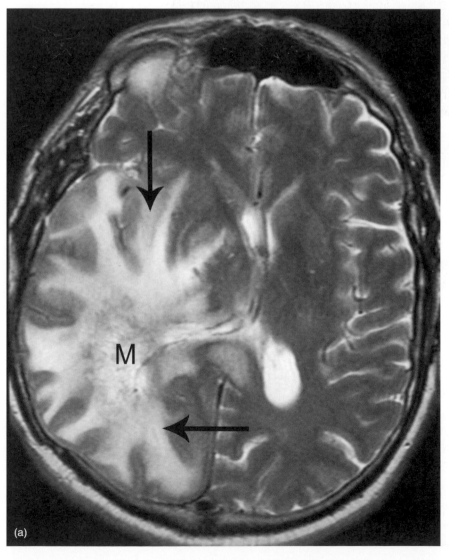

Fig. 14.13 *Malignant brain tumour (glioblastoma multiforme): magnetic resonance imaging. (a) T2-weighted transverse scan of the brain shows a high-signal mass (M) surrounded by high-signal oedema (arrows).*

(a)

Suspected space-occupying lesion: adult

- Signs of raised intracranial pressure.
- Headache, worse in the morning.
- Confusion; focal neurology: hemiparesis, focal seizures.
- Investigation of choice: MRI (Fig. 14.13(a) and (b)).
- CT if MRI contraindicated or difficult to obtain.

Suspected space-occupying lesion: child

- New onset headache, sleep related.
- No family history of migraine.
- Papilloedema.
- Investigation of choice: MRI.

Suspected dissection of carotid or vertebral artery

- Sudden-onset unilateral headache.
- Neck pain; ipsilateral Horner's syndrome.
- History of trauma or neck manipulation.
- Investigation of choice: MRI and MRA.

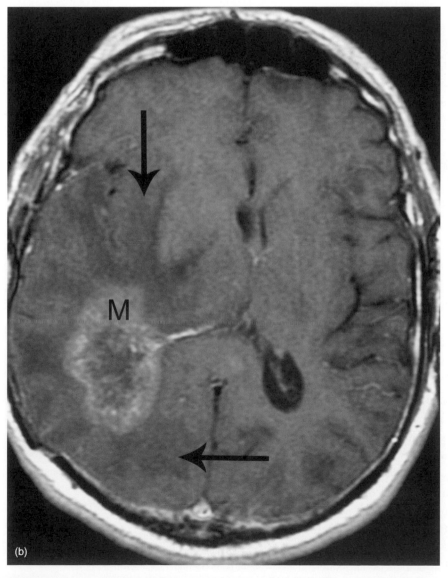

Fig. 14.13 *(b) T1-weighted contrast enhanced scan at the same level as (a). The oedema is low signal on this sequence (arrows). The tumour shows enhancement with contrast and is easier to differentiate from the surrounding oedema than on the T2-weighted scan. Lack of enhancement of the centre of the tumour is caused by necrosis.*

Suspected temporal arteritis

- New headache in an elderly patient (>60).
- Temporal tenderness.
- Increased erythrocyte sedimentation rate (ESR).
- Investigation of choice: MRI.

Suspected intracranial infection

- New headache with fever.
- Neck stiffness with meningitis.
- Reduced consciousness with encephalitis.
- History of sinusitis or middle ear infection.
- History of immune compromise, including human immunodeficiency virus (HIV).
- Investigation of choice: MRI with contrast material (gadolinium).
- CT if MRI not available, though less sensitive than MRI for meningitis and encephalitis.

OTHER COMMON INDICATIONS FOR IMAGING IN THE CENTRAL NERVOUS SYSTEM

EPILEPSY

Epilepsy is a common chronic condition that may be genetic or acquired, and characterized by predisposition to recurrent seizures. Seizures are characterized by abnormal electrical discharges in brain cells producing finite events of cerebral function. Classification of seizure type is important as this will help to guide the need for further investigation and subsequent management and counselling. There are two broad categories of seizure type: primary generalized and partial. Primary generalized seizures originate simultaneously from both cerebral hemispheres and produce bilateral clinical symptoms. Partial seizures originate from a localized area of the brain, based on clinical manifestations and electroencephalogram (EEG) findings. Clinical manifestations of partial seizures may include focal motor or sensory disturbance, psychiatric symptoms, or autonomic

signs or symptoms. Partial seizures are further classified as simple or complex. Complex partial seizures are associated with loss of consciousness; simple partial seizures are not.

Most generalized seizure disorders are idiopathic. Most patients will receive imaging for a first generalized seizure and in most cases this will not show an underlying abnormality. Partial seizures are more commonly associated with an underlying structural lesion. These may include vascular malformations, tumours, brain injury, and developmental abnormalities. In particular, developmental abnormalities of the temporal lobe and hippocampal formation are a common cause of partial complex seizures. These may include sclerosis and atrophy of the hippocampal formation and cortical dysplasia, characterized by abnormal areas of grey matter.

Magnetic resonance imaging is the imaging investigation of choice for the assessment of seizure disorders. Assessment should include high-resolution images of the temporal lobes in the coronal plane to search for developmental abnormalities, some of which may be extremely subtle (Fig. 14.14).

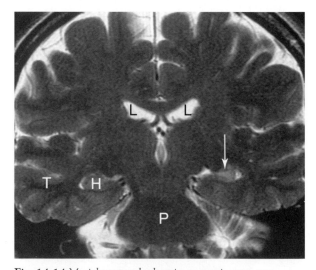

Fig. 14.14 *Mesial temporal sclerosis: magnetic resonance imaging (MRI). A T2-weighted coronal scan through the temporal lobes (T) in a patient with complex partial seizures. Note the normal right hippocampus seen as an oval-shaped structure (H). The left hippocampus shows reduced size and increased signal indicating mesial temporal sclerosis (arrow). Note also the pons (P) and lateral ventricles (L).*

DEMENTIA

The term dementia refers to deterioration of cognitive and intellectual functions not caused by impaired consciousness or perception. Dementia should be differentiated from delirium (acute transient confusion), psychiatric illness such as depression, and specific brain lesions leading to restricted function such as aphasia. Much research is currently directed at potential therapies for various types of dementia, making classification and accurate diagnosis increasingly important. Accurate diagnosis is also important for counselling of the patient and their family. The commonest causes of dementia are Alzheimer's disease (up to 80 per cent of cases) and multi-infarct dementia (10 per cent). Less commonly dementia may be caused by communicating hydrocephalus or chronic subdural haematoma, with rare causes such as Pick's disease and Creutzfeldt–Jakob disease also described.

Computed tomography (CT) and MRI are the primary imaging investigations of the patient with dementia. Magnetic resonance imaging is more accurate than CT, particularly for subtle changes and is the investigation of choice. Alzheimer's disease is suggested clinically by insidious onset of dementia after the age of 60 years, with progressive worsening. In particular, there is prominent loss of memory, especially of new material, with no focal neurological signs on examination. Signs of Alzheimer's disease on MRI include cortical atrophy in the parietal and temporal lobes with marked volume loss of the hippocampal formation. Atrophy of the hippocampal formation is best documented by coronal plane MRI through the temporal lobes. Multi-infarct dementia occurs in patients with risk factors for atheromatous disease and stroke, such as tobacco smoking, hypertension and diabetes. Multi-infarct dementia is characterized clinically by a sudden onset of cognitive decline with a step-wise deterioration in function. There are often accompanying focal signs on neurological examination such as weakness of an extremity or gait disturbance. Magnetic resonance imaging and CT show multiple infarcts involving the basal ganglia, white matter and cortical grey matter (Fig. 14.11, page 224).

Occasionally, diagnostic difficulty may arise with differentiating Alzheimer's disease from multi-infarct dementia on MRI. This is particularly the case where mixed patterns are seen. In such cases, scintigraphy may be useful. Scintigraphy may be performed to assess focal glucose metabolism with fluorodeoxyglucose positron-emission tomography (FDG-PET) or regional cerebral blood flow with ^{99m}Tc-hexamethylpropyleneamine oxime (HMPAO). FDG-PET shows reduced glucose metabolism in the temporal and parietal lobes in Alzheimer's disease; ^{99m}Tc-HMPAO shows reduced blood flow in these regions. In multi-infarct dementia, FDG-PET shows focal areas of reduced cortical and white matter metabolism.

MULTIPLE SCLEROSIS

Multiple sclerosis (MS) is a chronic central nervous system (CNS) disease of young adults characterized by the presence in the brain and spinal cord of focal lesions of demyelination, known as plaques. The plaques of MS occur in the white matter of the brain and in the spinal cord. In the brain, MS has a fairly characteristic distribution, with plaques tending to occur along the walls of the cerebral ventricles as well as the corpus callosum and posterior fossa. Plaques may also be seen in the spinal cord. The clinical presentation is extremely variable and may include double or impaired vision caused by optic neuritis, weakness, numbness and tingling in the limbs, and gait disturbance. Clinical findings often reflect the multifocal nature of the disease. In addition, the time course and nature of progression of the disease are quite variable.

Because of the importance of achieving a correct diagnosis in young adults, diagnostic criteria have been developed. Known as the 'McDonald criteria', these were released in 2001 and revised in 2005. The McDonald criteria use a combination of clinical factors, CSF findings (oligoclonal IgG bands) and MRI appearances to diagnose MS. Magnetic resonance imaging is certainly the imaging investigation of choice for the diagnosis of MS. Computed tomography is not sensitive for the demonstration of MS plaques. Specific MRI

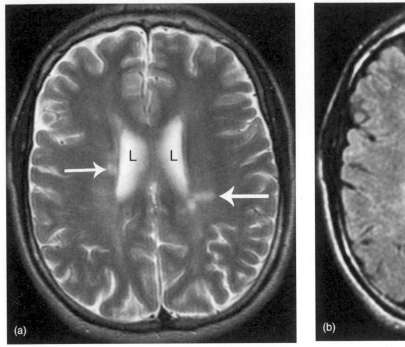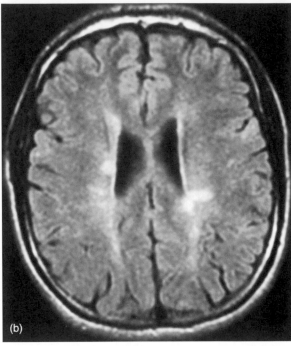

Fig. 14.15 *Multiple sclerosis: magnetic resonance imaging. (a) T2-weighted transverse scan at the level of the lateral ventricles (L) shows multiple areas of high signal in a periventricular distribution (arrows). These are the typical plaques seen in multiple sclerosis.(b) FLAIR (fluid attenuated inversion recovery) transverse scan at the same level as A. The high signal plaques are much easier to see than on the T2-weighted scan.*

sequences are required. The FLAIR (fluid attenuated inversion recovery) sequence shows CSF as black and MS plaques as focal white lesions. This allows accurate demonstration of subtle periventricular plaques (Fig. 14.15). Contrast material injection is also performed as so-called 'active' plaques may show enhancement. On follow-up studies the plaques may vary in appearance, with, for example, 'active' plaques becoming non-enhancing. This variation of appearances with time is an important factor in the McDonald criteria.

The topic of head and neck imaging covers a wide range of pathologies of the face and orbits, skull base, and neck. Head and neck imaging encompasses a number of specialties including ophthalmology, ear, nose and throat (ENT), neurology, neurosurgery and endocrinology. The more common indications for head and neck imaging are outlined in this chapter.

FACIAL TRAUMA

For notes on head trauma see Chapter 14.

MAXILLARY AND ZYGOMATIC FRACTURES

The Le Fort classification is used to describe fractures of the maxilla:
- Le Fort I: fracture line through the lower maxillary sinuses and nasal septum with separation of the lower maxilla.
- Le Fort II: fracture lines extend from the nasal bones in the midline through the medial and inferior walls of the orbits and the lateral walls of the maxillary sinuses, giving a large triangular separate fragment.
- Le Fort III: fracture lines run horizontally through the orbits and the zygomatic arches, causing complete separation of the facial bones from the cranium.

Zygomatic fractures occur in four places:
- Inferior orbital margin.
- Lateral wall of the maxillary sinus.
- Zygomatic arch.
- Lateral wall of orbit (usually diastasis of the zygomatico-frontal suture).

Plain radiographs using lateral, anteroposterior (AP) and angulated projections are usually performed in the

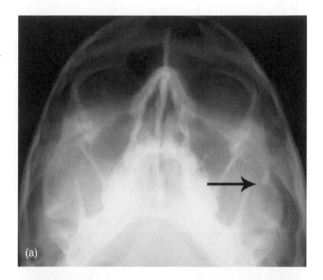

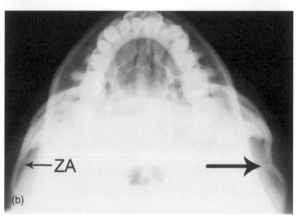

Fig. 15.1 *Zygomatic arch fracture: two examples. (a) Facial radiograph showing a depressed fracture of the left zygomatic arch (arrow). (b) Angulated view of (a) to show the zygomatic arches. Note the normal right zygomatic arch (ZA) and the fractured left arch (arrow).*

initial assessment of facial trauma (Fig. 15.1). In addition to bony changes other radiographic signs associated with facial fractures include soft-tissue swelling, opacification or fluid levels in the maxillary sinuses, and air in the orbit or other soft tissues. Computed tomography

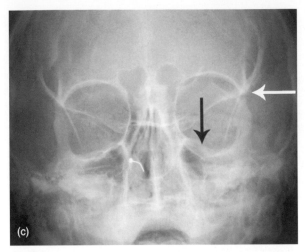

Fig. 15.1 (continued) (c) Facial radiograph showing diastasis of the left zygomaticofrontal articulation (white arrow) plus a fracture of the orbital floor (black arrow). Note the fluid level in the left maxillary sinus due to blood. (The metal object is a nose stud.)

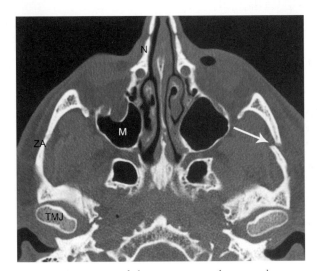

Fig. 15.2 Zygomatic arch fracture: computed tomography (CT). Transverse CT scan showing a fracture of the left zygomatic arch (arrow). Note also the normal right zygomatic arch (ZA), temporomandibular joint (TMJ), maxillary sinus (M) and nasal bones (N).

(CT) is also often used to define precisely the anatomy of facial fractures (Figs 15.2 and 15.3).

ORBITAL TRAUMA

The commonest type of orbital fracture seen is a blow-out type fracture. This is usually the result of a direct blow with sudden increase of intraorbital pressure, producing a fracture of the orbital floor. Radiographs may show a soft-tissue mass in the shape of a 'teardrop' in the roof of the maxillary sinus (Fig. 15.4). This is caused by downward herniation of orbital fat through the orbital floor fracture. The actual fracture is usually quite difficult to see unless displaced. Coronal CT shows the fractures as well as herniation of orbital structures into the maxillary sinus (Fig. 15.5). Usually only orbital fat is involved, however, other structures such as the inferior rectus and inferior oblique muscles may also herniate.

The CT signs of direct ocular trauma include deformity of the eyeball and intraocular haemorrhage seen as an irregular area of raised attenuation in the vitreous. The CT signs of extraocular trauma include optic nerve transection, retrobulbar haematoma and extraocular muscle damage.

ORBITAL FOREIGN BODIES

Radiographs may be used to diagnose radio-opaque foreign bodies and to localize these with respect to the bony margins of the orbit. Eye movement films give an idea of the position of a foreign body. Ultrasound (US) may also be used for foreign bodies. This provides accurate localization except for very small bodies lying posteriorly in the orbit. A foreign body shows as a dense localized echo, usually with shadowing. Computed tomography also provides accurate localization of orbital foreign bodies.

MANDIBULAR FRACTURES

Numerous views may be needed, including OPG (orthopantogram), which gives a panoramic view of the tooth-bearing part of the mandible. Being U-shaped the mandible often fractures in two places. The following areas must be fully imaged in suspected mandibular trauma: midline, body, angle, ramus, condyle and coronoid process (Fig. 15.6, page 234).

IMAGING OF THE ORBIT

Imaging of orbital trauma is discussed above. Ophthalmologists and allied professionals diagnose most disorders

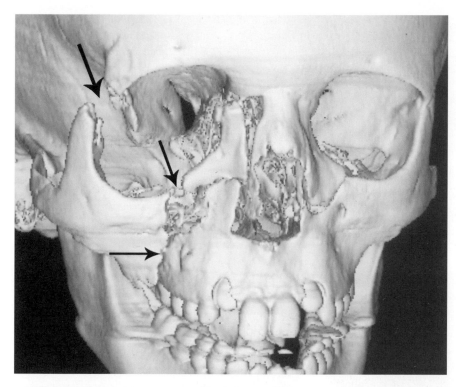

Fig. 15.3 *Complex facial fractures: computed tomography. A three-dimensional reconstructed image of the facial bones shows multiple maxillary and zygomatic fractures (arrows), including diastasis of the zygomaticofrontal articulation producing a gap in the lateral wall of the right orbit.*

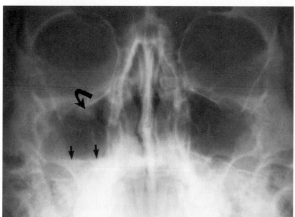

Fig. 15.4 *Orbital floor fracture. Frontal radiograph showing a fracture of the floor of the right orbit (curved arrow) with a round teardrop-shaped opacity in the roof of the maxillary sinus due to downward herniation of orbital fat. Note also the fluid level in the maxillary sinus owing to blood (straight arrows).*

Fig. 15.5 *Orbital floor fracture: computed tomography (CT). Coronal CT image through the orbits (O) showing a fracture of the right orbital floor with downward herniation of orbital fat (arrow) into the maxillary sinus (MS).*

of the eye and orbit without the need for imaging. Imaging is reserved for particular clinical indications. These indications include sudden loss of visual acuity, sudden onset of diplopia, and exophthalmos, especially when acute and progressive, painful or pulsatile. In these cases imaging is performed to diagnose orbital masses or fluid collections as well as intracranial lesions of the visual pathways or third, fourth and sixth cranial nerves. Imaging may also be used to assess orbital changes of underlying syndromes such as neurofibromatosis, or

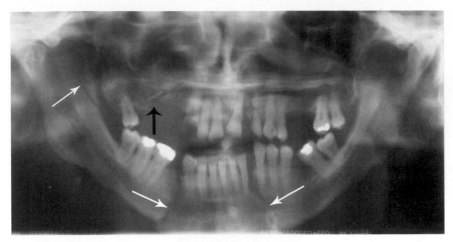

Fig. 15.6 *Mandible fractures: orthopantogram (OPG). A panoramic radiograph of the mandible, shows multiple fractures of the mandible (white arrows) as well as a fracture of the right maxilla (black arrow).*

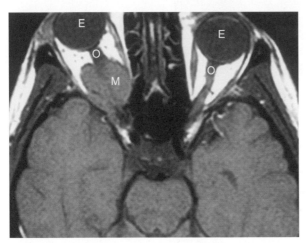

Fig. 15.7 *Orbital meningioma: magnetic resonance imaging. T1-weighted transverse scan through the orbits shows the eyes (E) and optic nerves (O). A mass arising from the dural sheath of the right optic nerve has the typical appearance of a meningioma.*

to assess the extent of a known orbital tumour. Common orbital tumours include:

- Malignant tumours: retinoblastoma in children; ocular melanoma in adults; optic nerve glioma; lymphoma.
- Optic nerve sheath meningioma (Fig. 15.7).
- Lacrimal gland tumours.
- Vascular lesions: haemangioma; varix.

Computed tomography and magnetic resonance imaging (MRI) are the investigations of choice for orbital imaging. Both modalities have excellent natural contrast provided by the bony orbital margins and the orbital fat surrounding the optic nerve and extra-ocular muscles. They often perform complementary roles in the imaging of orbital pathology: CT is more accurate for assessment of the bony margins of the orbit and for detecting calcification in vascular lesions and meningiomas, whereas MRI has superior soft-tissue contrast and is more accurate for delineating intracranial lesions of the visual pathways and cranial nerves.

IMAGING OF THE PARANASAL SINUSES

The paranasal sinuses are air-filled spaces in the medullary cavities of skull and facial bones. Named from the bones in which they occur the paranasal sinuses consist of the frontal, ethmoid, maxillary and sphenoid sinuses. These sinuses drain by small ostia into the nasal cavities. Mucociliary action within the sinuses pushes debris toward the draining ostia. While a variety of congenital anomalies and tumours may affect the paranasal sinuses, the most common indication for imaging is inflammation. Paranasal sinus inflammation may be acute or chronic. There is commonly associated disease in the nasal passages, in particular nasal polyposis in association with allergic sinusitis.

Acute sinusitis is usually viral or bacterial and presents clinically with facial pain and headache, nasal

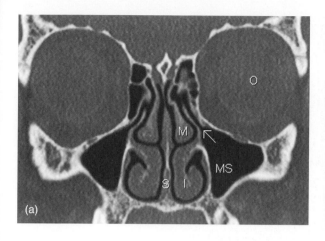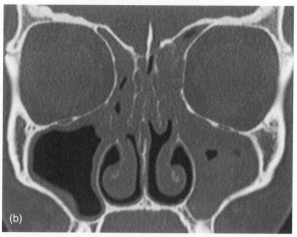

Fig. 15.8 *Computed tomography (CT) of the maxillary sinuses. (a) Normal sinuses: coronal CT through the osteomeatal unit. Note orbit (O), maxillary sinus (MS), sinus drainage pathway through maxillary ostium (arrow), middle turbinate (M), inferior turbinate (I) and nasal septum (S). (b) Paranasal sinus disease: CT through the same level as (a). Note mucosal thickening on the right and almost complete opacification of the left maxillary sinus. Mucosal thickening is occluding both maxillary ostia. Compare this appearance with (a).*

discharge and fever. Diagnosis is usually made on clinical grounds and may be confirmed with nasal cultures or minimally invasive procedures such as endoscopic paranasal sinus aspiration. Imaging is seldom required in the acute situation. Radiographs of the facial sinuses may show fluid levels in the maxillary sinuses or sinus opacification. Similarly, CT may show fluid in the sinus cavities. Acute bacterial frontal sinusitis may be complicated by meningitis, subdural empyema or cerebral abscess.

Chronic sinusitis is defined as sinus inflammation of over 12 weeks duration. The clinical presentation may include facial pain, nasal obstruction, and reduced sense of smell. Chronic sinusitis may be bacterial, allergic or fungal. Functional endoscopic sinus surgery (FESS) is performed for cases that do not respond to medical therapy. Imaging is performed to quantify disease and to define relevant underlying anatomical anomalies that may restrict sinus drainage, as well as to assist in presurgical planning and postoperative follow-up. Computed tomography is the investigation of choice and with multislice CT multiplanar reconstructions of this complex region may be performed. The key images in assessing chronic sinusitis and planning FESS are coronal CT scans of the osteomeatal unit. The osteomeatal unit is the region of the drainage pathways of the maxillary, frontal and anterior ethmoid sinuses (Fig. 15.8).

IMAGING OF THE TEMPORAL BONE

The temporal bone is an extremely complex structure. It contains the external auditory canal, middle and inner ear structures, and transmits the seventh cranial (facial) nerve. A number of congenital anomalies may occur as well as inflammatory conditions and tumours, most of which are beyond the scope of a student text. Two of the more common indications for imaging are to define fractures of the temporal bone and to 'rule out acoustic neuroma'.

Fractures of the temporal bone are usually discovered at the time of initial CT for assessment of head injury. Less commonly they may present with hearing loss or cerebrospinal fluid (CSF) leak following recovery from acute injuries. Temporal bone fractures are best seen on transverse CT scans. Fractures are classified as transverse or longitudinal, depending on the relationship of the fracture line to the axis of the temporal bone. Longitudinal temporal bone fractures run parallel to the long axis of the temporal bone, roughly in the coronal plane (Fig. 15.9). Longitudinal fractures tend not to involve the inner ear structures. They may present with conductive hearing loss owing to disruption of middle ear ossicles. Transverse temporal

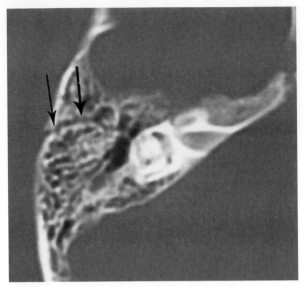

Fig. 15.9 *Temporal bone fracture (arrows): computed tomography.*

bone fractures run in the sagittal plane, perpendicular to the long axis of the temporal bone. These fractures often disrupt inner ear structures causing sensorineural hearing loss. Transverse fractures may also involve the facial nerve canal producing ipsilateral facial weakness.

One of the most common imaging investigations in ENT is CT or MRI to rule out acoustic neuroma. Acoustic neuroma refers to a nerve sheath tumour of the eighth cranial nerve. These usually involve the vestibular component of this nerve so that a more pathologically correct term for this tumour is vestibular schwannoma. These tumours usually present in adults with slowly progressive unilateral sensorineural hearing loss. There may be associated tinnitus and vertigo. Vertigo without hearing loss is usually not caused by vestibular schwannoma. Clinical screening of patients with unilateral sensorineural hearing loss is usually performed with brainstem electrical response audiometry. Imaging is indicated if this indicates a retrocochlear cause for hearing loss.

The seventh and eighth cranial nerves exit the brainstem and pass laterally across a CSF-filled space known as the cerebellopontine angle (CPA). They enter the internal auditory canal (IAC), which carries

these nerves laterally through the temporal bone to the facial nerve canal, cochlea and vestibule. Vestibular schwannomas vary in size and are often quite small. Imaging for their diagnosis centers on the pathways of the eighth cranial nerve through the CPA and IAC. Magnetic resonance imaging is the imaging investigation of choice. High-definition scans are able to display the anatomy of these small structures in exquisite detail (Fig. 15.10). Where MRI is contraindicated, CT may be performed, though is less accurate for small tumours.

INVESTIGATION OF A NECK MASS

The anatomy of the neck is extremely complex and beyond the scope of this book. A few introductory comments may serve to set the roles of imaging of neck masses in perspective. Multiple muscles, blood vessels and nerves course through the neck, with the airway in the centre and the spine posterior. Several organs are also present, including the salivary glands and thyroid gland. To make sense of this anatomy and to narrow the differential diagnosis for pathologies, the neck is divided by the hyoid bone into the suprahyoid and infrahyoid neck. The suprahyoid neck is further subdivided into various anatomical spaces, including the parapharyngeal, masticator, parotid, carotid, retropharyngeal and perivertebral spaces. Spaces of the infrahyoid neck include visceral, anterior cervical, posterior cervical, carotid, retropharyngeal and perivertebral spaces. These anatomical spaces are all definable on CT and MRI, and to a lesser extent on US.

Lymphadenopathy is a common cause of neck mass. Causes of neck lymphadenopathy include:
- Infection.
- Head and neck malignancy such as squamous cell carcinoma (SCC) of the larynx or oral cavity.
- Systemic malignancy, including lymphoma.

Some of the other more common neck masses that may be encountered are outlined below:
- Abscess: usually occur in close relation to the airway in the parapharyngeal or retropharyngeal spaces.

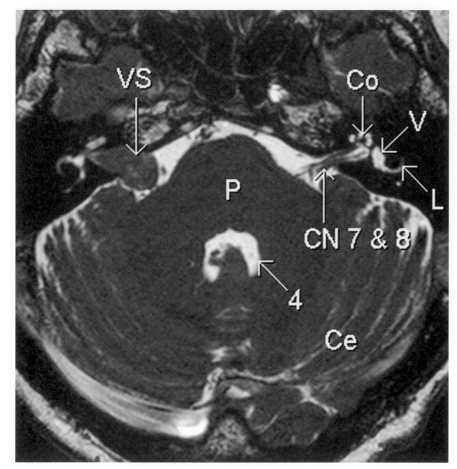

Fig. 15.10 *Vestibular schwannoma ('acoustic neuroma'): magnetic resonance imaging. High-resolution T2-weighted transverse scan through the posterior fossa shows the following: right vestibular schwannoma (VS), pons (P), fourth ventricle (4), cerebellum (Ce), normal left seventh and eighth cranial nerves (CN 7 & 8), cochlea (Co), vestibule (V), lateral semicircular canal (L). (See also Fig. 1.36, page 24.)*

- Second branchial cleft cyst: presents in young adults with a mass of the upper neck anterior to the sternomastoid muscle.
- Thyroglossal duct cyst: cyst of remnants of the thyroglossal duct occurring anteriorly in the midline.
- Cystic hygroma (lymphatic malformation):
  (i) Occurs in infants and young children;
  (ii) Complex cystic mass of the lower lateral neck;
  (iii) Associated with Turner's syndrome.
- Dermoid cyst: midline cyst containing fat in the floor of the mouth.
- Carotid body tumour: paraganglioma located in the bifurcation of the common carotid artery.

A mass may also be shown to be arising in one of the salivary glands, either parotid or submandibular. Common benign salivary gland tumours include pleomorphic adenoma and adenolymphoma (Warthin's tumour). Malignant salivary gland tumours are much less common and include adenoid cystic carcinoma (cylindroma) and mucoepidermoid carcinoma. Other soft-tissue tumours that may occur in the parotid gland include lipoma, neuroma and melanoma.

Masses and diffuse diseases of the thyroid gland are considered separately below.

The roles of imaging in the investigation of neck masses are to define the following:
- Localization of the mass:
  (i) Suprahyoid or infrahyoid;
  (ii) Specific anatomical space;
  (iii) Organ of origin: thyroid, salivary glands.
- Features of the mass:
  (i) Cystic or solid;
  (ii) Calcification or fat;

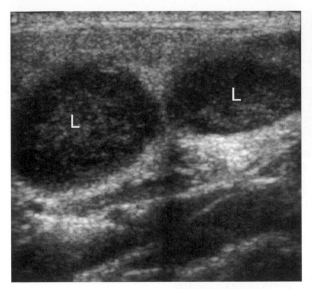

Fig. 15.11 *Cervical lymphadenopathy: ultrasound (US). Enlarged neoplastic lymph nodes seen on US as round hypoechoic masses (L).*

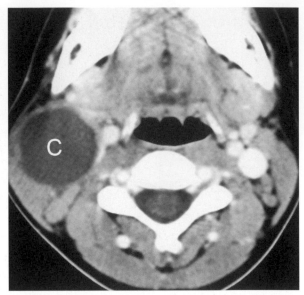

Fig. 15.12 *Second branchial cleft cyst (C): computed tomography.*

    (iii) Enhancement with intravenous contrast
           material.
  • Anatomical relations:
    (i) Position relative to the great vessels, thyroid
         gland, laryngeal cartilages;
    (ii) Retrosternal extension.
  • Evidence of malignancy:
    (i) Invasion of surrounding structures;
    (ii) Lymphadenopathy.

Ultrasound is an accurate and non-invasive screening test for initial localization and characterization of a neck mass (Fig. 15.11). It will usually differentiate cystic from solid lesions. A specific diagnosis may often be made, particularly for cystic lesions such as branchial cleft cyst and thyroglossal cyst. For solid lesions, US provides an excellent modality for guidance of fine needle aspiration (FNA) or biopsy.

   Depending on local availability and expertise, CT or MRI may be used to further delineate neck masses. This is particularly true for deep masses or for complex and multifocal pathologies such as extensive lymphadenopathy. Both CT and MRI provide good localization of the plane of origin of a mass, plus definition of

anatomical relations (Figs 15.12 and 15.13). Complications such as invasion of surrounding structures and lymphadenopathy are well seen.

INVESTIGATION OF A SALIVARY GLAND CALCULUS

Most salivary calculi are visible on plain radiographs. Specific views are used for the gland of interest, such as intraoral films to show the submandibular ducts (Fig. 15.14). Sialography is indicated for suspected salivary gland calculus in the parotid and submandibular ducts and glands. Plain films are first performed as above. The opening of the salivary duct is then cannulated with a fine catheter and oil-based or water-soluble contrast medium injected. A calculus appears as a filling defect within a localized expansion of the salivary duct, and the proximal duct may be dilated. Other findings that may be seen on sialography include strictures, dilated ducts (sialectasis) and cavities within the gland, some of which may contain calculi. Sialography is contraindicated in the presence of acute salivary gland infection. When performed carefully by an experienced

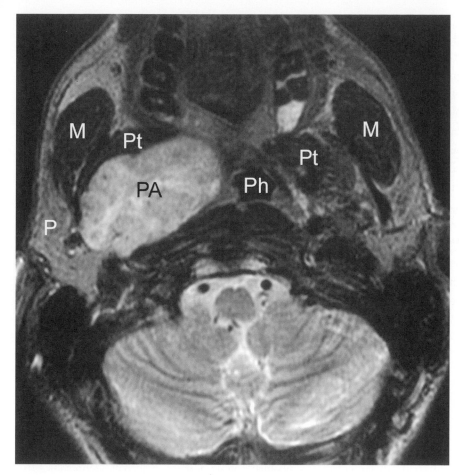

Fig. 15.13 *Pleomorphic adenoma: magnetic resonance imaging. T2-weighted transverse scan through the oropharynx shows a mass (PA) arising from the deep lobe of the right parotid gland. Note also the superficial lobe of the right parotid gland (P), masseter muscles (M), oropharynx (Ph) and pterygoid muscles (Pt) compressed on the right by the mass.*

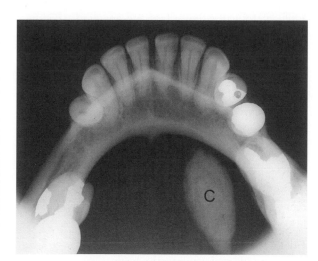

Fig. 15.14 *Submandibular calculus. A dental radiograph of the anterior floor of the mouth shows a large calculus (C) in the left submandibular duct.*

operator, US is a highly accurate technique for the non-invasive diagnosis of parotid calculi. A small US probe placed in the mouth may be used to diagnose calculi of the submandibular glands and ducts.

STAGING OF CARCINOMA OF THE LARYNX

Squamous cell carcinoma of the larynx is most common in male adults, particularly those with a history of heavy smoking and alcohol use. Depending on the relationship of the tumour to the vocal cords, SCC of the larynx is classified as supraglottic, glottic or subglottic. Clinical presentation may include sore throat, hoarse voice or stridor. Squamous cell carcinoma of the larynx spreads by local invasion through the laryngeal mucosa to the laryngeal cartilages and beyond. Lymph node metastases are common, particularly with supraglottic tumours. Distant metastases may occur in the lungs.

Laryngoscopy is used for assessment of the laryngeal mucosal surface. Computed tomography is the imaging investigation of choice for further staging of SCC of the larynx. Squamous cell carcinoma of the larynx appears on CT as a high-attenuation mass causing asymmetry of the airway and anatomical distortion with obliteration of surrounding fat planes. Complicating factors that may be seen include invasion of surrounding structures such as laryngeal cartilages and cervical lymphadenopathy. Magnetic resonance imaging may be used in a problem-solving role in the confirmation of laryngeal cartilage invasion. Fluorodeoxyglucose positron-emission tomography (FDG-PET) is most useful in the post-laryngectomy patient where CT is suspicious for recurrent SCC.

THYROID IMAGING

With the development of high-resolution US, FNA techniques, and accurate laboratory tests including cytopathology, the diagnostic evaluation of thyroid disease has evolved over the past few years. Imaging of the thyroid is indicated in the assessment of diffuse thyroid diseases and of thyroid nodules and masses. Computed tomography may be used to outline the anatomy of large goitres prior to surgical removal.

DIFFUSE THYROID DISEASES

For diffuse thyroid diseases such as Graves' disease, Hashimoto's thyroiditis, subacute thyroiditis and multinodular goitre the diagnosis is often achieved by clinical history and examination, plus laboratory tests for thyroid function and antibodies. These may be complemented by thyroid scintigraphy with ^{99m}Tc and by US, including colour Doppler. In particular, in the assessment of a patient with hyperthyroidism scintigraphy and US may be helpful in distinguishing Graves' disease from thyroiditis, or from multinodular goitre.

Imaging appearances of the common diffuse thyroid diseases are as follows:
- Graves' disease (diffuse toxic goitre):
  (i) ^{99m}Tc scintigraphy: intensely increased uptake;
  (ii) US with colour Doppler: enlarged, hypoechoic and hypervascular thyroid.
- Hashimoto thyroiditis (chronic lymphocytic thyroiditis):
  (i) ^{99m}Tc scintigraphy: reduced uptake;
  (ii) US with colour Doppler: hypoechoic and hypervascular thyroid.
- Subacute (De Quervain) thyroiditis:
  (i) ^{99m}Tc scintigraphy: reduced uptake;
  (ii) US with colour Doppler: mildly enlarged and hypervascular thyroid.
- Multinodular goitre:
  (i) ^{99m}Tc scintigraphy: patchy uptake;
  (ii) US with colour Doppler: enlarged thyroid with multiple solid nodules.

THYROID NODULES AND MASSES

A thyroid nodule is defined as a discrete mass lesion in the thyroid gland, distinguishable from thyroid parenchyma on US. The most common thyroid nodules are benign colloid nodules. Follicular adenoma is a true benign neoplasm of the thyroid gland. Thyroid carcinoma is usually of epithelial origin and is classified into papillary, follicular, medullary and anaplastic. Papillary carcinoma is the most common type (75–80 per cent). It has an excellent prognosis with a 30-year survival rate of 95 per cent.

Thyroid nodules are extremely common, being found in up to 40 per cent of adults on US examination. Conversely, thyroid cancer is quite uncommon. It follows that the majority of thyroid nodules are benign. Thyroid nodules may be assessed clinically and with imaging, the aim being to decide which nodules may be malignant. Clinical factors associated with an increased likelihood of a nodule being malignant include:
- Family history of thyroid cancer.
- History of irradiation to the neck.
- Patient age <20 years or >60 years.
- Rapid growth of the nodule.

- Fixation to adjacent structures.
- Vocal cord paralysis.
- Adjacent lymphadenopathy.

Ultrasound is the imaging investigation of choice for characterization of thyroid nodules. Relevant US features of thyroid nodules include:

- Size: the incidence of cancer in nodules smaller than 1 cm is extremely low.
- Composition: cystic, solid or mixed.
- Margins: well-defined margin or 'halo'; irregular margins.
- Calcification: coarse or fine.
- Vascularity.

The three US features most associated with malignancy are:

1 The nodule is solid or predominantly solid
2 Fine calcifications
3 Increased vascularity, particularly if centrally in the nodule.

Fine needle aspiration of thyroid nodules is usually definitive. Under direct palpation FNA is often the first and only diagnostic procedure performed for a palpable thyroid nodule. Ultrasound-guided FNA is used for non-palpable nodules and increasingly for palpable nodules (Fig. 15.15). Ultrasound-guided FNA has several advantages over palpation-directed FNA. It is generally safer and more accurate. With the use of colour Doppler, the needle tip may be directed toward less vascular areas. This reduces the risk of haemorrhage following the procedure. It also provides a less bloodstained specimen, which increases the accuracy of cytology.

Given that thyroid nodules are so common, it would be impractical and undesirable to FNA all of them. As such, criteria have been developed and released in a consensus statement by the Society of Radiologists in Ultrasound. Their recommendations are summarized below. Fine needle aspiration is indicated for solitary nodules with the following features:

- >1.0 cm with fine calcifications.
- >1.5 cm if predominantly solid or with coarse calcifications.
- >2.0 cm if mixed solid and cystic components.

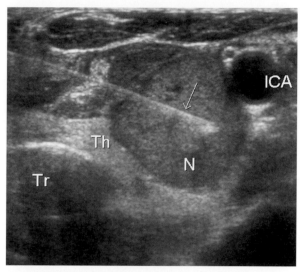

Fig. 15.15 *Fine-needle aspiration of a thyroid nodule: ultrasound (US) guidance. A transverse US image shows a fine needle (arrow) entering a nodule (N) in the left lobe of the thyroid (Th). Note also the trachea (Tr) in the midline and the internal carotid artery (ICA) lateral to the nodule.*

Where multiple nodules are present, each nodule is judged on its merits using the criteria above. Nodules not meeting the above criteria may still be referred for FNA if there is suspicion of malignancy on clinical grounds.

PRIMARY HYPERPARATHYROIDISM

Primary hyperparathyroidism is the most common indication for imaging of the parathyroid glands. The causes of primary hyperparathyroidism are as follows:

- Solitary parathyroid adenoma: 80 per cent.
- Multiple parathyroid adenomas: 7 per cent.
- Parathyroid hyperplasia: 10 per cent.
- Parathyroid carcinoma: 3 per cent.

Preoperative imaging for localization of parathyroid adenoma is not always performed, as in some centres it is felt unlikely to improve the rate of surgical success. However, where the surgeon requires preoperative localization, US is the investigation of first choice. Ultrasound with high-resolution equipment has a high

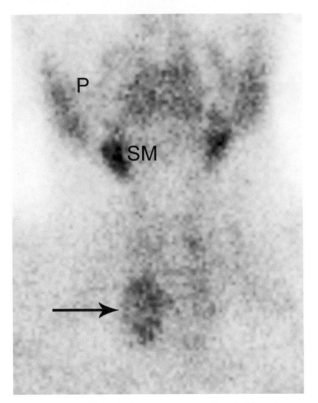

Fig. 15.16 *Parathyroid adenoma: scintigraphy. A delayed image from a sestamibi scan shows a large mass in the right lower neck (arrow) in a patient with hypercalcaemia. Note normal physiological uptake of sestamibi by the parotid (P) and submandibular (SM) glands.*

sensitivity (80–90 per cent) for the detection of parathyroid adenoma. The US appearance of parathyroid adenoma is a well-defined hypoechoic mass, usually of around 1.0–1.5 cm diameter. The principal cause of a false negative US is ectopic adenoma, which may be present in up to 10 per cent of cases.

Where US is negative, further imaging may be performed (i.e. scintigraphy, CT and MRI).

The imaging technique chosen will reflect local expertise and availability. Computed tomography and MRI are particularly useful for ectopic adenoma located in the mediastinum. Scintigraphy with ^{99m}Tc-sestamibi shows a high rate of uptake in parathyroid adenoma (Fig. 15.16). It is especially useful for ectopic or multiple adenomas.

Postoperative imaging for recurrent or persistent hyperparathyroidism is best performed with US complemented by sestamibi scintigraphy.

Paediatric radiology is an extremely diverse subject encompassing many subspecialty areas. Some topics are considered beyond the scope of a student text. These include congenital heart disease, imaged with echocardiography and magnetic resonance imaging (MRI), and congenital brain disorders, imaged with MRI. For further information on these topics the reader is referred to more specialized texts. This chapter will introduce some of the more common paediatric problems that require imaging.

NEONATAL RESPIRATORY DISTRESS: THE NEONATAL CHEST

The normal neonatal chest X-ray (see Fig. 3.3b) has the following features:
- Thymus may be prominent.
- Heart shadow is quite prominent and globular in outline; normal cardiothoracic ratio up to 65 per cent.
- Air bronchograms may be seen in the medial third of the lung fields.
- Diaphragms normally lie at the level of the sixth rib anteriorly.
- Ossification of the proximal humeral epiphysis occurs at 36 weeks gestation; visible ossification of this centre implies a term gestation.

The differential diagnosis of neonatal respiratory distress involves only a few abnormalities, which tend to give quite typical radiographic patterns as described below. When assessing a neonatal chest X-ray (CXR) the clinical setting should always be borne in mind. For example, in the premature infant with respiratory distress, hyaline membrane disease will be the most likely diagnosis. In a distressed term infant following caesarean delivery retained lung fluid will be most likely. For a term delivery with meconium-stained liquor, consider meconium aspiration syndrome.

Finally, it should be remembered that acutely ill neonates may have various tubes and vascular catheters visible on CXR and it is important to check that these are correctly positioned:
- Endotracheal tube: tip above carina.
- Nasogastric tube: end few cm curled in stomach.
- Umbilical artery catheter: tip in lower thoracic aorta away from renal artery origins.
- Umbilical vein catheter: tip in lower right atrium.

CHEST X-RAY APPEARANCES OF COMMON NEONATAL DISORDERS

Hyaline membrane disease

Hyaline membrane disease (HMD) is a generalized lung condition caused by insufficient surfactant production. It occurs most commonly in premature infants. The presentation is usually respiratory distress and cyanosis soon after birth. The CXR changes of hyaline membrane disease include reduced lung volume, granular pattern throughout the lungs, air bronchograms and poor pulmonary expansion (Fig. 16.1).

There have been major advances in the treatment of prematurity over the last 10–15 years. These include the antenatal administration of steroids to accelerate lung maturity plus the development of therapeutic surfactant. Surfactant therapy produces marked improvement of respiratory distress accompanied by resolution of the radiographic abnormalities. Failure of resolution of the radiographic changes of HMD after a couple of days may imply an added abnormality such as persistent

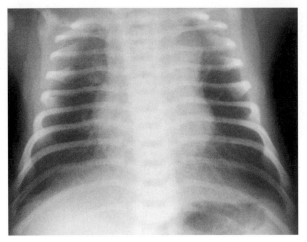

Fig. 16.1 *Mild hyaline membrane disease (HMD). Note a fine granular pattern throughout both lungs. With improved treatment methods HMD often presents quite subtle radiographic changes, as shown in this example.*

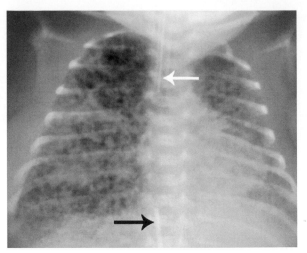

Fig. 16.2 *Hyaline membrane disease complicated by pulmonary interstitial emphysema. Note the presence of multiple small air bubbles throughout both lungs, more obvious on the right. Note also an endotracheal tube (white arrow) and umbilical artery catheter (black arrow).*

ductus arteriosus (PDA) or infection. New or worsening airspace consolidation may indicate a pulmonary haemorrhage. This is a recognized complication of surfactant therapy. Other complications of HMD that may be seen on CXR relate to air leaks and include pulmonary interstitial emphysema (PIE) (Fig. 16.2), pneumothorax (Fig. 16.3) and pneumomediastinum.

Transient tachypnoea of the newborn

This self-limiting condition is also known as retained fetal lung fluid or wet-lung syndrome. Transient tachypnoea of the newborn (TTN) is caused by persistence of fetal lung fluid at birth. It usually presents with respiratory distress in a term infant following a prolonged labour or caesarean section. The CXR signs of TTN include increased lung volume, prominent linear pattern with thickening of lung fissures (Fig. 16.4) and small pleural effusions. These changes usually resolve rapidly within 24 hours.

Meconium aspiration syndrome

Meconium aspiration may be seen with meconium-stained liquor. Passage of meconium *in utero* is a response

to fetal distress. Meconium aspiration syndrome therefore occurs in distressed neonates. The CXR signs of meconium aspiration include increased lung volume, dense, patchy opacities in central lungs and complications such as pneumonia or pneumothorax.

Pulmonary oedema: cardiac failure

Specific patterns of cardiac enlargement and alterations of the cardiac outline may be seen with congenital heart disease. These are beyond the scope of this book. Suspected congenital heart disease is assessed with echocardiography and MRI. Cardiomegaly is certainly a feature of cardiac failure, though it is not a reliable sign in neonates. More commonly, cardiac failure shows a combination of alveolar and interstitial opacification bilaterally. Pleural effusions are also seen with pleural fluid commonly extending up the lateral chest wall.

Neonatal pneumonia

Neonatal pneumonia may produce a variety of CXR appearances including lobar consolidation or patchy widespread consolidation. Dense bilateral consolidation may mimic the appearances of HMD.

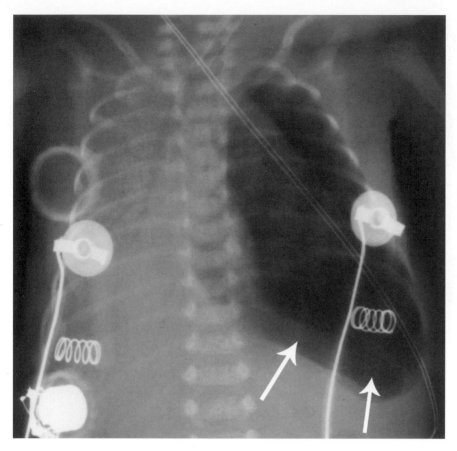

Fig. 16.3 *Hyaline membrane disease complicated by a left tension pneumothorax. Note increased volume of the left hemithorax with shift of the mediastinum to the right. Also, as the infant is supine most of the pneumothorax lies anteriorly and inferiorly producing lucency of the inferior left chest and upper abdomen (arrows).*

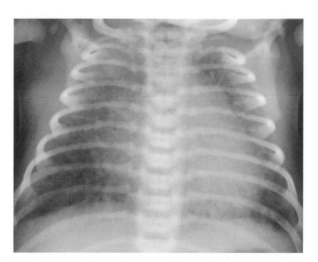

Fig. 16.4 *Transient tachypnoea of the newborn (TTN; retained fetal lung fluid). Chest X-ray shows widespread linear opacities throughout both lungs. There is no evidence of a granular pattern or of air bronchograms, which helps distinguish TTN from hyaline membrane disease.*

Chronic lung disease

Previously known as bronchopulmonary dysplasia, chronic lung disease occurs in premature infants. The incidence of chronic lung disease increases with low birth weight, early gestational age and duration of pulmonary ventilation. The radiological changes of chronic lung disease evolve over time. In the first 3 days the CXR signs are those of HMD. Over the next week there is increased opacification of both lungs. This is followed by the development of a 'bubbly' pattern through the lungs. This consists of air-filled 'bubbles' separated by irregular lines. After the first month these 'bubbles' expand, producing increased lung volumes. Most infants with chronic lung disease will survive but with a high incidence of poor neurological development. The CXR changes generally resolve over time, though often with some minor residual pulmonary overexpansion and linear stranding.

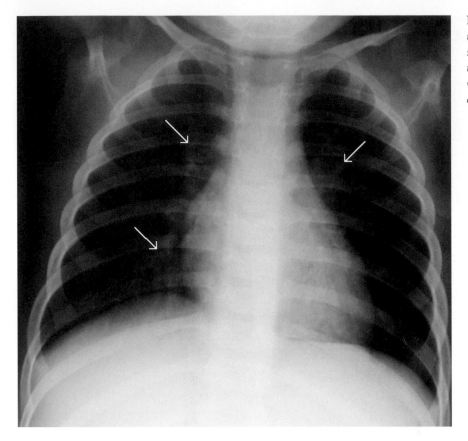

Fig. 16.5 *Viral lower respiratory tract infection. Chest X-ray shows bronchial wall thickening in the parahilar regions (arrows) with no focal areas of airspace consolidation.*

PATTERNS OF PULMONARY INFECTION IN CHILDREN

Most pulmonary infections in children are due to viruses such as respiratory syncytial virus (RSV), influenza, parainfluenza and adenovirus, or mycoplasma pneumonia. These infections tend to be seasonal and occur in epidemics. Less commonly, bacterial infections may occur. These tend to be sporadic and less seasonal. Bacteria that commonly cause pulmonary infections in children include *Streptococcus pneumoniae*, *Staphylococcus aureus*, and *Haemophilus influenzae*. Although there is some overlap, viruses tend to produce an interstitial pattern while bacteria tend to produce alveolar consolidation. Mycoplasma may produce an interstitial or alveolar pattern, or a combination of the two. The most important question on the chest X-ray of a child with a lower respiratory infection is therefore: 'Is alveolar consolidation present?' If the answer is 'No', then treatment will usually consist of supportive measures without the use of antibiotics. If the answer is 'Yes', then a bacterial aetiology is suspected and antibiotics may be required.

PATTERNS OF VIRAL INFECTION

The child with a viral lower respiratory tract infection usually presents with a couple of days of malaise, tachypnoea and cough. The most common CXR pattern seen with viral pulmonary infection is bilateral parahilar infiltration (Fig. 16.5). This consists of irregular linear opacity extending into each lung from the hilar complexes, with bronchial wall thickening a prominent feature. Hilar lymphadenopathy may increase the amount of hilar opacification. Atelectasis caused by mucous plugs and bronchial inflammation will commonly complicate this pattern. Atelectasis may involve whole lobes, or it may be seen as linear opacities that may be multiple, and that may be transient and migratory on serial films. It is

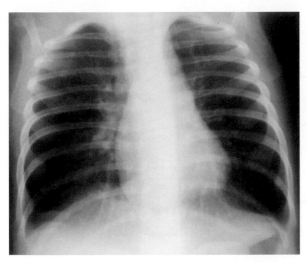

Fig. 16.6 *Bronchiolitis. Chest X-ray in a 6-month-old child with fever and respiratory distress shows overexpansion of both lungs with flattening of the hemidiaphragms. There are no focal areas of airspace consolidation to indicate bacterial infection.*

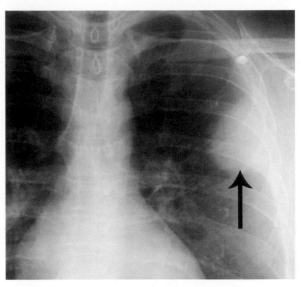

Fig. 16.7 *Round pneumonia. Round opacity with slightly blurred margins in the left upper lobe (arrow). This resolved rapidly with antibiotic therapy.*

important to recognize the lung volume loss associated with atelectasis, as this will differentiate it from consolidation. Consolidation may rarely complicate viral infection. It is thought to be caused by haemorrhagic bronchiolitis rather than a genuine exudate.

BRONCHIOLITIS

Although caused by viral infection, bronchiolitis represents a distinct clinical entity. Affected children present with tachypnoea, dyspnoea, cough, and cyanosis. Bronchiolitis is usually caused by the respiratory syncytial virus, with a peak incidence at around 6 months of age. The usual CXR pattern seen is overexpansion of the lungs as a result of bilateral air trapping. Severe cases may be complicated by atelectasis (Fig. 16.6). Where bronchiolitis is recurrent or prolonged, underlying asthma or cystic fibrosis should be considered.

BACTERIAL INFECTION

Children with a bacterial pulmonary infection usually present with abrupt onset of malaise, fever and cough. The typical CXR pattern of bacterial infection is alveolar consolidation. The appearance of alveolar consolidation is as described in Chapter 3 (i.e. fluffy opacity

with air bronchograms that may be lobar or patchy in distribution). A common pattern of early infection in children is round pneumonia. This is seen on CXR as a dense round opacity, which may be mistaken for a mass (Fig. 16.7). The clinical setting should provide the diagnosis and a follow up CXR in 6–24 hours will usually show evolution of the round opacity to a more lobar pattern. Round pneumonia is much less common in adults.

Established cases of bacterial infection are usually easily diagnosed on CXR. Difficulties may arise with early infections where the consolidation may be extremely subtle. Overlying structures may obscure certain parts of the lung. Consolidation in these areas may be very difficult to see. Particular attention should be given to the following:

- Apical segments of the lower lobes, which are obscured by the hilar complexes.
- The lung bases, which are obscured by the diaphragms.
- The left lower lobe, which lies behind the heart (Fig. 16.8).
- The apical segments of the upper lobes, which are obscured by overlying ribs and clavicles.

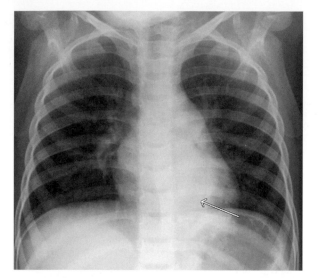

Fig. 16.8 *Left lower lobe pneumonia. A small area of airspace consolidation is seen behind the heart in the posterior basal segment of the left lower lobe (arrow).*

For further notes on interpretation of chest X-rays, see Chapter 3.

URINARY TRACT INFECTION

Urinary tract infection (UTI) is one of the most common indications for imaging in paediatrics. The diagnosis of UTI is based on analysis of urine. Using a 'best catch' method to obtain a midstream urine specimen, UTI is defined as $>10^5$ colony-forming units per millilitre (CFU/mL). Where urine is obtained by catheter UTI is defined as $>5 \times 10^4$ CFU/mL. Specimens obtained by leaving a bag on the child and awaiting micturition are notoriously unreliable, leading to overdiagnosis due to contamination. Urinary tract infection is more common in young children. In infants it occurs with equal incidence in males and females and usually presents with signs of generalized sepsis, including fever, vomiting and anorexia. In children older than 6 months it is more common in females. The clinical presentation is usually more specific with fever, frequency and dysuria. Flank pain may indicate pyelonephritis, though the differentiation of pyelonephritis from cystitis in a child with UTI may be very difficult on clinical grounds.

IMAGING THE CHILD WITH URINARY TRACT INFECTION

Most guidelines have indicated that all children with urinary tract infection should be investigated radiologically. This orthodoxy is being questioned because of a number of controversies, as will be discussed below. The purposes of the imaging investigation of the child with UTI are to:

- Diagnose underlying urinary tract abnormalities.
- Diagnose and grade vesicoureteric reflux (VUR).
- Differentiate cystitis (UTI confined to the bladder) from pyelonephritis (UTI involving one or both kidneys).
- Document renal damage.
- Establish a baseline for subsequent evaluation of renal growth.
- Establish the prognosis.

Most children are initially investigated with ultrasound (US) and micturating cystourethrogram (MCU). Depending on the results of these tests, as well as the clinical situation, further imaging may be performed to document renal function and diagnose renal scars.

Ultrasound is performed to detect abnormalities of the urinary tract that may predispose the child to the development of recurrent UTI. The more common abnormalities that may be detected with US include hydronephrosis (see below), neurogenic bladder (usually associated with congenital neurological abnormalities such as spina bifida), and renal duplex.

Renal duplex is a single kidney with two separate collecting systems. (The term 'renal duplication' should be reserved for cases where there are two separate kidneys on one side). The part of the kidney drained by each collecting system of a duplex kidney is referred to as a moiety. The term 'duplex kidney' refers to a range of anomalies from a bifid renal pelvis to complete duplication of the ureters. The most common pattern is of two separate ureters that exit the kidney and join to form a single ureter that enters the bladder. With complete ureteric duplication the ureter draining the upper moiety usually inserts inferior and medial to the ureter from the lower moiety (Weigert–Meyer rule). It may enter the inferior bladder or may have an ectopic insertion. Sites of ectopic insertion include the bladder neck, urethra, vagina or perineum in females, or the prostatic urethra and ejaculatory system in males. Regardless of the site of insertion the upper moiety ureter is prone to obstruction. Ureterocele may also complicate the insertion of the upper moiety ureter. Ureterocele is a cyst-like expansion

of the distal end of the ureter projecting into the bladder. (It should be noted that ectopic insertion and uretero-cele might be seen with a single ureter.) The ureter draining the lower moiety of a duplex kidney is prone to reflux rather than obstruction (Figs 16.9 and 16.10).

Micturating cystourethrogram is performed primarily to diagnose vesicoureteric reflux and grade its severity as follows (Fig. 16.11):

- Grade 1: reflux into non-dilated ureter.
- Grade 2: reflux into non-dilated collecting system.
- Grade 3: reflux into mildly dilated collecting system.

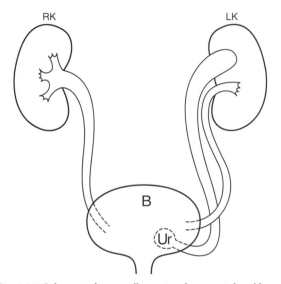

Fig. 16.9 *Schematic diagram illustrating the potential problems of a duplex renal collecting system. For orientation note the right kidney (RK), left kidney (LK) and bladder (B). The ureter from the upper moiety implants lower than that from the lower moiety and is sometimes complicated by ureterocele (Ur) and obstruction. The ureter from the lower moiety implants higher and is prone to reflux.*

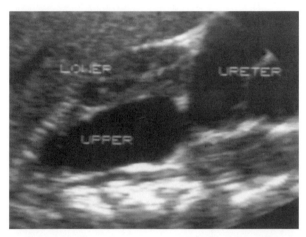

Fig. 16.10 *Duplex collecting system: ultrasound. This shows dilated loops of ureter, dilated upper moiety collecting system and normal lower moiety.*

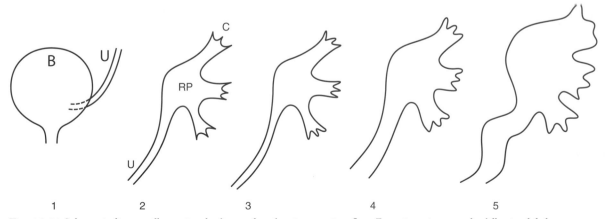

Fig. 16.11 *Schematic diagram illustrating the five grades of vesicoureteric reflux. For orientation note the following labels: bladder (B), ureter (U), renal pelvis (RP) and calyces (C).*

- Grade 4: reflux into moderately dilated collecting system.
- Grade 5: reflux into grossly dilated collecting system with dilated, tortuous ureter.

Micturating cystourethrography may be performed radiographically or with scintigraphy. Both methods involve catheterization of the child. The principal advantage of the radiographic method is that it provides more precise anatomical imaging of the urinary tract, including the urethra. Radiographic MCU may therefore be helpful in documenting the site of insertion of the ureter as well as diagnosing underlying anomalies such as posterior urethral valves in males (Fig. 16.12). Once the diagnosis of VUR is established, scintigraphic reflux studies may be performed for follow-up. The main advantage of the scintigraphic method is a lower radiation dose than with radiographic MCU. The principal disadvantage is lack of anatomical resolution (Fig. 16.12c).

When moderate to severe reflux is diagnosed, or in the presence of underlying urinary tract anomalies, further imaging studies may be required. Scintigraphy with ^{99m}Tc-mercaptoacetylglycine (MAG3) or ^{99m}Tc-diethylenetriamine pentaacetic acid (DTPA) may be performed to differentiate obstructive from non-obstructive hydronephrosis and to quantify differential renal function. Differential renal function is expressed as the percentage of overall renal function contributed by each kidney. Scintigraphy with ^{99m}Tc-dimercapto-succinic acid (DMSA) is much more sensitive than US for the documentation of renal scars (Fig. 16.13). It is taken up by cells of the proximal convoluted tubule and so outlines the renal cortex. ^{99m}Tc-DMSA

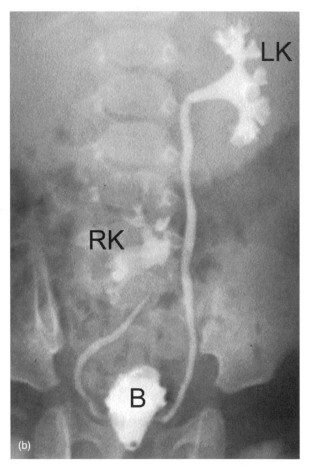

Fig. 16.12 *Vesicoureteric reflux (VUR). (a) Micturating cystourethrogram (MCU) in a female infant shows contrast material filling the bladder (B) and outlining the urethra (U). There is bilateral grade 3 VUR. Note the reduced number of calyces on the left (LK) compared with the right (RK) indicating reflux into the lower moiety of a duplex collecting system. (b) Bilateral grade 2 VUR. Note that the right kidney (RK) is malpositioned in the pelvis (pelvic kidney).*

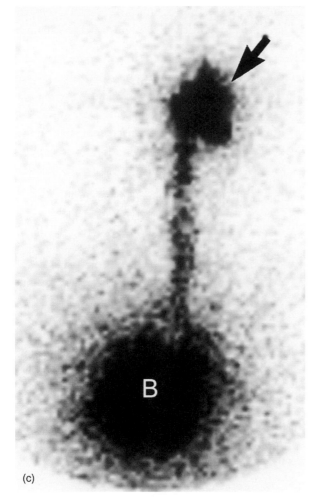

(c)

Fig. 16.12 *(c) Scintigraphic MCU shows reflux of radionuclide from the bladder (B) into the left kidney (arrow). Note the relative lack of anatomical definition compared with the radiographic studies shown in (a) and (b).*

scans are also used to diagnose pyelonephritis, seen as focal areas of reduced tracer uptake in an acutely febrile child. With UTI confined to the bladder (cystitis) a DMSA study shows normal bilateral renal tracer uptake.

CONTROVERSIES IN THE IMAGING OF CHILDREN WITH URINARY TRACT INFECTION

The logic behind the investigation and treatment of childhood UTI has been based on the following. In

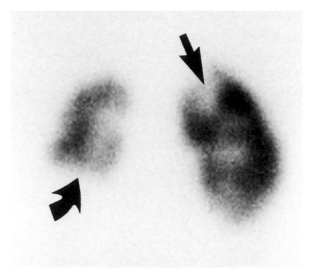

Fig. 16.13 *Renal scarring: Dimercaptosuccinic acid (DMSA) scan. This scan shows extensive right renal scarring, especially of the lower pole (curved arrow), with a smaller scar of the left upper pole (straight arrow).*

children with UTI, VUR is associated with infection of the kidney (pyelonephritis). Infection of the lower urinary tract (cystitis) is generally regarded as less serious than pyelonephritis. Pyelonephritis may be associated with an increased incidence of subsequent renal scarring. This scarring is most marked at the renal poles and leads to chronic renal disease or reflux nephropathy. This in turn may lead to an increased incidence of hypertension and end-stage renal failure. To prevent these complications, children with UTI and known vesicoureteric reflux are generally treated with long-term antibiotics. Based on more recent studies many of these long-standing beliefs about childhood UTI are in dispute.

In the 1950s, when it was discovered that VUR was associated with renal scars, a causative role was assumed. It is now known that around 50 per cent of cases of acute pyelonephritis in children are not associated with VUR. Children with non-VUR associated pyelonephritis have the same risk of developing renal scars as those with VUR. Furthermore it has been shown that scarring may be seen with only a single UTI and that some scars may predate UTI. An evolving concept is that some renal 'scars' are in fact a form of renal dysplasia caused by a mesenchymal induction defect that also causes high-grade VUR. This form of anomaly is more common in male infants and is present at birth. True acquired scars with focal fibrotic lesions in the kidney secondary to pyelonephritis are more common in females and usually do not develop beyond the age of 4 years.

There are also controversies in the management of childhood UTI and VUR. There is no evidence that antibiotic prophylaxis has any effectiveness in preventing renal scarring and long-term complications. In a world where antibiotic resistance is endemic this is a very important point. The trend in management of childhood UTI is toward antibiotic treatment of each UTI and away from antibiotic prophylaxis. It is well known that VUR, even when high grade, usually resolves spontaneously. Most cases of VUR are now managed conservatively, with surgery reserved for cases where there is proven progressive renal scarring or recurrent infections.

RECOMMENDATIONS FOR IMAGING CHILDREN WITH URINARY TRACT INFECTION

Based on the above a few recommendations can be made as to which children with UTI should be investigated:

- Males of any age with a first UTI.
- Females under 3 years of age with a first UTI.
- Females older than 3 years with recurrent UTI or with other factors, including family history of UTI and VUR, abnormal voiding, poor growth or hypertension.

Recommendations may also be made as to the use of the various imaging modalities:

- US as the first line investigation in all (MAG3 scan if obstruction suspected on US).
- MCU for children younger than 1 year.
- DMSA for young males and recurrent UTI in others (may also be used to make the specific diagnosis of pyelonephritis if this will alter management).
- More aggressive investigation for recurrent or complicated cases.

HYDRONEPHROSIS

Hydronephrosis is the most common cause of a neonatal abdominal mass. Hydronephrosis may also present with urinary tract infection (see below), or may be detected on prenatal screening US. In fact, the advent of virtually universal prenatal US screening has led to a marked increase in the early diagnosis of hydronephrosis. Mild asymptomatic hydronephrosis may be followed with serial US examination. More severe cases may require treatment, including surgical correction. The more common causes of hydronephrosis in children are:

- Pelviureteric junction (PUJ) obstruction.
- Vesicoureteric junction (VUJ) obstruction.
- VUR.
- Primary megaloureter.
- Duplex kidney with upper pole ureterocele.

Ultrasound and scintigraphy are the main imaging modalities for assessment of hydronephrosis. The roles of imaging of hydronephrosis are:

- Document severity of urinary tract dilatation.
- Differentiate obstructive from non-obstructive causes.
- Define level of obstruction.
- Diagnose underlying anatomical anomalies.

Ultrasound (US) is the initial imaging modality of choice in the investigation of hydronephrosis. Signs of hydronephrosis on US are dilated renal pelvis and calyces. A round, markedly dilated renal pelvis is seen in PUJ obstruction (Fig. 16.14). In VUJ obstruction the dilated ureter can be followed on US. Long-standing cases of hydronephrosis may show thinning of the renal cortex. Underlying anomalies such as ureterocele or duplex collecting system are usually well seen on US.

Diuretic scintigraphy with ^{99m}Tc-MAG3 or ^{99m}Tc-DTPA is used to differentiate mechanical urinary tract obstruction from non-obstructive causes of hydronephrosis. Furosemide is injected after the renal collecting system is filled with isotope. The rate of 'washout' of isotope is then assessed. With mechanical obstruction such as PUJ obstruction, isotope continues to accumulate in the collecting system following diuretic

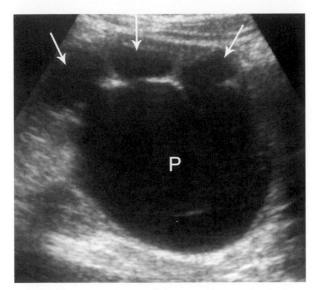

Fig. 16.14 *Hydronephrosis caused by pelviureteric junction obstruction: ultrasound. This shows a markedly dilated renal pelvis (P) communicating with dilated calyces (arrows).*

injection (Fig. 16.14). With non-mechanical obstruction such as congenital megaloureter, isotope is rapidly washed out of the dilated collecting system. Scintigraphy is also used to quantify differential renal function and to show the level of obstruction at either PUJ or VUJ.

Vesicoureteric reflux is suspected when scintigraphy shows a non-obstructive hydronephrosis. Micturating cystourethrogram is used to document VUR and to diagnose underlying anomalies such as posterior urethral valves.

INVESTIGATION OF AN ABDOMINAL MASS

A child with an abdominal mass may present in a number of ways. The attending paediatrician often finds congenital masses that are present at birth. Hydronephrosis and other congenital masses are also frequently diagnosed on obstetric US. In older children, an abdominal mass may produce a visible bulge or may be felt by a parent. Depending on location, there may be specific signs or symptoms such as jaundice or intestinal obstruction.

Common causes of abdominal masses in children are as follows:
- Renal:
    (i) Hydronephrosis (considered separately above);
    (ii) Multicystic dysplastic kidney;
    (ii) Polycystic renal conditions;
    (iii) Nephroblastoma.
- Neuroblastoma.
- Hepatic:
    (i) Hepatoblastoma;
    (ii) Hepatocellular carcinoma;
    (iii) Haemangioendothelioma.

It is also important to remember that a distended large bowel in a child with chronic constipation may mimic an abdominal mass.

IMAGING OF THE CHILD WITH AN ABDOMINAL MASS

The roles of imaging for an abdominal mass are:
- Diagnosis of a mass.
- Define organ of origin.
- Characterize mass:
    (i) Margins: well-defined or infiltrative;
    (ii) Contents: calcification, necrosis, cyst formation, fat.
- Diagnose complications and evidence of malignancy:
    (i) Metastases;
    (ii) Lymphadenopathy;
    (iii) Invasion of surrounding structures;
    (iv) Vascular invasion.
- Pretreatment planning.
- Guidance of percutaneous biopsy or other interventional procedures such as nephrostomy.
- Follow-up: response to therapy, diagnosis of recurrent tumour.

Abdomen X-ray (AXR) and CXR are often performed in the initial work-up of a child with an abdominal mass. Signs of an abdominal mass on AXR include a soft-tissue opacity causing displacement of bowel loops. Neuroblastoma has a high incidence of calcification.

Signs that may be seen on CXR relate to metastatic spread and include pleural effusion, lymphadenopathy (mediastinal and paravertebral), and pulmonary metastases. Ultrasound is the first investigation of choice in children for assessing the site of origin of a mass and as guidance for further investigations. It is an excellent screening tool in children where lack of mesenteric and retroperitoneal fat allows good definition of organs and blood vessels.

With its fast scanning times, multidetector row computed tomography (MDCT) is particularly advantageous in children. It provides accurate characterization of an abdominal mass and its organ of origin, and is highly sensitive for the presence of calcification and fat. Computed tomography (CT) is also used to diagnose complications of malignancy, as above, including local invasion and metastatic disease.

Magnetic resonance imaging has several advantages in children and in many centres is performed in preference to CT for the assessment of an abdominal mass. It uses no radiation and no iodinated contrast media. The multiplanar scanning capabilities of MRI are particularly useful. Coronal scanning may be useful in hydronephrosis for detecting the level of obstruction. Coronal images also demonstrate liver, adrenal and renal tumours very well. Magnetic resonance imaging provides excellent imaging of blood vessels. Renal vein invasion by nephroblastoma can be detected without the use of iodinated contrast media. The principal disadvantage of MRI compared with CT is its relatively long scanning time that necessitates longer general anaesthetics in young children and infants. Where CT is more widely used, MRI may be used to define specific clinical problems, such as spinal invasion by neuroblastoma.

Renal scintigraphy complements US in the assessment of benign renal conditions that may present as an abdominal mass. ^{99m}Tc-DTPA or ^{99m}Tc-MAG3 may be used. MAG3 has more efficient renal extraction than DTPA and is more widely used in paediatric patients. Renal scanning with DTPA or MAG3 provides physiological information such as differential renal function

and diuretic 'wash-out', as well as anatomical information such as level of obstruction. Bone scintigraphy with ^{99m}Tc-MDP is performed for suspected skeletal metastases. Iodine-labelled metaiodobenzylguanidine (^{123}I-MIBG) is a specialized agent occasionally used for staging of neuroblastoma.

IMAGING FINDINGS OF COMMON ABDOMINAL MASSES

Multicystic dysplastic kidney

Multicystic dysplastic kidney (MCDK) is the second most common cause of an abdominal mass in a neonate, after hydronephrosis. In MCDK multiple cysts of varying size replace the kidney. There is associated absence of the ipsilateral ureter and the renal artery is hypoplastic. Congenital abnormality of the contralateral kidney occurs in 30 per cent of cases. This is usually a pelvi-ureteric junction obstruction. Bilateral MCDK is not compatible with life. The natural history of MCDK is involution. Surgical removal is no longer routinely performed.

Ultrasound shows the kidney replaced by a lobulated collection of variably sized non-communicating cysts (Fig. 16.15). Scintigraphy with ^{99m}Tc-MAG3 or ^{99m}Tc-DTPA shows absence of renal function on early scans. Later scans may show minor peripheral activity with no evidence of central migration of isotope.

Polycystic renal conditions

Various hereditary syndromes including tuberous sclerosis and von Hippel–Lindau disease may be associated with renal cysts. Polycystic renal conditions are classified according to genetic inheritance, pathological findings, and clinical presentation.

Autosomal recessive polycystic kidney disease (ARPKD) refers to a spectrum of disorders with associated liver disease, with infantile and juvenile forms described. In infantile cases, the renal disease tends to be more severe with less hepatic involvement; in older children the liver disease is the dominant feature. Ultrasound shows symmetrically enlarged kidneys that are markedly hyperechoic.

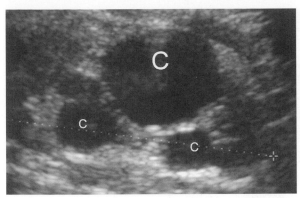

Fig. 16.15 *Multicystic dysplastic kidney: ultrasound. The left kidney is replaced by a collection of non-communicating cysts (C).*

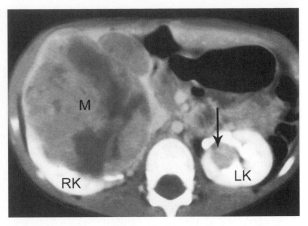

Fig. 16.16 *Wilms tumour (nephroblastoma): computed tomography (CT). Transverse CT scan shows a large mass (M) arising from and distorting the right kidney (RK). Note also a small mass (arrow) arising in the left kidney indicating bilateral disease.*

Autosomal dominant polycystic kidney disease (ADPKD) usually presents in middle age with enlarged kidneys and hypertension. At this time the enlarged kidneys contain cysts of varying size. However, ADPKD may rarely present in childhood with bilateral enlarged kidneys; this may be asymmetrical. On US examination, the kidneys are of increased echogenicity because of multiple cysts that are too tiny to be seen individually. Occasionally, separate small anechoic cysts are seen. (See also Fig. 9.2, page 131 for an example of ADPKD in an adult.)

Nephroblastoma (Wilms tumour)

Nephroblastoma is the most common solid intra-abdominal tumour in childhood. Most cases occur between the ages of 1 year and 5 years. The usual presentation is an asymptomatic renal mass, though there may be associated haematuria or abdominal pain. Fifteen per cent of nephroblastomas are associated with congenital anomalies including non-familial aniridia, congenital hemihypertrophy, and Weidemann–Beckwith syndrome.

On US nephroblastoma appears as a hyperechoic mass with hypoechoic areas due to necrosis. The mass tends to replace renal parenchyma with progressive enlargement and distortion of the kidney. Computed tomography or MRI shows a renal mass with distortion of kidney. The mass shows less intense contrast enhancement than functioning renal tissue (Fig. 16.16).

Complications that may be seen on CT or MRI include lymphadenopathy, invasion of renal vein and inferior vena cava (IVC), liver metastases and invasion of surrounding structures. Further staging is performed with chest CT. Chest CT is more accurate than CXR for the initial diagnosis of pulmonary metastases. Although less accurate than CT for initial diagnosis, a CXR should always be performed to establish a baseline for follow-up examinations.

Neuroblastoma

Neuroblastoma is a malignant childhood tumour arising from primitive sympathetic neuroblasts of the embryonic neural crest. Sixty per cent occur in the abdomen; of these, two-thirds arise in the adrenal gland. Other common abdominal sites are the periaortic sympathetic ganglia and ganglia at the aortic bifurcation. The peak age of incidence is 2 years with most neuroblastomas occurring at less than 5 years. A less common subgroup is congenital neuroblastoma in infants. This tumour has a better prognosis because of its tendency to spontaneous regression.

Ultrasound shows a mass usually with a heterogeneous texture due to areas of necrosis, haemorrhage and calcification. Computed tomography or MRI shows a heterogeneous mass with displacement or invasion of

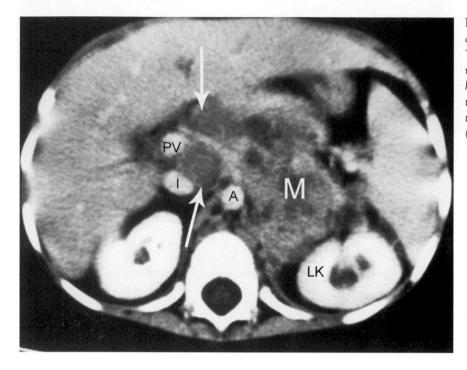

Fig. 16.17 *Neuroblastoma: computed tomography (CT). Transverse CT scan shows a large mass (M) anterior to the left kidney (LK) with extension across the midline (arrows). Note also the aorta (A), inferior vena cava (I) and portal vein (PV).*

the kidney (Fig. 16.17). Calcification is seen on CT in most cases. Neuroblastoma tends to spread across the midline to encase or displace major blood vessels. Other complications seen on CT or MRI include invasion of surrounding structures, including vertebral invasion, lymphadenopathy and liver metastases. Further staging is performed with chest CT for pulmonary metastases and bone scintigraphy with ^{99m}Tc-MDP. Occasionally, scintigraphy with ^{123}I-MIBG may be performed for staging. However, MIBG is expensive and relatively difficult to obtain and is usually reserved for difficult cases.

Hepatoblastoma

Hepatoblastoma is the most common hepatic tumour in children. Hepatoblastoma has an increased incidence in Weidemann–Beckwith syndrome, hemihypertrophy and biliary atresia; it is not associated with cirrhosis. Most hepatoblastomas occur under the age of 3 years. Ultrasound of hepatoblastoma shows a well-circumscribed mass of higher echogenicity than surrounding liver. Computed tomography shows a hepatic mass of equal or reduced attenuation compared with adjacent liver tissue.

Areas of necrosis, calcification and occasionally fat may be seen. Hepatoblastoma may invade the portal vein or IVC. Vascular invasion may be seen on CT as a filling defect within an enlarged portal vein or IVC.

Hepatocellular carcinoma

Hepatocellular carcinoma is uncommon in children, with an increased incidence in chronic liver diseases, such as cirrhosis, biliary atresia or tyrosinaemia. Ultrasound shows an ill-defined hypoechoic mass in the liver. Computed tomography may show a solitary low attenuation mass or multiple confluent masses.

Haemangioendothelioma

Haemangioendothelioma is a highly vascular benign multicentric liver tumour that may be associated with cutaneous haemangiomas. It usually presents in infancy with hepatomegaly, cardiac failure, or acute haemorrhage. Ultrasound shows multiple discrete hyperechoic masses in the liver. Computed tomography shows multiple low attenuation hepatic masses with occasional calcification.

INTUSSUSCEPTION

Intussusception refers to prolapse or telescoping of a segment of bowel (referred to as the intussusceptum) into the lumen of more distal bowel (the intussuscepiens). The most common form of intussusception is ileo-colic (i.e. prolapse of distal small bowel into the colon). The ileo-ileal form is much less common. Intussusception occurs most commonly in young children, usually from 6 months to 2 years of age, with a peak incidence at around 9 months. At this age intussusception is usually regarded as idiopathic, although enlarged lymph nodes secondary to viral infection are thought to be responsible in most cases. In older children, a lead point should be strongly suspected. Such causes include Meckel diverticulum, mesenteric cyst and lymphoma. Intussusception may also occur in adults with underlying causes, including benign small bowel tumours such as lipoma, Meckel diverticulum and foreign body.

Common signs and symptoms of intussusception include vomiting, blood stained stool, colicky abdominal pain, listlessness and palpable abdominal mass. Imaging consists of an abdomen X-ray (AXR) followed by ultrasound (US). Contrast enema is usually not required for diagnosis of intussusception. In suitable cases intussusception may be reduced under radiological guidance.

Signs of intussusception on AXR include:

- 'Target' lesion in right upper quadrant caused by swollen hepatic flexure seen end-on with layers of peritoneal fat within and surrounding the intussusception.
- Meniscus sign resulting from air outlining intussusceptum (Fig. 16.18).
- Relatively gasless right side of abdomen.
- Small bowel obstruction.
- Free air indicates intestinal perforation.

Ultrasound of intussusception show a characteristic appearance of a kidney-shaped multilayered mass. This consists of a hypoechoic rim surrounding hyperechoic concentric rings due to layers of oedematous bowel

wall and mesentery. In older children, US may occasionally show a lead point such as lymphoma or duplication cyst.

Intussusception is a surgical emergency and early involvement of radiological and surgical teams is mandatory. There are two contraindications to radiological reduction. The first of these is shock; the child must be adequately hydrated before attempting reduction. The second contraindication to radiological reduction is intestinal perforation, as indicated by clinical signs of peritonism and/or visualization of free air on AXR. Symptoms of greater than 12 hours duration or small bowel obstruction make radiological reduction more difficult and so decrease the likelihood of success, but are not of themselves absolute contraindications.

Reduction is most commonly performed under X-ray screening with various operators using a variety of contrast agents including barium, water-soluble contrast and gas. Gas reduction is now widely used and has several advantages. It is relatively quick and clean, and if perforation does occur it is safer than with barium. Some centres use US-guided liquid reduction. A post-evacuation AXR is usually performed after reduction to exclude early recurrence. Recurrences occur in 5–10 per cent of cases and should lead to repeat enema reduction. With multiple recurrences or a suspected pathological lead point, surgical intervention is mandatory.

HYPERTROPHIC PYLORIC STENOSIS

Hypertrophic pyloric stenosis refers to idiopathic hypertrophy of the circular muscle fibres of the pylorus, which produces progressive gastric outlet obstruction. The condition is most common in first-born male infants and the peak age of presentation is at around 6 weeks. Clinical presentation is usually with forceful non-bile stained vomiting leading to dehydration and hypokalaemic alkalosis. Palpation of a pyloric muscular mass in the right upper quadrant of an infant with a typical clinical history is diagnostic of hypertrophic pyloric stenosis and imaging is not required in such cases. Imaging is useful in infants with equivocal symptomatology, or with typical symptoms where a mass cannot be palpated.

Ultrasound is highly accurate for the diagnosis of pyloric stenosis and is the investigation of choice. The thickened pylorus is seen on US as a round target-like lesion in cross-section. A rim of hypoechoic thickened muscle with a hyperechoic centre produces the target appearance. The stomach is usually distended and no gastric contents are seen to pass through the thickened pylorus on real-time scanning. The thickened

pylorus may be measured with hypertrophic pyloric stenosis indicated by the following US measurements:

- Total pyloric diameter >13 mm.
- Pyloric muscle thickness >3 mm.
- Pyloric length >16 mm (Fig. 16.19).

OESOPHAGEAL ATRESIA AND TRACHEO-OESOPHAGEAL FISTULA

During early embryological development the foregut develops into a ventral respiratory component (lungs

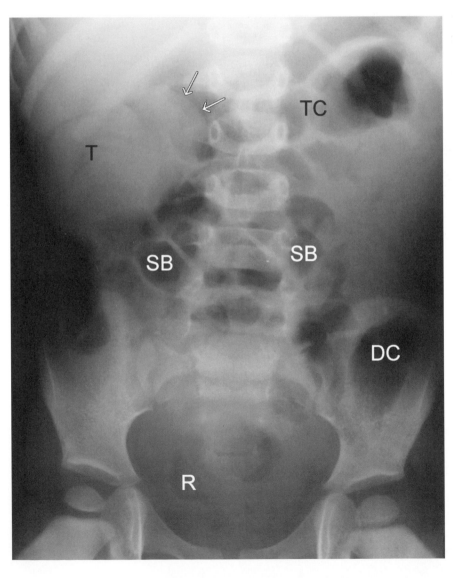

Fig. 16.18 *Intussusception. Abdomen X-ray shows normal rectum (R) and descending colon (DC) with a few moderately distended loops of small bowel (SB). A round soft-tissue opacity (arrows) is seen projecting into the transverse colon (TC). This is the leading edge of the intussusception. Note also a target-shaped 'mass' (T) in the right upper abdomen resulting from multiple thickened layers of bowel seen 'end-on'.*

and trachea) and a dorsal digestive component (oeso-phagus and stomach). Congenital foregut malforma-tions caused by failure of complete separation of dorsal and ventral foregut components occur in 1:3000 live births. These malformations are classified as shown in Fig. 16.20. With the widespread use of obstetric US oesophageal atresia and tracheo-oesophageal fistula (TOF) may be suspected prenatally. Findings on obstet-ric US may include polyhydramnios, and absence of a normal fluid-filled fetal stomach.

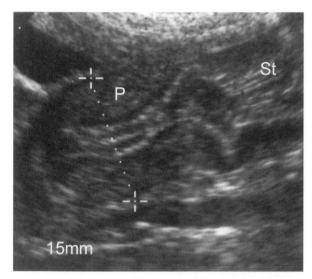

Fig. 16.19 *Pyloric stenosis: ultrasound. There is thickening of the wall of the pylorus (P) with failure of passage of fluid from the stomach (St).*

Most cases of oesophageal atresia and TOF may be diagnosed with plain films (CXR and AXR) of the neonate. Radiographic findings depend on the type of lesion present. The most common form, oesophageal atresia with distal TOF, shows the following radio-graphic signs:

- Air in the blind-ending upper oesophageal pouch posterior to trachea.
- Nasogastric tube curled in pouch.
- Air in gastrointestinal tract implies a distal fistula (Fig. 16.21).

A gasless abdomen is seen with no TOF or a proximal TOF. In all forms, signs of aspiration pneumonia may be seen on the CXR.

Contrast studies are not usually needed except for the diagnosis of 'H-Type' TOF. In this uncommon variant, the oesophagus is formed normally with no oesophageal atresia. The upper oesophagus is joined to the trachea by a thin fistula. Plain films are often nor-mal, apart from possible signs of aspiration pneumo-nia. Contrast studies are important as the fistula may be very small and difficult to image. Water-soluble contrast material is injected through a feeding tube placed in the upper oesophagus.

Associated anomalies occur in approximately 25 per cent of cases of oesophageal atresia and TOF. These anomalies include:

- Vertebral anomalies.
- Anorectal atresia.

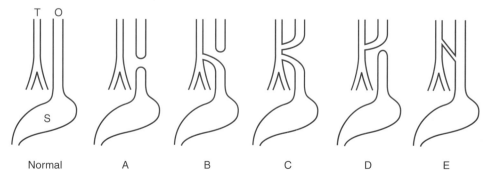

Fig. 16.20 *Schematic diagram illustrating the classification and relative incidences of oesophageal atresia and tracheo-oesophageal fistula. Note the normal orientation of trachea (T), oesophagus (O) and stomach (S). (a) Oesophageal atresia with no fistula: 9 per cent. (b) Oesophageal atresia with distal fistula: 82 per cent. (c) Oesophageal atresia with proximal and distal fistulas: 2 per cent. (d) Oesophageal atresia with proximal fistula: 1 per cent. (e) Fistula without oesophageal atresia ('H' type fistula): 6 per cent.*

- Duodenal atresia.
- Renal anomalies, such as MCDK and renal agenesis.
- Cardiac anomalies, such as ventricular septal defect (VSD), atrial septal defect and PDA.
- Radial dysplasia and other limb anomalies.

Given these associations all patients with a TOF should have a renal ultrasound and an echocardiogram. The plain films of the chest and abdomen should be scrutinized for vertebral anomalies. Also, a right-sided aortic arch is seen in 5 per cent of cases. It is important to diagnose right-sided aortic arch pre-operatively, as the surgical approach may have to be amended.

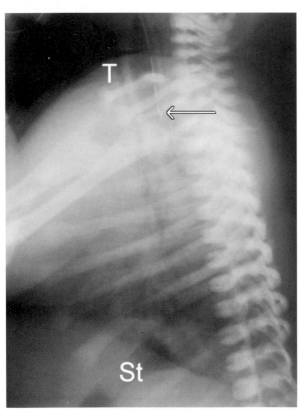

Fig. 16.21 *Oesophageal atresia and tracheo-oesophageal fistula. Lateral view shows a nasogastric tube in the blind-ending upper oesophageal segment (arrow). Gas in the stomach (St) indicates the presence of a fistula from trachea to the distal oesophagus. Note also that the trachea (T) is narrowed because of tracheomalacia, which is commonly associated with oesophageal atresia.*

GUT OBSTRUCTION AND/OR BILE-STAINED VOMITING IN THE NEONATE

Neonatal gut obstruction with or without bile-stained vomiting is a common clinical problem with a wide differential diagnosis. In some cases such as duodenal obstruction, AXR alone is sufficient for diagnosis. In other conditions such as malrotation the AXR may be normal. In other cases such as Hirschsprung disease the AXR may show non-specific appearances such as dilated bowel loops. Contrast studies such as upper GI series and contrast enema are often required for diagnosis, particularly for malrotation and large bowel disorders.

DUODENAL OBSTRUCTION

Duodenal atresia is the most common cause of congenital duodenal obstruction. Other causes include duodenal stenosis or web. A rare cause of congenital duodenal obstruction is annular pancreas. This is caused by a congenital anomaly whereby pancreatic tissue encircles and constricts the second part of the duodenum. Thirty per cent of patients with duodenal atresia have Down syndrome. Other associated anomalies include oesophageal atresia, imperforate anus, renal anomalies and congenital heart disease.

Duodenal atresia may be suspected on prenatal ultrasound with polyhydramnios plus a fluid-filled double bubble in the fetal abdomen resulting from a dilated fluid-filled stomach and duodenal cap.

Abdomen X-ray of the neonate with duodenal atresia shows the classic 'double bubble' sign caused by gas in distended stomach and duodenal cap (Fig. 16.22). There is associated absence of gas in distal bowel. Occasionally a 'triple bubble' may be seen on AXR, with gas in the gallbladder producing a third bubble.

JEJUNO-ILEAL ATRESIA

Atresia of the small bowel most commonly occurs in the proximal jejunum. Abdomen X-ray shows a few dilated small bowel loops in the left upper quadrant.

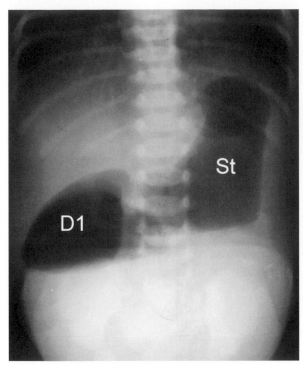

Fig. 16.22 *Duodenal atresia. Abdomen X-ray shows the characteristic 'double bubble' caused by gas filling the stomach (St) and first part of the duodenum (D1). Gas is unable to pass more distally because of atresia of the second part of the duodenum.*

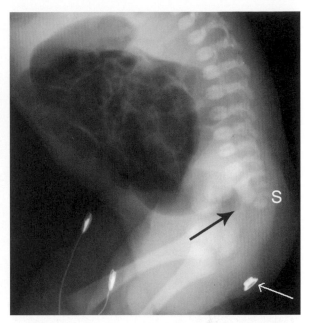

Fig. 16.23 *Anorectal atresia. Lateral radiograph showing the high termination of the distal large bowel (black arrow), marker placed on perineum (white arrow) and failure of formation of distal sacral segments (S).*

Occasionally, widespread calcification throughout the abdomen due to meconium peritonitis may be seen.

ANORECTAL ATRESIA

Absence of an anus indicates anorectal atresia. Anorectal atresia is classified as either a low or high anomaly. The key anatomical feature in classification of anorectal atresia is the levator sling. With a low anomaly the bowel ends below the levator sling. With a high anomaly the bowel ends above the levator sling, and is usually associated with a fistula into the vagina or posterior urethra.

A lateral rectal radiograph is performed to classify anorectal atresia by assessing the relationship of the most distal part of the bowel to the pelvic floor (Fig. 16.23). Gas in the bladder or vagina indicates the presence of a fistula. Associated sacral anomalies may also be seen including failure of sacral segmentation or sacral agenesis. Ultrasound of the perineum may be used to determine the distance between the anal dimple on the perineal surface and the distal bowel end, thus aiding surgical planning.

HIRSCHSPRUNG DISEASE

Hirschsprung disease involves an aganglionic segment of distal large bowel. This occurs during embryological development owing to arrest of normal craniocaudal migration of neuroblasts. A distal short aganglionic segment is the most common form. This causes distal obstruction with dilatation of normally innervated bowel proximal to the aganglionic segment. Total colonic aganglionosis occurs in 5 per cent. Hirschsprung disease usually presents in neonates with abdominal distension and constipation. Less commonly it may be a cause of chronic constipation in an older child.

An AXR in Hirschsprung disease may show dilated bowel loops. Contrast enema is definitive when it shows an abrupt transition zone from the small distal aganglionic segment to dilated normally innervated bowel.

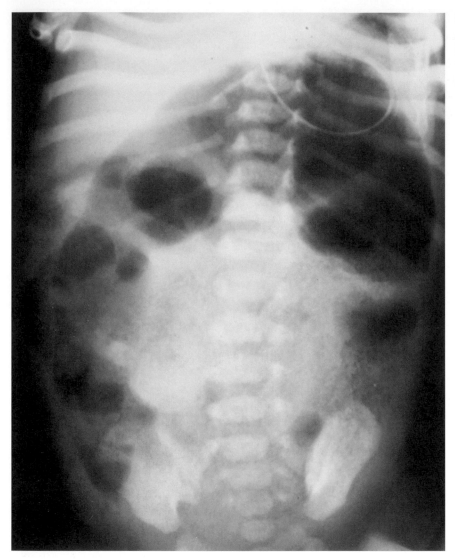

Fig. 16.24 *Meconium ileus. Abdomen X-ray shows distended large bowel with a characteristic 'soap-bubble-appearance on both sides of the abdomen.*

MECONIUM ILEUS

Meconium ileus is caused by viscous meconium impacted in the distal ileum. Meconium ileus occurs in association with cystic fibrosis (mucoviscidosis). Obstetric US may show polyhydramnios and hyperechoic contents in fetal small bowel. An AXR of the neonate may show a 'soap bubble' appearance in right lower quadrant due to complex retained meconium in the distal small bowel. There may also be dilated small bowel loops of variable calibre with no fluid levels on the erect view (Fig. 16.24). Contrast enema shows a small colon (microcolon) plus a large distal ileum with filling defects due to meconium. Contrast enema may be therapeutic in that it can disimpact the viscous meconium.

MECONIUM PLUG SYNDROME

Meconium plug syndrome refers to inspissated meconium causing distal large bowel obstruction. It is not related to meconium ileus. An AXR usually shows non-specific dilated small bowel loops. Contrast enema is often therapeutic. It shows a dilated rectum with large filling defects in the colon.

MALROTATION AND MIDGUT VOLVULUS

All of the small bowel from the second part of duodenum plus the proximal large bowel to the distal transverse colon is formed from the embryological midgut in several stages. Up to the week 6 of gestation the midgut lies within the abdominal cavity. From the weeks 6 to 10 of gestation the midgut develops outside the abdominal cavity (physiological herniation). By week 10 the midgut returns to the abdominal cavity. During these various stages of embryological development the midgut rotates through 270 degrees. This produces the final normal orientation of the small bowel mesentery and bowel loops. Specifically, the junction of the fourth part of the duodenum with the jejunum lies to the left of midline at the level of the first part of the duodenum. Proximal small bowel loops lie to the left and the caecum lies in the right lower abdomen.

Malrotation refers to a wide spectrum of anatomical variants, the common feature being abnormal rotation of the midgut. These anatomical variations include:

- Duodenum and duodenojejunal flexure to the right of midline.
- Colon to the left of midline.
- Caecum in the left upper abdomen.
- Transverse colon lying posterior to the superior mesenteric artery.
- Peritoneal (Ladd) bands: fibrous bands that cross the duodenum and may cause compression.
- Internal paraduodenal hernia.
- Shortened small bowel mesenteric attachment.

These anatomical variants may produce clinically significant complications, including volvulus of the small bowel and duodenum, and intestinal obstruction by Ladd bands or paraduodenal hernia. These complications lead to two common types of clinical presentation:

- Severe bile-stained vomiting in neonates.
- Intermittent symptoms in older children: vomiting, nausea, and abdominal pain.

Imaging investigation of suspected malrotation consists of AXR plus a contrast study of the upper gastrointestinal tract (GIT). As well as examining the upper GIT, contrast material may be followed through to the caecum and colon.

The AXR in a child with malrotation is often normal, particularly if performed when the child is asymptomatic. The AXR may show non-specific signs such as dilatation of the duodenum. The upper GIT contrast study is usually definitive in the diagnosis or exclusion of malrotation. The key finding is malposition of the duodenojejunal junction. As mentioned above, this junction should lie to the left of midline. Positioning of the duodenojejunal junction to the right or in the midline indicates malrotation. Other signs of malrotation that may be seen on the contrast study include:

- Duodenal obstruction
- Proximal jejunum lying in the right abdomen
- 'Corkscrew' appearance of small bowel loops (Fig. 16.25)
- Abnormally high caecum on follow-through films.

NON-ACCIDENTAL INJURY

Non-accidental injury is a distressing condition for all involved. The importance of making an early diagnosis cannot be overstated and plain films of affected areas, plus skeletal survey (radiographs of the ribs, skull, and long bones) are important in the diagnostic workup. In considering the diagnosis of non-accidental injury, one should be alert for:

- Fractures inconsistent with the history.
- Multiple fractures at different stages of healing.
- Fractures at unusual sites such as sternum or scapula.

The following patterns of skeletal injury are suggestive of non-accidental injury:

- Long bones:
  - (i) Periosteal new bone formation related to prior fractures;
  - (ii) Metaphyseal or epiphyseal plate fractures (Fig. 16.26, page 265);
  - (iii) Spiral diaphyseal fractures.

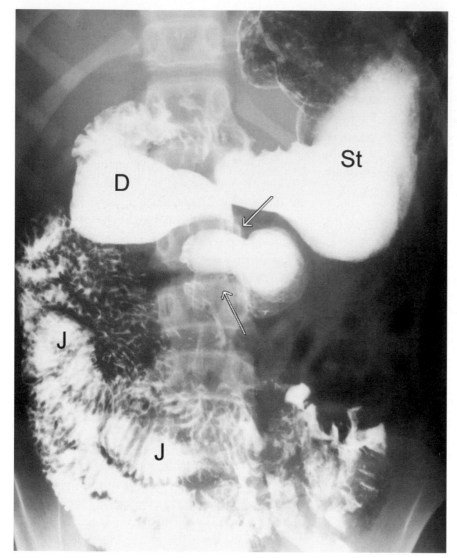

Fig. 16.25 *Malrotation: barium study. Note: normally located stomach (St), duodenum (D) does not pass across the midline to the left, 'corkscrew' configuration of proximal small bowel (arrows) and jejunum (J) located abnormally on the right.*

- Ribs:
  - (i) Up to 80 per cent of rib fractures are occult and may only become visible with healing (Fig. 16.27);
  - (ii) Posterior rib fractures are particularly suspicious;
- Skull:
  - (i) Accidental skull fractures tend to be thin and linear;
  - (ii) Non-accidental skull fractures tend to have the following features: multiple/complex; depressed fractures, especially in the occipital bone; wide fractures i.e. >5 mm.

A wide range of soft-tissue injuries may also occur in non-accidental injury, including hepatic, splenic and renal damage. Brain injuries are common. Subdural haematoma along the falx cerebri in the midline usually indicates severe shaking of the child.

Differential diagnosis of non-accidental injury includes birth-related trauma and conditions causing abnormally fragile bones such as osteogenesis imperfecta.

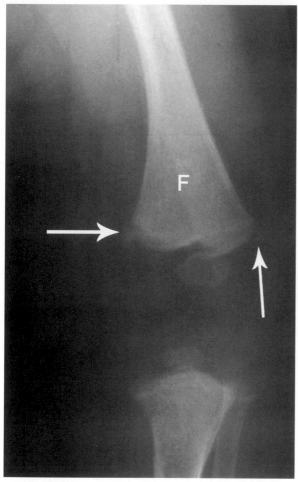

Fig. 16.26 *Non-accidental injury. Radiograph of the femur (F) shows typical metaphyseal corner fractures (arrows).*

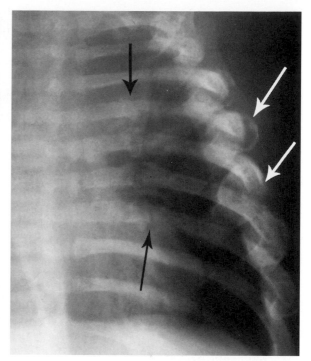

Fig. 16.27 *Non-accidental injury. Chest X-ray (CXR) showing multiple posterior (black arrows) and lateral (white arrows) rib fractures.*

If non-accidental injury is suspected, a radiologist expert in paediatric imaging should report the radiographs.

HIP PROBLEMS IN CHILDREN

DEVELOPMENTAL DYSPLASIA OF THE HIP

Developmental dysplasia of the hip (DDH) occurs in one or two per 1000 births. It involves females more commonly than males by a ratio of 8:1. The left hip is much more commonly involved than the right. Previously known as congenital hip dislocation, the term DDH more accurately reflects the underlying disorder, which is dysplasia of the acetabulum. This may lead to varying degrees of hip joint subluxation, dislocation and dysfunction. Risk factors for the development of DDH include family history, breech presentation, neuromuscular disorders and foot deformities.

Early diagnosis is essential, as conservative management such as splinting for a few weeks is usually successful in all but the most severe cases. Clinical tests such as Ortolani and Barlow manoeuvres may be helpful. Imaging assessment has in the past consisted of a pelvis radiograph. This has limited accuracy, especially below the age of 6 months as most of the essential structures such as the femoral head and acetabular rim are composed of cartilage and cannot be seen radiographically.

Ultrasound is the investigation of choice for suspected DDH in infants (Fig. 16.28). It has a number of advantages, including lack of ionizing radiation. The

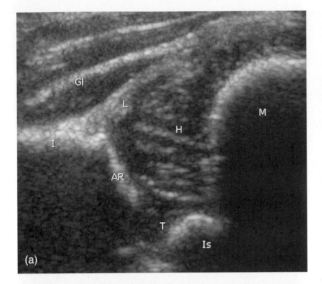

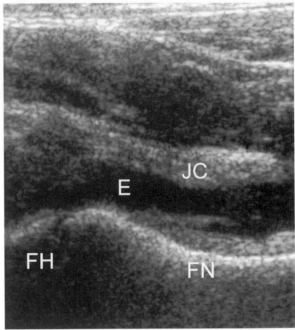

Fig. 16.29 *Hip joint effusion: ultrasound. The image was obtained with the probe parallel to the femoral neck (FN), with the round surface of the femoral head (FH) seen medially. The effusion is seen as anechoic fluid (E) elevating the joint capsule (JC).*

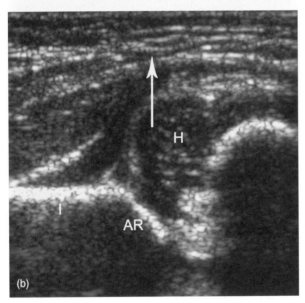

Fig. 16.28 *Developmental dysplasia of the hip (DDH): ultrasound (US). (a) Coronal US of a normal infant hip showing the following: lateral wall of the ilium (I), acetabular roof (AR) femoral head (H), femoral metaphysis (M), labrum (L), triradiate cartilage (T), ischium (Is) and gluteal muscles (Gl). (b) Coronal US of DDH showing a shallow angle between the acetabular roof and ilium, plus displacement of the femoral head out of the acetabulum (arrow).*

cartilage structures are well seen and reproducible measurements of the angle of the acetabular roof and the position of the femoral head may be taken and used in follow-up examinations. Dynamic real-time

US may be used to assess hip stability, and the position of the hip in a splint may be confirmed.

Radiographic assessment is used in children over 9 months of age. At this age US is less accurate because of ossification of the femoral head obscuring the deeper structures of the acetabulum.

The child with missed DDH may present with late walking or a limp. Permanent acetabular dysplasia and delayed femoral head ossification may occur with long-term complications, including limp, early and severe osteoarthritis, and tearing of the acetabular labrum.

SEPTIC ARTHRITIS OF THE HIP

Septic arthritis of the hip most commonly presents before the age of 3 years. It is usually caused by haematogenous spread from respiratory or urinary tract infection. Plain films are insensitive and early scintigraphy may be negative. Ultrasound is the investigation of choice to diagnose the presence of a hip

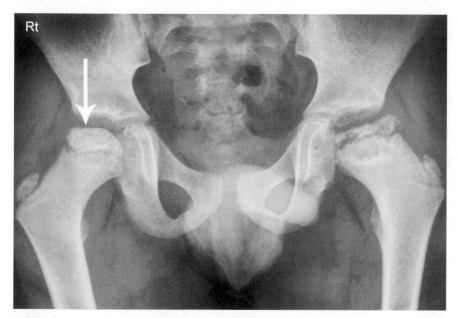

Fig. 16.30 *Perthes disease. Advanced changes of Perthes disease on the left with flattening, irregularity and sclerosis of the femoral epiphysis, widening of the metaphysis and widening of the hip joint. There are much more subtle early changes on the right with slight irregularity and flattening of the femoral head (arrow).*

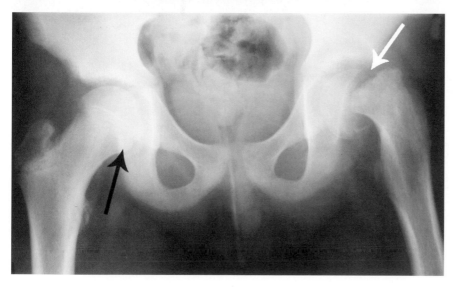

Fig. 16.31 *Slipped capital femoral epiphysis. Marked slip of the left capital femoral epiphysis (white arrow). Note the normal metaphyseal overlay sign on the right side producing a white triangle where the lower corner of the femoral metaphysis overlays the acetabulum (black arrow). This appearance is lost on the left because of the metaphysis being pushed laterally.*

joint effusion (Fig. 16.29). Diagnostic aspiration may be safely performed under US control.

TRANSIENT SYNOVITIS (IRRITABLE HIP)

Transient synovitis is a benign, self-limiting hip disorder. Peak age is 4–10 years, with males more commonly affected than females. A limp develops rapidly over 1–2 days. There is often a history of a recent viral illness and mild fever. Full blood count and erythrocyte sedimentation rate (ESR) are performed followed

by bed rest, with imaging usually not required. Plain films are usually normal with signs of joint effusion such as joint-space widening being quite insensitive. If imaging is required, US is the investigation of choice to diagnose a joint effusion.

PERTHES DISEASE

Perthes disease of the hip has a peak age of incidence of 4–7 years, with females more commonly affected than males. Ten per cent of cases are bilateral, with changes often being asymmetric. It is therefore important to carefully scrutinize both hip joints, even if only one is symptomatic. Plain films are often normal early. Scintigraphy may show a photopenic spot due to ischaemia. Early radiographic signs of Perthes disease include reduced size and sclerosis of the femoral epiphysis with joint-space widening. A subchondral fracture may be seen producing a linear lucency deep to the articular surface of the femoral head. Radiographic signs later in the course of Perthes disease include delayed maturation and fragmentation of the femoral head with cyst formation in the femoral neck. These signs may be accompanied by flattening of the femoral head (coxa plana) and widening of the femoral neck (coxa magna) (Fig. 16.30).

SLIPPED CAPITAL FEMORAL EPIPHYSIS

Slipped capital femoral epiphysis (SCFE) is a disorder of adolescent males. It is bilateral in 20 per cent of cases. Associations of SCFE include obesity and avascular necrosis. The capital femoral epiphysis undergoes posteromedial slip, producing hip pain and a limp. Radiographic signs are best appreciated on a lateral projection, where the slip of the femoral head is well seen. Signs on the anteroposterior (AP) film may be more difficult to appreciate and include widening and irregularity of the femoral growth plate and reduced height of the epiphysis (Fig. 16.31).

Index